AF676736

Sensor Data Analytics for Intelligent Healthcare Delivery

This book explores the transformative potential of sensor data analytics in healthcare, focusing on both real-time and streaming analytics applications in clinical and non-clinical environments. It introduces the foundations of sensor data collection and analytics, delving into data acquisition techniques, mining challenges, and the integration of wearable technologies. It addresses key methodologies and real-world use cases, illustrating how sensor data can improve healthcare delivery, optimize operations, and enhance patient outcomes. It includes topics from algorithmic approaches to practical implementations across a variety of medical domains.

Key Features:

- Covers fundamental concepts of sensor data acquisition, preprocessing, and real-time analysis for healthcare systems.
- Examines the role of wearables in continuous monitoring and their analytics use in clinical workflows.
- Addresses the challenges and techniques for handling streaming data in dynamic healthcare environments.
- Explores machine learning and data mining algorithms tailored to healthcare sensor data.
- Provides examples across hospital operations, patient monitoring, diagnostics, and healthcare management.

This book is for researchers and practitioners in data science, healthcare informatics, biomedical engineering, and healthcare management.

Advances in Digital Technologies for Smart Applications

Series Editor:
Saad Motahhir

The *Advances in Digital Technologies for Smart Applications* series publishes leading-edge research on innovative digital technologies and their application in smart systems. Key topics include AI, IoT, blockchain, and their integration into various sectors, including finance, healthcare, and public governance.

Data Analytics for Finance Using Python
Nitin Jaglal Untwal and Utku Kose

Big Data and Blockchain Technology for Secure IoT Applications
Shitharth Selvarajan, Gouse Baig Mohammad, Sadda Bharath Reddy, and Praveen Kumar Balachandran

Technology-Based Teaching and Learning in Pakistani English Language Classrooms
Muhammad Mooneeb Ali

Medical Knowledge Paradigms for Enabling the Digital Health Ecosystem
Usha Desai, Vivek P Chavda, Ankit Vijayvargiya, and Ravichander Janapati

Soft Computing in Renewable Energy Technologies
Najib El Ouanjli, Mahmoud A. Mossa, Mariya Ouaissa, Sanjeevikumar Padmanaban, and Said Mahfoud

Leveraging the Potential of Artificial Intelligence in the Real World: Smart Cities and Healthcare
Tien Anh Tran, Edeh Michael Onyema, and Arij Naser Abougreen

eGovernment Whole-of-Government Approach for Good Governance: The Back-Office Integrated Management IT Systems
Said Azelmad

Advances in Digital Marketing in the Era of Artificial Intelligence: Case Studies and Data Analysis for Business Problem Solving
Moez Ltifi

NanoRevolution: Unveiling the Future of Energy through Advanced Materials and Digital Technologies
Abderrahman Abbassi

Quantum Computing and Artificial Intelligence in Logistics and Supply Chain Management
By Pushan Kumar Dutta, Pronaya Bhattacharya, Jai Prakash Verma, Ashok Chopra, Neel Kanth Kundu, and Khursheed Aurangzeb

Sensor Data Analytics for Intelligent Healthcare Delivery
By G. S. Karthick

For more information about this series, please visit: https://www.routledge.com/Advances-in-Digital-Technologies-for-Smart-Applications/book-series/ADT

Sensor Data Analytics for Intelligent Healthcare Delivery

Edited by
G. S. Karthick

CRC Press
Taylor & Francis Group
Boca Raton London New York

CRC Press is an imprint of the
Taylor & Francis Group, an **informa** business
A CHAPMAN & HALL BOOK

Designed cover image: Shutterstock

First edition published 2026
by CRC Press
2385 NW Executive Center Drive, Suite 320, Boca Raton FL 33431

and by Chapman and Hall/CRC Press
4 Park Square, Milton Park, Abingdon, Oxon, OX14 4RN

CRC Press is an imprint of Taylor & Francis Group, LLC

© 2026 selection and editorial matter G. S. Karthick; individual chapters, the contributors

Reasonable efforts have been made to publish reliable data and information, but the author and publisher cannot assume responsibility for the validity of all materials or the consequences of their use. The authors and publishers have attempted to trace the copyright holders of all material reproduced in this publication and apologize to copyright holders if permission to publish in this form has not been obtained. If any copyright material has not been acknowledged please write and let us know so we may rectify in any future reprint.

Except as permitted under U.S. Copyright Law, no part of this book may be reprinted, reproduced, transmitted, or utilized in any form by any electronic, mechanical, or other means, now known or hereafter invented, including photocopying, microfilming, and recording, or in any information storage or retrieval system, without written permission from the publishers.

For permission to photocopy or use material electronically from this work, access www.copyright.com or contact the Copyright Clearance Center, Inc. (CCC), 222 Rosewood Drive, Danvers, MA 01923, 978-750-8400. For works that are not available on CCC please contact mpkbookspermissions@tandf.co.uk

Trademark notice: Product or corporate names may be trademarks or registered trademarks and are used only for identification and explanation without intent to infringe.

ISBN: 9781032775463 (hbk)
ISBN: 9781032781884 (pbk)
ISBN: 9781003486640 (ebk)

DOI: 10.1201/9781003486640

Typeset in Times
by codeMantra

Contents

Preface

Background

In recent years, the integration of sensor technologies in healthcare has revolutionized patient monitoring and treatment strategies. With the advent of IoT devices and wearable sensors, healthcare providers now have access to vast amounts of real-time data, enabling proactive and personalized healthcare delivery. This book explores the transformative potential of sensor data analytics in enhancing healthcare outcomes and addresses the challenges and opportunities in this rapidly evolving field.

About this Book

Sensor Data Analytics for Intelligent Healthcare Delivery delves into the intricacies of analyzing sensor data to improve patient care. It covers a wide range of topics, including data acquisition techniques, advanced analytics algorithms, and real-world applications across various medical domains. This book is designed to serve as a comprehensive guide for researchers, healthcare professionals, and technologists interested in leveraging sensor data for optimizing healthcare services.

Target Audience

This book is intended for researchers, practitioners, and students in the fields of healthcare informatics, biomedical engineering, data science, and healthcare management. It is also valuable for healthcare policymakers and industry professionals looking to understand the potential of sensor data analytics in reshaping the future of healthcare.

Organization of the Book

This book is organized into 16 chapters, each contributed by esteemed researchers and practitioners in the field of healthcare sensor data analytics. These chapters collectively address fundamental concepts, advanced methodologies, and real-world applications that shape the landscape of intelligent healthcare delivery. By highlighting cutting-edge advancements and practical insights, this book showcases how sensor data analytics can revolutionize healthcare practices.

The summary of the chapter contents is depicted as follows:

Chapter 1 provides foundational concepts and architectures of healthcare sensor data analytics, emphasizing its pivotal role in modern healthcare systems.

Chapter 2 explores statistical approximation techniques for enhancing analytics of streaming sensor data in healthcare applications.

Chapter 3 offers comprehensive insights into transformative healthcare solutions facilitated by sensor data analytics.

Chapter 4 discusses real-time anomaly detection in healthcare sensor data, crucial for early intervention and improved patient outcomes.

Chapter 5 covers basic principles and essential techniques in healthcare sensor data analytics.

Chapter 6 details the design and development of physiotherapy robots for human upper-limb rehabilitation, integrating sensor technologies for enhanced medical practice.

Chapter 7 focuses on mortality prediction in non-alcoholic fatty liver disease using machine learning, showcasing predictive analytics applications in clinical settings.

Chapter 8 presents a machine learning framework for predicting cognitive impairment through handwriting analysis, aiding clinical decision-making.

Chapter 9 optimizes deep learning algorithms for pneumonia diagnosis using chest X-ray data, demonstrating the application of AI in medical diagnostics.

Chapter 10 discusses melanoma detection using deep convolutional neural networks, highlighting image-based approaches for skin cancer diagnosis.

Chapter 11 explores advanced skin cancer classification using deep learning architectures, focusing on dermatoscopic image analysis for clinical applications.

Chapter 12 introduces a neuro-fuzzy multimodal ensemble algorithm for Alzheimer's disease prediction, leveraging hybrid AI techniques in healthcare.

Chapter 13 unveils insights from fine-tuning BERT for medical healthcare, enhancing question answering systems for efficient clinical decision support.

Chapter 14 utilizes cosine wavelet geometric guided sparse representation transform for lossless medical image compression, enhancing diagnostic image quality.

Chapter 15 offers a comprehensive analysis of advanced techniques in healthcare sensor data analytics, exploring innovative approaches and methodologies.

Chapter 16 explores the Internet of Medical Things (IoMT) in healthcare, focusing on connected devices for patient care and monitoring.

Each chapter contributes unique perspectives and practical knowledge, aiming to empower researchers, healthcare professionals, and policymakers with the latest advancements in sensor data analytics for intelligent healthcare delivery.

G. S. Karthick
Department of Software Systems,
PSG College of Arts & Science, Coimbatore, Tamil Nadu, India

Acknowledgments

Writing this part is probably the most difficult task. Although the list of people to thank heartily is long, making this list is not the hard part. The difficult part is to search for the words that convey the sincerity and enormity of our gratitude and love.

First of all, I would like to thank the almighty.

Acknowledgment when sincerely given is a reward without price. I am thankful to the publishing team of Taylor & Francis for accepting to publish this edited book. I would like to thank the entire development team for helping us in bringing this project to a successful end.

I would like to express our deepest appreciation to the Editorial Advisory Board members for extending their valuable suggestions and support to accomplish the task in a successful manner.

I would like to express appreciation and thank the reviewers for their careful reading of our manuscript and their many perceptive comments and suggestions. I want to acknowledge the authors for their valuable contributions, and hereby, I convey my sincere thankfulness.

I owe my sincere thanks to my grandparents who are always blessing me from heaven. I express my deepest gratitude to my parents Mr. G. Selvaraj and Mrs. S. Saraswathi for their moral support, blessings, and encouragement throughout my life. Above all, I would like to thank my wife Mrs. K. Haripriya for her constant support and for keeping me sane.

I am extremely thankful to the Management, Principal, Secretary, and Vice-Principal of PSG College of Arts & Science, Coimbatore, for providing encouragement and support to complete this project. I am greatly indebted to my family members and friends for their constant support in every aspect of life and for encouraging me to finish this book.

G. S. Karthick
Department of Software Systems
PSG College of Arts & Science, Coimbatore, Tamil Nadu, India

About the Editor

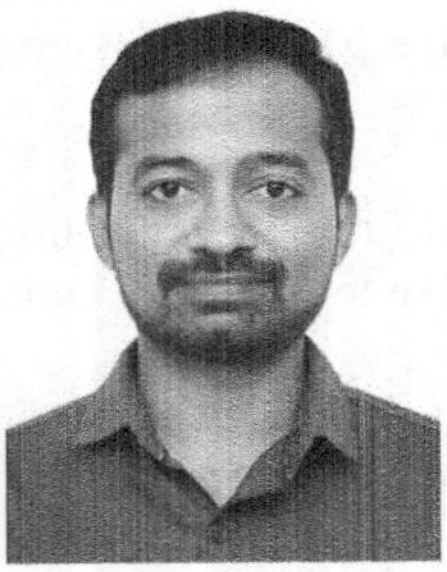

G. S. Karthick is currently working as an Assistant Professor in the Department of Software Systems, PSG College of Arts & Science, Coimbatore, India. Previously, he worked as a Research Fellow under the DST-ICPS Project from April 2019 to March 2022 in the Department of Computer Science, School of Computer Science and Engineering, Bharathiar University, Coimbatore, India. Also, he worked as an Assistant Professor in the Department of Computer Science, Sri Ramakrishna College of Arts and Science, Coimbatore, India. He received his Ph.D. in Computer Science from Bharathiar University (University Department) in February 2023. He topped the Post-Graduation with a Gold Medal in 2017 from Bharathiar University, Coimbatore, India. He topped the Under-Graduation with an exemplary performance from SNR Sons College, Coimbatore, India, and also aced three subjects to receive gold medals in 2015. He qualified for UGC-NET Computer Science and Applications in December 2020. Further, he has visited many institutions and universities as a resource person at various events. He has received an Indian Patent Grant for his innovative contribution to the field of wireless networks and the Internet of Things. He has published research papers in international journals and presented papers at international and national conferences. He has published many book chapters, and in addition, he has edited four books and authored two books. He is an Associate Editor of *IJHISI*, *IJITN*, and *IJEHMC*. Also, he is an active reviewer in high-standard journals of Elsevier, IEEE, Springer, IGI Journals, and many peer-reviewed journals. He has received many awards and rewards for his achievements in academic and research careers. His areas of specialization are machine learning, the Internet of Things, wireless sensor networks, and analysis of algorithms. His current research interests focus on the recent developments in the healthcare Internet of Things and machine learning algorithms.

Contributors

Hady Abdalla
Department of Applied Computer Science
Canadian International College (CIC)
Cairo, Egypt

Wafaa Abdelgawad
Department of Applied Computer Science
Canadian International College (CIC)
Cairo, Egypt

Jyoti Anand
Department of Computer Science and Engineering
Techno International New Town
Kolkata, India

U. V. Anbazhagu
Department of Computing Technologies
SRM Institute of Science and Technology
Kattankulathur, India

Aadharsh B
Department of Electronics and Communication Engineering
Coimbatore Institute of Technology
Coimbatore, India

Anitha B
Department of Electronics and Communication Engineering
KIT-Kalaignarkarunanidhi Institute of Technology
Coimbatore, Tamil Nadu, India

Arunpriya C
Department of Computer Applications
PSG College of Arts & Science
Coimbatore, India

S. Chidambaram
Department of Information Technology
National Engineering College
Kovilpatti, India

Mani Deepak Choudhry
Department of Computing Technologies
School of Computing
SRM Institute of Science and Technology
Kattankulathur, India

Dhanushiya D
Department of Nursing
PSG College of Nursing
Coimbatore, India

Esraa Darwish
Department of Applied Computer Science
Canadian International College (CIC)
Cairo, Egypt

Elakkiya E
Department of Computer Science and Engineering
SRM University
Andhra Pradesh, India

Mohammed Hassan El-tohamy
Department of Applied Computer Science
Canadian International College (CIC)
Cairo, Egypt

Mukul Kumar Gupta
Department of Electronics and Instrumentation Engineering
MJP Rohilkhand University
Bareilly, India

V. Harish
Department of Management Sciences
PSG Institute of Management, PSG College of Technology
Coimbatore, India

Anubhav Jaiswal
Department of Computer Science and Engineering
Techno International New Town
Kolkata, India

S. Janarthanam
School of Science and Computer Studies
CMR University
India

S. Jeevanandham
Department of Information Technology
Sri Ramakrishna Engineering College
Coimbatore, India

Akshya Jothi
Department of Computational Intelligence
School of Computing
SRM Institute of Science and Technology
Kattankulathur, India

Umapathi K
Department of Biomedical Engineering
KIT-Kalaignarkarunanidhi Institute of Technology
Coimbatore, India

Ramdas Kapila
Department of Computer Science and Engineering (Data Science)
B V Raju Institute of Technology
Telangana, India

G. S. Karthick
Department of Software Systems
PSG College of Arts & Science
Coimbatore, India

Mitraansh Raaj Khanna
Department of Computer Technologies
SRM Institute of Science and Technology
Kattankulathur, India

P. Kirubanantham
Department of Computing Technologies
SRM Institute of Science and Technology
Kattankulathur, India

Ankush Kumar
Department of Computer Science and Engineering
Techno International New Town
Kolkata, India

Roushan Kumar
School of Engineering, Mechanical Department
University of Petroleum and Energy Studies
Dehradun, India

Ajanthaa Lakshmanan
Department of Computing Technologies
SRM Institute of Science and Technology
Kattankulathur, India

Jayasheela M
Department of Electronics and Communication Engineering
KIT-Kalaignarkarunanidhi Institute of Technology
Coimbatore, India

Marwan Makhlouf
Department of Applied Computer Science
Canadian International College (CIC)
Cairo, Egypt

T. Mathankumar
Department of Computer Science
Bharathiar University
Coimbatore, India

Youssef M. Nassar
Department of Applied Computer Science
Canadian International College (CIC)
Cairo, Egypt

Anandarupa Neogi
Department of Computer Science and Engineering
Techno International New Town
Kolkata, India

B. Prakash
SRM Institute of Science and Technology
Kattankulathur, India

K. Premalatha
Bannari Amman Institute of Technology
Sathyamangalam, India

N. Priyanka
School of Computer Science and Engineering (SCOPE)
Vellore Institute of Technology
Vellore Campus, India

S. Poornima
Department of Computer Technologies
SRM Institute of Science and Technology
Kattankulathur, India

Sowrabh S
Design Engineer, Software Department
Kawasaki Robotics
Coimbatore, India

Bikash Sadhukhan
Department of Computer Science and Engineering
Techno International New Town
Kolkata, India

Sumalatha Saleti
Department of Computer Science and Engineering
SRM University
Andhra Pradesh, India

Gehad Ismail Sayed
Department of Applied Computer Science
Canadian International College (CIC)
Cairo, Egypt

Prakhar Kunwar Sinha
Department of Computer Technologies
SRM Institute of Science and Technology
Chennai, India

C. Sivamathi
Department of Computer Science
PSG College of Arts & Science
Coimbatore, India

G. Subbulakshmi
Department of Physics
Shree Venkateshwara Arts and Science (Co-Education) College
Kugalur, India

Alluri Sai Sunanda
Department of Computer Science and Engineering
SRM University
Andhra Pradesh, India

M. Sundarrajan
Department of Networking and Communications
School of Computing
SRM Institute of Science and Technology
Kattankulathur, India

P. Swathypriyadharsini
Department of Computer Science and Engineering
Bannari Amman Institute of Technology
Sathyamangalam, India

Varnita Verma
Department of Interdisciplinary Research
Indian Institute of Technology (IIT)
Delhi, India

S. Vijayarani
Department of Computer Science
Bharathiar University
Coimbatore, India

N. Sriyani
School of Computer Science and Engineering
(SCOPE)
Vellore Institute of Technology
Vellore Campus, India

S. Poornima
Department of Computing Technologies
SRM Institute of Science and Technology
Kattankulathur, India

Sowrabh S.
[illegible]
[illegible]
Ernakulam, India

Rakesh Sadanandan
Department of Computer Science and
Engineering
Institute of Engineering and Management, New Town
Kolkata, India

Subalakshmi Ravi
Department of Computer Science and
Engineering
SRM University
Andhra Pradesh, India

Gohar Rashid Sofed
Department of Applied Computer Science
[illegible]
[illegible]

Prabhat Kumar Sinha
Department of Computer Technologies
SRM Institute of Science and Technology
Chennai, India

L. Sujatha
Department of Computer Science
PSG College of Arts and Science
Coimbatore, India

R. Sathish Kumar
Department of Physics
Sri Venkateswara [illegible]
of Educational Colleges
Erode, India

Abhijeet Shrivastava
Department of Computer Science and
Engineering
SRM University
Andhra Pradesh, India

M. Sundarrajan
Department of Networking and
Communications
School of Computing
SRM Institute of Science and Technology
Kattankulathur, India

T. Venugopal
Department of Computer Science and
Engineering
Santhiram Engineering College
[illegible], India

Vaibhav Verma
Department of [illegible]
Indian Institute of Technology (IIT)
Delhi, India

S. [illegible]
Department of [illegible]
Bharathiar University
Coimbatore, India

1 Healthcare Sensor Data Analytics

Foundational Concepts, Architecture, Data Analysis Techniques, Data Quality, Errors, and Applications

G. S. Karthick

1.1 INTRODUCTION TO SENSOR DATA ANALYTICS

Sensor data analytics refers to the process of collecting, processing, and analyzing data generated by sensors to extract meaningful insights and make informed decisions. Sensors are devices that detect and measure physical properties such as temperature, pressure, motion, or biological signals like heart rate or glucose levels. In healthcare, sensor data analytics involves leveraging these technologies to monitor patients' health status, diagnose conditions, predict outcomes, and personalize treatments.

The core of sensor data analytics lies in transforming raw sensor data into actionable information. This process typically includes data preprocessing (cleaning, filtering), feature extraction (identifying relevant patterns), and applying advanced analytics techniques such as machine learning and statistical modeling (Banaee et al. 2013). This enables healthcare professionals to derive insights that aid in clinical decision-making, improve patient outcomes, and enhance operational efficiency.

1.2 IMPORTANCE OF SENSOR DATA ANALYTICS IN HEALTHCARE

Sensor data analytics plays a pivotal role in modern healthcare systems, offering several crucial benefits (Lu et al. 2020):

1. **Remote Patient Monitoring:** Sensors enable continuous monitoring of patients' vital signs and health parameters outside traditional clinical settings. This capability is particularly valuable for managing chronic diseases like diabetes or cardiovascular conditions, where real-time data can prompt timely interventions and reduce hospitalizations.
2. **Early Detection and Diagnosis:** By continuously monitoring physiological data, sensors can detect subtle changes indicative of health deterioration or disease onset. This early detection facilitates timely diagnosis and proactive healthcare management, potentially improving treatment outcomes and reducing healthcare costs.
3. **Personalized Medicine:** Sensor data analytics supports personalized treatment plans tailored to individual patient profiles. By analyzing data on patients' physiological responses and behaviors, healthcare providers can optimize treatment strategies, adjust medication dosages, and recommend lifestyle modifications based on real-time insights.

DOI: 10.1201/9781003486640-1

4. **Enhanced Healthcare Delivery:** Integrating sensor data analytics into healthcare delivery systems enhances efficiency and quality of care. Automated data collection and analysis streamline workflows, reduce manual errors, and enable healthcare providers to focus more on patient care and less on administrative tasks.
5. **Research and Innovation:** Sensor data contributes to medical research by providing large-scale, real-world data sets for epidemiological studies, clinical trials, and population health analytics. This data-driven approach fuels innovation in healthcare technology and facilitates the development of new diagnostics, therapies, and preventive strategies.
6. **Patient-Centric Care:** Access to personal health data empowers patients to actively participate in their own care. Wearable sensors and mobile health apps enable individuals to track their fitness levels, monitor chronic conditions, and make informed decisions about their health behaviors, fostering a proactive approach to wellness.

1.3 SENSORS IN HEALTHCARE

In healthcare, sensors are indispensable tools that enable the precise measurement and monitoring of physiological parameters and environmental conditions. These sensors are designed to capture data from both the human body and the surrounding environment, providing healthcare professionals with valuable insights for diagnosis, treatment, and patient care (Forkan and Khalil 2017).

1.3.1 Physiological Sensors

Physiological sensors are specifically designed to monitor various biological parameters related to human health. These sensors play a crucial role in continuous health monitoring, early detection of medical conditions, and management of chronic diseases. Here are some of the commonly used physiological sensors:

Electrocardiogram (ECG) Sensors: ECG sensors detect and record the electrical activity of the heart. They are used to assess cardiac function, diagnose arrhythmias, detect myocardial ischemia, and monitor the effectiveness of cardiac treatments.

Blood Glucose Monitors: These sensors measure glucose levels in the blood, essential for managing diabetes. They enable diabetic patients to monitor their blood sugar levels regularly, adjust insulin doses, and make informed decisions about diet and exercise.

Pulse Oximeters: Pulse oximeters measure oxygen saturation levels in arterial blood. They are critical for monitoring respiratory function, assessing the severity of lung diseases (e.g., COPD), and evaluating patients during anesthesia or in intensive care settings.

Blood Pressure Monitors: Blood pressure monitors measure systolic and diastolic blood pressure. They are used to diagnose hypertension, assess cardiovascular health, and monitor the effects of medications and lifestyle interventions.

Temperature Sensors: Temperature sensors monitor body temperature variations. They are used to detect fevers, monitor patients recovering from infections, and ensure thermal comfort in clinical environments.

1.3.2 Environmental Sensors

Environmental sensors are designed to monitor external factors that can affect health outcomes, such as air quality, radiation levels, and ambient conditions. These sensors provide valuable data for assessing environmental risks, ensuring workplace safety, and improving public health. Here are some of the commonly used environmental sensors:

Air Quality Sensors: Air quality sensors measure concentrations of pollutants such as particulate matter (PM), carbon monoxide (CO), nitrogen dioxide (NO_2), and volatile organic compounds (VOCs). They are used to assess indoor and outdoor air quality, identify sources of pollution, and mitigate respiratory health risks.

Radiation Detectors: Radiation detectors monitor levels of ionizing radiation in medical imaging (e.g., X-rays, CT scans), nuclear medicine procedures, and occupational settings. They ensure patient and healthcare worker safety by preventing excessive radiation exposure.

Humidity Sensors: Humidity sensors measure atmospheric moisture levels. They are used in healthcare settings to control indoor air quality, prevent fungus growth, and maintain optimal conditions for patients with respiratory conditions.

1.4 HIGH-LEVEL ARCHITECTURE OF HEALTHCARE SENSOR DATA ANALYTICS

The architecture of healthcare sensor data analytics integrates advanced technologies to harness real-time data from sensors deployed across healthcare facilities (Ahmad et al. 2018). structured framework encompasses data acquisition, streaming data processing, robust storage solutions, analytics modules, machine learning capabilities, user interfaces, and automated control applications, which has been shown in Figure 1.1. By leveraging these components, healthcare providers can monitor patient health metrics, optimize medical equipment performance, and enhance operational efficiency, ultimately improving patient care outcomes and driving healthcare innovation.

Data Acquisition and Transmission: In healthcare sensor data analytics, data acquisition begins with various sensors and smart devices deployed across healthcare facilities. These sensors capture real-time data from patients, medical equipment, and environmental conditions (Akhbarifar et al. 2020). This data is transmitted securely through field and cloud

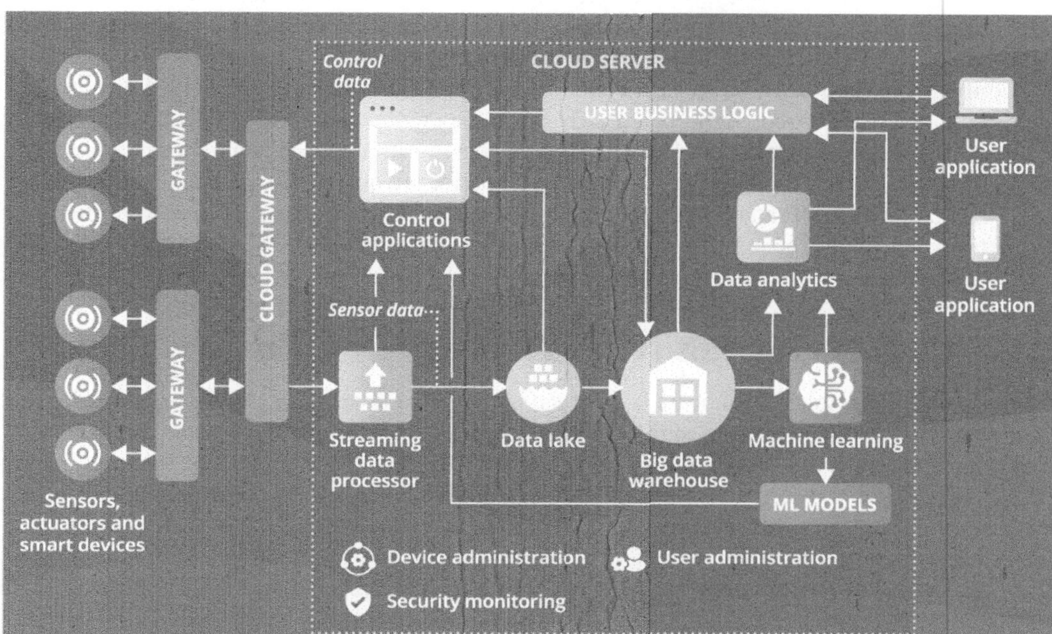

FIGURE 1.1 High-level architecture of healthcare sensor data analytics.

gateways to ensure continuous connectivity and reliability. It forms the foundational layer for subsequent processing and analysis, vital for monitoring patient health metrics and operational parameters in healthcare settings.

Streaming Data Processing: Once sensor data reaches the system, the streaming data processor undertakes initial processing tasks. This includes data validation, aggregation, and filtering to manage the high volume of incoming data efficiently. Real-time analytics capabilities enable the immediate detection of anomalies or critical events, such as irregular patient vital signs or equipment malfunctions, prompting timely interventions and ensuring patient safety.

Data Storage and Management: In healthcare, a robust architecture involves storing sensor data in a data lake for scalability and flexibility. Structured data (e.g., vital signs, medical records) and unstructured data (e.g., images, videos) are stored until needed for analysis. Transformed and cleaned data, along with essential metadata like patient demographics and sensor configurations, resides in a big data warehouse. This ensures high-quality data storage, optimized for advanced analytics, long-term insights, and regulatory compliance in healthcare environments.

Analytics and Machine Learning Modules: Analytics modules in healthcare sensor data analytics leverage stored data to uncover trends, dependencies, and correlations critical for patient care and operational efficiency. These modules generate scheduled and ad hoc reports, forecast patient outcomes, and offer actionable insights to healthcare providers. Optional machine learning modules continuously refine predictive models, enhancing decision-making capabilities based on evolving patient data and operational contexts.

User Applications and Interfaces: User applications play a pivotal role in healthcare sensor data analytics by providing healthcare professionals with intuitive interfaces to monitor patient health statuses, review medical equipment performance, and assess environmental conditions. Users can interact with the system to send manual commands for adjusting medical device settings or environmental controls based on real-time sensor data. Customizable features allow users to fine-tune machine learning models, generate personalized reports, and optimize healthcare delivery strategies.

Control Applications: Control applications automate actions based on predefined thresholds or anomaly detection within healthcare sensor data (Syed et al. 2019). These applications autonomously adjust medical device settings (e.g., insulin dosage, ventilator parameters) or environmental controls (e.g., room temperature, air quality) to optimize patient care outcomes and operational efficiency. This proactive approach ensures timely responses to dynamic healthcare environments, enhancing patient safety and healthcare delivery effectiveness.

1.5 SENSOR DATA ACQUISITION TECHNIQUES

Sensor data acquisition in healthcare is a critical process that involves capturing, transmitting, and processing data from sensors designed to monitor physiological parameters and environmental conditions (Mustafa and Varol 2020). These sensors utilize various acquisition techniques, including direct wiring and wireless communication. Direct wiring ensures stable, interference-free data transmission, suitable for high-precision measurements in clinical settings. In contrast, wireless communication, using technologies like Bluetooth and Wi-Fi, facilitates remote monitoring and real-time data transmission, essential for applications such as wearable health devices and telehealth.

The acquisition techniques specified in Table 1.1 are essential for ensuring accuracy, reliability, and real-time monitoring capabilities in healthcare sensor data management. Cloud-based data storage plays a pivotal role by enabling the transmission of sensor data to secure cloud servers. This method supports scalability, accessibility, and collaborative healthcare efforts across different

TABLE 1.1
Overview of Sensor Data Acquisition Techniques in Healthcare

Acquisition Technique	Description	Applications
Direct wiring	Sensors are physically connected to data acquisition systems via cables, ensuring stable and interference-free data transmission suitable for high-precision clinical measurements.	Clinical & Laboratory Environments
Wireless communication	Utilizes wireless technologies (e.g., Bluetooth, Wi-Fi) for remote data transmission, enabling real-time monitoring and flexibility in sensor deployment.	Wearable Health Devices, Telehealth Applications
Cloud-based storage	Sensor data is transmitted to secure cloud servers for storage, facilitating scalability, accessibility, and integration with electronic health records (EHRs) across healthcare facilities.	Remote Patient Monitoring, Collaborative Healthcare
Edge computing	Data processing and analysis occur locally on edge devices before transmission to centralized systems or the cloud, reducing latency and optimizing bandwidth usage.	Real-Time Analytics, Data Privacy Enhancement

facilities and remote locations. It also facilitates advanced analytics and integration with electronic health records (EHRs) for comprehensive patient management and data-driven decision-making.

Edge computing complements these methods by processing and analyzing data locally on edge devices before transmitting it to centralized systems or the cloud. This approach reduces latency, optimizes bandwidth usage, and enhances data privacy by limiting data transmission to essential information. These acquisition techniques are crucial considerations in healthcare to ensure accuracy, reliability, and real-time monitoring capabilities, while also addressing security, interoperability, scalability, and cost-efficiency challenges inherent in sensor data management and integration within healthcare systems.

1.6 DATA PREPROCESSING TECHNIQUES

Data preprocessing is essential in healthcare sensor data analysis to enhance data quality, reduce noise, and prepare data for accurate modeling and interpretation. This process involves several techniques, including noise reduction and filtering, as well as data normalization and scaling, each playing a crucial role in improving the reliability and effectiveness of healthcare analytics (Joshi et al. 2018).

1.6.1 Noise Reduction and Filtering Techniques

Noise in sensor data can arise from various sources, including environmental interference, sensor imperfections, or transmission errors. Noise reduction techniques aim to mitigate these disturbances to ensure that the data accurately reflects the underlying physiological or environmental signals.

Moving Average Filter: The moving average filter computes the average of the last N data points to smooth out short-term fluctuations, reducing high-frequency noise. It is effective for noise reduction in continuous data streams such as heart rate monitoring or temperature measurements.

$$\text{Filtered Value at Time } t = \frac{1}{N} \sum_{i=t-N+1}^{t} x_i \tag{1.1}$$

Median Filter: The median filter replaces each data point with the median value within a sliding window of size *N*, effectively reducing outliers and impulsive noise. It is suitable for removing spikes and sudden fluctuations in physiological data, improving signal clarity.

$$\text{Filtered Value at Time } t = \text{median}\left(x_{t-N+1}, x_{t-N+2}, \ldots, x_t\right) \tag{1.2}$$

1.6.1.1 An Illustrated Example

Consider a simple sample dataset given in Table 1.2, collected from wearable sensors monitoring heart rate (HR), body temperature (Temp), and oxygen saturation (SpO_2) of patients:

This dataset shows heart rate (HR), body temperature (Temp), and oxygen saturation (SpO_2) recorded over time. Notice an anomaly in the heart rate at the 4-second mark, which is likely due to noise.

Noise is a common problem in sensor data, caused by factors such as sensor inaccuracies or external environmental interference. To clean the data, we apply noise reduction techniques such as Moving Average Filtering and Median Filtering.

Moving Average Filter: The moving average filter smooths the data by averaging a certain number of previous data points. For example, for a window size of 3, the moving average for heart rate (HR) at time *t* would be:

$$\text{HR}_{\text{FILTERED}}(t) = \frac{\text{HR}(t-2) + \text{HR}(t-1) + \text{HR}(t)}{3} \tag{1.3}$$

After applying a moving average filter to the heart rate data is shown in Table 1.3:

TABLE 1.2
Dataset from Wearable Device

Time (s)	HR (bpm)	Temp (°C)	SpO_2 (%)
1	80	36.5	98
2	82	36.7	97
3	85	36.8	99
4	300	36.6	96
5	78	36.5	98
6	81	36.9	97

TABLE 1.3
Applying Moving Average Filter to Heart Rate Data

Time (s)	HR (bpm)	Moving Avg (HR)
1	80	N/A
2	82	N/A
3	85	82.33
4	300	155.67
5	78	154.33
6	81	153.00

TABLE 1.4
Applying Median Filter to Heart Rate Data

Time (s)	HR (bpm)	Median (HR)
1	80	N/A
2	82	N/A
3	85	82
4	300	85
5	78	82
6	81	81

Notice that the moving average has smoothed the data, but the extreme outlier (300 bpm) still skews the result. To handle such anomalies better, a median filter can be used.

Median Filter: A median filter replaces each data point with the median of surrounding values within a sliding window. This technique is effective for removing outliers. For a window size of 3, the results of applying the median filter to the heart rate data are shown in Table 1.4:

The extreme heart rate value (300 bpm) is effectively replaced by the median of its surrounding values, providing a more realistic heart rate trend.

1.6.2 Data Normalization and Scaling Techniques

Normalization and scaling techniques adjust the range and distribution of data to ensure consistency and comparability across different features or datasets (Kakria et al. 2015). These techniques are particularly important in sensor data analysis to standardize variables and enhance the performance of machine learning algorithms.

Min-Max Normalization: Scales data to a fixed range [0, 1] by subtracting the minimum value and dividing by the range (maximum – minimum). It ensures all features have the same scale, which is useful for algorithms like k-nearest neighbors (KNN) and neural networks.

$$x_{\text{norm}} = \frac{x - \min(X)}{\max(X) - \min(X)} \tag{1.4}$$

Z-Score Standardization: Standardizes data to have a mean (μ) of 0 and standard deviation (σ) of 1. It is useful when data follows a Gaussian distribution, facilitating the interpretation of coefficients in regression models and improving convergence in optimization algorithms.

$$x_{\text{std}} = \frac{x - \mu}{\sigma} \tag{1.5}$$

1.6.2.1 An Illustrated Example

Sensor data often contains features with different ranges. For example, heart rate is measured in beats per minute (bpm) and can range from 60 to 200, while body temperature is measured in degrees Celsius (°C) and typically ranges from 35 °C to 40 °C. In machine learning models, having features in different ranges can skew the results. Therefore, normalization and scaling are essential.

Min-Max Normalization: Min-max normalization scales the data to a specific range, typically [0, 1]. The formula for min-max normalization is:

$$x_{\text{norm}} = \frac{x - \min(X)}{\max(X) - \min(X)} \tag{1.6}$$

For example, the results of applying min-max normalization to the heart rate (HR) data is shown in Table 1.5:

$$\text{HR}_{\text{norm}} = \frac{\text{HR} - 78}{300 - 78} \tag{1.7}$$

After normalization, heart rate data is scaled between 0 and 1, making it easier to compare with other features, like body temperature or SpO_2.

Z-Score Standardization: *Z*-score standardization (also called standard scaling) transforms the data to have a mean of 0 and a standard deviation of 1. The formula for *z*-score standardization is:

$$x_{\text{std}} = \frac{x - \mu}{\sigma} \tag{1.8}$$

Where μ is the mean and σ is the standard deviation of the feature.

If the mean heart rate is $\mu = 117.67$ bpm and the standard deviation is $\sigma = 92.94$ bpm, then standardize the heart rate data as shown in Table 1.6:

TABLE 1.5
Applying Min-Max Normalization to Heart Rate Data

Time (s)	HR (bpm)	Normalized HR
1	80	0.0092
2	82	0.0184
3	85	0.0321
4	300	1.0000
5	78	0.0000
6	81	0.0138

TABLE 1.6
Applying *Z*-Score Standardization to Heart Rate Data

Time (s)	HR (bpm)	Standardized HR
1	80	−0.405
2	82	−0.384
3	85	−0.347
4	300	1.962
5	78	−0.427
6	81	−0.395

This transformation allows us to compare features with different units and magnitudes in a more standardized way, which is important for machine learning algorithms that assume normally distributed data.

1.7 FEATURE EXTRACTION AND SELECTION

In healthcare sensor data analytics, feature extraction and selection are critical steps to ensure that relevant information is captured from raw data and that only the most important features are used for building predictive models (Nubenthan and Ravichelvan 2017). This process helps improve model accuracy, reduce complexity, and avoid overfitting, which is essential when dealing with vast amounts of data generated by healthcare sensors.

1.7.1 Feature Extraction in Healthcare Sensor Data

Feature extraction involves transforming raw sensor data into meaningful representations that capture the essential patterns and characteristics of the data. These extracted features serve as inputs for machine learning algorithms (Hartmann et al. 2019). In healthcare, common features extracted from sensor data include time-domain, frequency-domain, and statistical features, depending on the type of data and application.

1.7.1.1 Time-Domain Features

Time-domain features are directly extracted from the raw sensor signal and provide information about the signal's behavior over time.

Mean (Average Value): The mean value of a signal over a time window is often used as a simple representation of a sensor's average behavior.

$$\text{Mean} = \frac{1}{N}\sum_{i=1}^{N} x_i \tag{1.9}$$

where N is the number of samples and x_i is the value of the sensor data at time i.

Standard Deviation (SD): The standard deviation measures the variability of the sensor data, which is important for understanding fluctuations in physiological signals.

$$\text{SD} = \sqrt{\frac{1}{N}\sum_{i=1}^{N} (x_i - \mu)^2} \tag{1.10}$$

where μ is the mean of the signal.

Peak-to-Peak Amplitude: Measures the difference between the maximum and minimum values of the signal.

$$\text{Peak-to-Peak} = \max(x) - \min(x) \tag{1.11}$$

1.7.1.2 Frequency-Domain Features

Frequency-domain features provide insights into the periodic components of the sensor signal, which can be particularly useful for analyzing physiological signals such as ECG or EEG data.

Fourier Transform (FT): The Fourier Transform converts the time-domain signal into its frequency components. It is often used to analyze the dominant frequencies in physiological signals.

$$X(f) = \sum_{n=0}^{N-1} x(n) e^{-j2\pi fn/N} \tag{1.12}$$

where $X(f)$ is the frequency-domain representation of the signal and $x(n)$ is the time-domain signal.

Power Spectral Density (PSD): The PSD measures the power distribution of a signal across frequencies. It is particularly useful for identifying rhythmic patterns or irregularities in signals like EEG or heart rate variability.

$$\text{PSD}(f) = \frac{|X(f)|^2}{N} \tag{1.13}$$

1.7.1.3 Statistical Features

Statistical features capture the underlying statistical properties of the sensor data and are often used to summarize the signal over a certain window.

Skewness: Skewness quantifies the asymmetry of the data distribution.

$$\text{Skewness} = \frac{N}{(N-1)(N-2)} \sum_{i=1}^{N} \left(\frac{x_i - \mu}{\sigma} \right)^3 \tag{1.14}$$

Kurtosis: Kurtosis measures the "tailedness" or the extremity of values in the data distribution.

$$\text{Kurtosis} = \frac{N(N+1)}{(N-1)(N-2)(N-3)} \sum_{i=1}^{N} \left(\frac{x_i - \mu}{\sigma} \right)^4 - \frac{3(N-1)^2}{(N-2)(N-3)} \tag{1.15}$$

1.7.2 Feature Selection in Healthcare Sensor Data

Feature selection aims to choose the most relevant features from the extracted set, which improves model performance by eliminating redundant or irrelevant features (Esposito et al. 2018). In healthcare, this process is particularly important to avoid overfitting, reduce computational complexity, and ensure interpretability.

1.7.2.1 Filter Methods

Filter methods rank features based on their statistical relationship with the target variable, independent of any machine learning model. Common filter methods include (Dyskin et al. 2018):

Correlation Coefficient: Measures the linear relationship between each feature and the target variable. Features with a high correlation are preferred.

$$r = \frac{\sum (x_i - \mu_x)(y_i - \mu_y)}{\sqrt{\sum (x_i - \mu_x)^2} \sqrt{\sum (y_i - \mu_y)^2}} \tag{1.16}$$

where r is the correlation coefficient, x_i represents feature values, and y_i represents target values.

Mutual Information: Mutual information measures the amount of information shared between a feature and the target variable. Features with higher mutual information scores are considered more informative.

$$I(X;Y) = \sum_{x \in X} \sum_{y \in Y} p(x,y) \log\left(\frac{p(x,y)}{p(x)p(y)}\right) \tag{1.17}$$

1.7.2.2 Wrapper Methods

Wrapper methods evaluate the performance of different feature subsets by training and testing machine learning models. These methods use search algorithms like Forward Selection or Backward Elimination to identify optimal feature sets (Jeon et al. 2014).

- **Forward Selection:** Begins with an empty set of features and iteratively adds the feature that improves model performance the most until no further improvement is observed.
- **Backward Elimination:** Starts with all features and iteratively removes the least important feature based on model performance until an optimal subset is reached.
- **Recursive Feature Elimination (RFE):** RFE is a wrapper method that recursively removes the least significant feature, based on model coefficients, to select an optimal feature subset. It is often combined with machine learning models like Support Vector Machines (SVM) or Random Forest.

1.7.2.3 Embedded Methods

Embedded methods incorporate feature selection as part of the training process of machine learning models (Baig and Gholamhosseini 2013). These methods automatically select features that contribute the most to the model's predictive power.

Lasso Regression (L1 Regularization): Lasso regression adds a penalty term proportional to the absolute values of the model coefficients, forcing some coefficients to become zero, effectively selecting a subset of important features.

$$\text{Lasso Loss} = \sum_{i=1}^{N} \left(y_i - \hat{y}_i + \lambda \sum_{j=1}^{p} |w_j| \right) \tag{1.18}$$

where λ controls the strength of the regularization, and w_j represents the model coefficients.

Tree-Based Feature Importance: Decision tree algorithms (like Random Forests) rank features based on their contribution to reducing uncertainty (entropy or variance) at each split.

$$\text{Feature Importance} = \frac{\sum (\Delta\text{Impurity})}{\text{Total Nodes}} \tag{1.19}$$

where ΔImpurity refers to the change in impurity (e.g., Gini impurity or entropy) at each split involving the feature.

1.7.2.4 Illustrated Example with Sample Dataset – Feature Extraction

In healthcare, sensor data analytics often involves working with vast amounts of raw data captured from sensors like wearable devices, medical monitors, or environmental sensors (Chang et al. 2018). To make this data useful for predictive models, feature extraction and selection techniques are employed. These processes help in converting raw data into meaningful features and then selecting the most relevant features that can significantly improve model performance. Let's explore these concepts using a simple sample dataset.

Consider a small dataset collected from a wearable sensor that monitors a patient's physiological parameters such as heart rate (HR), body temperature (Temp), and oxygen saturation (SpO_2). The dataset, captured every second over a 6-second window, is shown in Table 1.7:

Here, the heart rate (HR) has an anomaly at the 4-second mark, where the value spikes to 300 bpm, which is likely due to sensor noise.

Feature extraction is the process of deriving meaningful and informative metrics from raw sensor data. In our example, we can extract time-domain, frequency-domain, and statistical features to summarize the data effectively.

1.7.2.4.1 Time-Domain Features

Mean (Average Value): The mean gives the central tendency of the data, which is useful to understand the overall trend of the physiological measurements. For example, the mean heart rate (HR) is calculated as:

$$\text{Mean HR} = \frac{80+82+300+78+81}{6} = 117.67\,\text{bpm} \tag{1.20}$$

Standard Deviation (SD): The standard deviation measures how much the values deviate from the mean. A higher standard deviation indicates more variability in the data. For heart rate:

$$\text{SD HR} = \sqrt{\frac{(80-117.67)^{2} + (82-117.67)^{2} + \ldots}{6}} =\approx 92.94\,\text{bpm} \tag{1.21}$$

Peak-to-Peak Amplitude: The peak-to-peak value represents the difference between the maximum and minimum values of the sensor signal:

$$\text{Peak-to-Peak HR} = 300 - 78 = 222\,\text{bpm} \tag{1.22}$$

This feature is particularly helpful in identifying anomalies like the outlier at 300 bpm.

1.7.2.4.2 Frequency-Domain Features

Frequency-domain analysis is useful for understanding periodic patterns in physiological data, such as ECG signals or breathing rates. We can apply the Fourier Transform to convert the heart rate data into the frequency domain:

TABLE 1.7
Physiological Parameters Dataset from Wearable Sensor

Time (s)	HR (bpm)	Temp (°C)	SpO_2 (%)
1	80	36.5	98
2	82	36.7	97
3	85	36.8	99
4	300	36.6	96
5	78	36.5	98
6	81	36.9	97

$$X(f) = \sum_{n=0}^{N-1} x(n) e^{-j2\pi fn/N} \tag{1.23}$$

This would reveal the dominant frequencies in the signal, but for simplicity, we can summarize the frequency-domain information using Power Spectral Density (PSD), which quantifies the power distribution of the signal across different frequencies.

1.7.2.4.3 Statistical Features

Skewness: Skewness helps in determining the asymmetry of the data. In our dataset, the presence of an outlier like 300 bpm introduces positive skewness, indicating that the data is right-skewed.

$$\text{Skewness} = \frac{6}{(6-1)(6-2)} \sum_{i=1}^{6} \left(\frac{\text{HR}_i - 117.67}{92.94} \right)^3 \approx 1.35 \tag{1.24}$$

A skewness value greater than zero indicates that the distribution is skewed to the right.

Kurtosis: Kurtosis measures the "tailedness" of the distribution. A high kurtosis value means that the data has heavy tails or extreme values like the 300 bpm in our case.

$$\text{Kurtosis} \approx 3.1 \tag{1.25}$$

This shows that the heart rate data has a slightly higher than normal kurtosis, indicating the presence of extreme values or outliers.

1.7.2.5 Illustrated Example with Sample Dataset – Feature Selection

Feature selection involves selecting the most relevant features from the extracted set, improving model accuracy and reducing computational complexity. We now focus on methods to choose the optimal features from our dataset.

1.7.2.5.1 Filter Methods

Correlation Coefficient: This measures the linear relationship between each feature (e.g., HR, Temp, SpO_2) and the target variable, such as the likelihood of detecting a cardiac event. A high correlation coefficient indicates a strong relationship.

The formula for correlation between heart rate (HR) and a hypothetical target variable (e.g., cardiac event risk) is:

$$r = \frac{\sum (\text{HR}_i - \mu_{\text{HR}})(y_i - \mu_y)}{\sqrt{\sum (\text{HR}_i - \mu_{\text{HR}})^2} \sqrt{\sum (y_i - \mu_y)^2}} \tag{1.26}$$

In healthcare, features like HR and SpO_2 are often highly correlated with the likelihood of specific medical conditions, making them important candidates for model inputs.

Mutual Information: Mutual information quantifies the amount of information shared between a feature and the target variable. Features with higher mutual information scores provide more insight into the target outcome, such as identifying abnormal heart rates as early warning signs.

1.7.2.5.2 Wrapper Methods

Recursive Feature Elimination (RFE): RFE is a popular wrapper method that recursively removes the least important features based on their contribution to a machine learning model. For example, we might start with HR, Temp, and SpO_2, and iteratively eliminate features that do not contribute significantly to the model's performance.

For our sensor dataset, RFE might suggest that HR and SpO_2 are critical features, while Temp is less relevant for predicting the target health outcome (e.g., detecting a cardiac event).

1.7.2.5.3 Embedded Methods

Lasso Regression (L1 Regularization): Lasso regression adds a penalty for non-zero coefficients, driving some feature weights to zero, effectively selecting a subset of important features. The Lasso regression formula is:

$$\text{Lasso Loss} = \sum_{i=1}^{N} \left(y_i - \hat{y}_i + \lambda \sum_{j=1}^{p} |w_j| \right) \tag{1.27}$$

where λ controls the regularization strength. For our sensor data, Lasso might determine that HR is the most significant feature for predicting health outcomes, while Temp and SpO_2 contribute less.

After applying feature selection techniques, we might identify the following optimal features from our healthcare sensor dataset:

1. **Heart Rate (HR):** Highly correlated with the target health outcomes, especially after removing noise and normalizing.
2. **SpO_2:** Relevant for respiratory or cardiac conditions, especially when combined with HR.
3. **Skewness and Kurtosis of HR:** These statistical features may help in identifying abnormal patterns in heart rate, such as arrhythmias or outliers caused by sensor noise.

1.8 SENSOR DATA FUSION IN HEALTHCARE

Sensor data fusion is a crucial process in healthcare analytics that involves integrating data from multiple sensors to obtain a more accurate and comprehensive understanding of a patient's condition or environment (Otoom et al. 2013). By combining data from various sources, healthcare providers can enhance decision-making, improve patient monitoring, and enable better diagnostic capabilities. This section explores the integration of data from multiple sensors and discusses various fusion techniques and algorithms used in healthcare applications.

1.8.1 Integration of Data from Multiple Sensors

In healthcare, various types of sensors are used to collect a wide range of physiological and environmental data. For example, wearable devices may monitor heart rate, temperature, oxygen saturation, and physical activity levels simultaneously. Additionally, stationary sensors in a clinical setting can monitor vital signs such as blood pressure, ECG, and respiratory rate. The integration of data from these multiple sensors provides a more holistic view of a patient's health status.

The integration process involves several steps:

1. **Data Collection:** Data is gathered from various sensors, which may be distributed across different locations (e.g., home, clinic, hospital). Each sensor captures specific parameters relevant to the patient's health.
2. **Data Preprocessing:** Before fusion, data from different sensors often needs to be cleaned and standardized. This may involve noise reduction, normalization, and alignment of data streams to ensure that they are comparable.

3. **Data Fusion:** The core of sensor data fusion is the combination of information from different sensors. This can involve various fusion techniques, depending on the nature of the data and the goals of the analysis.
4. **Data Interpretation:** The fused data is then interpreted to provide actionable insights, such as early detection of health issues, trends in patient monitoring, or changes in environmental conditions affecting health.

1.8.2 Applications of Sensor Data Fusion in Healthcare

Sensor data fusion has several practical applications in healthcare, including:

- **Remote Patient Monitoring:** By integrating data from wearable devices, healthcare providers can continuously monitor patients' vital signs, allowing for timely interventions when anomalies are detected.
- **Disease Diagnosis and Prognosis:** Fusion techniques can help combine data from multiple sources to identify patterns and relationships that may indicate the presence of a particular disease or predict its progression.
- **Clinical Decision Support Systems:** Fusing data from various sensors provides comprehensive insights, assisting healthcare professionals in making informed decisions about patient care.
- **Smart Environments for Elderly Care:** In smart homes equipped with various sensors (e.g., motion detectors, health monitoring devices), data fusion can be used to detect changes in behavior that may indicate health issues, enabling timely assistance.

1.8.3 Illustrated Example with Sample Dataset – Sensor Data Fusion

Consider the following dataset given in Table 1.8, collected from two sensors: Sensor A (HR): measures heart rate in beats per minute (bpm), and Sensor B (SpO_2): measures blood oxygen saturation in percentage (%).

Sensor data fusion involves combining information from multiple sensors to create a more comprehensive dataset that provides a holistic view of the patient's physiological status.

Simple Averaging: A common method is to average the readings from both sensors at each time point.

Average HR (bpm)

$$\text{Average HR} = \frac{80+82+85+78+81}{5} = 81.2\,\text{bpm} \tag{1.28}$$

TABLE 1.8
Physiological Parameters Dataset

Time (min)	HR (Sensor A)	SpO_2 (Sensor B)
1	80	98
2	82	97
3	85	99
4	78	96
5	81	97

Average SpO_2 (%)

$$\text{Average HR} = \frac{97+98+99+96+97}{5} = 97.4\% \quad (1.29)$$

Combined dataset after averaging is shown in Table 1.9:

Weighted Averaging: Sometimes, sensors are weighted differently based on their reliability or importance. Assuming Sensor A (HR) is given more weight (70%) and Sensor B (SpO_2) is given less weight (30%):

$$\text{Weighted Average HR} = 0.7 * \text{HR} * 0.3 * \text{SpO}_2 \quad (1.30)$$

Calculating for each time point as,

$$\text{Weighted Average HR} = 0.7 * 80 * 0.3 * 98 = 85.4 \text{ bpm} \quad (1.31)$$

Repeat similarly for other time points.

Kalman Filtering: Kalman filtering can be applied to fuse the measurements from Sensor A and Sensor B to obtain a more accurate estimate of HR and SpO_2.

Define State Variables: Let x_k represent the state vector at time k. For our case, the state vector could be

$$x_k = \begin{bmatrix} \text{HR}_k \\ \text{SpO}_{2k} \end{bmatrix} \quad (1.32)$$

Measurement Model: Each sensor provides measurements related to the state vector with noise:

$$z_k = \begin{bmatrix} \text{HR}_k \\ \text{SpO}_{2k} \end{bmatrix} \quad (1.33)$$

Measurement noise v_k accounts for inaccuracies or noise in each sensor's measurements.

State Transition Model: Assume a simple model where the physiological parameters change smoothly over time. The state transition matrix F_k might be an identity matrix if we assume no significant dynamics between time steps.

Measurement Model: The measurement matrix H_k is typically an identity matrix, assuming direct measurement of HR and SpO_2.

Initial Conditions: Start with an initial estimate $\hat{x}_0$ based on the first measurements and an initial covariance matrix P_0.

TABLE 1.9
Combined Dataset After Simple Averaging of Sensor Readings

Time (min)	Combined HR (bpm)	Combined SpO_2 (%)
1	81.2	97.4
2	81.2	97.4
3	81.2	97.4
4	81.2	97.4
5	81.2	97.4

TABLE 1.10
Filtered HR and SpO_2 Measurements Using Kalman Filtering

Time (min)	Filtered HR (Sensor A)	Filtered SpO_2 (Sensor B)
1	80.000	98.000
2	81.795	97.318
3	83.984	97.738
4	82.799	97.179
5	82.948	97.148

Process and Measurement Noise: Determine appropriate process noise Q_k and measurement noise R_k covariances based on the characteristics of the sensors and expected noise levels.

Table 1.10 shows the filtered results using the Kalman Filtering for the provided dataset of HR and SpO_2 measurements:

1.9 DATA QUALITY DIMENSIONS

Data Quality Dimensions are fundamental metrics that underpin the integrity and usefulness of data in analytical processes across various domains. Ensuring high-quality data is essential for deriving accurate insights and making informed decisions. These dimensions—consistency, completeness, time-frame, and accuracy—act as benchmarks to evaluate and enhance the reliability of datasets.

Consistency: Consistency in data quality ensures that information remains coherent and aligned within its intended context. It pertains to the uniformity and reliability of data across different sources or over time. In analytical settings, consistency ensures that data interpretations and conclusions drawn from analyses are accurate and dependable. For instance, in IoT sensor data, consistency ensures that measurements from various sensors reflect the same environmental conditions or operational states consistently, despite potential environmental factors or device variations.

Completeness: Completeness refers to the extent to which all expected data values are present in a dataset. It ensures that no information or observations are missing, which could otherwise lead to gaps in analysis or biased conclusions. In datasets involving time-series data, such as patient health records or manufacturing sensor readings, completeness is critical to maintaining the integrity and reliability of historical trends and predictive models. Addressing completeness ensures that data-driven decisions are based on comprehensive and representative information.

Time-Frame: Time-frame in data quality pertains to the timeliness and synchronization of data capture and reporting. It ensures that data points are recorded within appropriate intervals and align with the intended temporal scope of analysis. In time-sensitive applications like financial markets or real-time monitoring systems, adherence to time-frame dimensions ensures that insights derived from data analytics are relevant and actionable. It also facilitates accurate trend analysis and performance evaluation by capturing data points at consistent intervals without delays or discrepancies.

Accuracy: Accuracy measures the closeness of data values to their true or expected values. It ensures that data collected and reported by sensors, devices, or systems are reliable and trustworthy for decision-making. In healthcare diagnostics or environmental monitoring, accuracy is crucial for ensuring that measurements reflect actual conditions or patient states accurately. Calibration, validation procedures, and quality control measures are essential to maintain data accuracy, minimizing errors and ensuring that analytical models produce reliable outcomes.

1.9.1 Illustrated Example with Sample Dataset – Data Quality Dimensions

Consider a dataset containing temperature readings from IoT sensors deployed across different locations over a week (Table 1.11):

In this dataset:

- **Timestamp**: Indicates the time when each temperature reading was recorded.
- **Location**: Specifies the sensor location or identifier (e.g., Sensor A, Sensor B, Sensor C).
- **Temperature (°C)**: Represents the recorded temperature in degrees Celsius at each timestamp and location.

Consistency: Consistency ensures that data is coherent and aligned with its context. In our example: all sensors should report temperatures consistently based on their location. If Sensor A consistently reports temperatures lower than Sensors B and C despite similar environmental conditions, it might indicate a calibration issue or environmental influence.

Completeness: Completeness checks if all expected data values are present. If Sensor B fails to report temperature readings for a few hours due to connectivity issues, there will be gaps in the dataset. Addressing missing data ensures a comprehensive dataset for accurate analysis.

Time-Frame: Time-frame ensures data is captured within an appropriate timeframe. If Sensor A reports a temperature at 08:00:00 and Sensor B reports the next reading at 08:15:00, the time interval between readings should be consistent across all sensors. Inconsistent intervals may affect time-series analysis accuracy.

Accuracy: Accuracy measures the closeness of sensor measurements to the true value. Calibration checks ensure that each sensor accurately measures temperature. If Sensor C consistently reports temperatures 2°C higher than the actual ambient temperature, it affects the accuracy of temperature predictions and analyses.

1.10 ERRORS IN SENSOR DATA

Errors in sensor data are fundamental challenges in the realm of modern data analytics and technology-driven applications (Islam et al. 2018). These errors, stemming from a variety of sources such as measurement inaccuracies, environmental factors, and technical limitations, can significantly impact the reliability and usability of data collected by sensors. Understanding and effectively managing these errors are critical for ensuring the accuracy of measurements and the validity of insights derived from sensor data across diverse domains.

TABLE 1.11
Temperature Readings from IoT Sensors

Timestamp	Location	Temperature (°C)
2024-10-01 08:00:00	Sensor A	22
2024-10-01 08:15:00	Sensor B	23
2024-10-01 08:30:00	Sensor C	24
2024-10-01 08:45:00	Sensor A	21
2024-10-01 09:00:00	Sensor B	22

Errors in sensor data encompass a range of deviations from true measurements. It includes uncertainties that arise due to inherent limitations in sensor precision, outliers that represent unexpected and potentially misleading data points, and systematic biases influenced by environmental conditions or sensor calibration issues (Malik and Malik 2020). Drifts in sensor readings over time, missing data points due to transmission failures, and anomalies caused by sensor malfunctions further complicate the reliability of sensor-derived information.

Addressing these challenges requires a multidisciplinary approach that integrates advanced sensor technologies, rigorous calibration procedures, robust data quality assurance methods, and sophisticated data processing techniques (Dias and Cunha 2018). By systematically identifying, quantifying, and mitigating these errors, organizations can enhance the accuracy, reliability, and utility of sensor data for critical applications in healthcare, environmental monitoring, industrial automation, and beyond.

1.10.1 Types of Errors in Sensor Data

Uncertainties: Uncertainties in sensor data arise from inherent limitations in measurement accuracy and precision. These errors stem from factors such as sensor sensitivity, calibration drifts, and environmental variability that introduce unavoidable variability in measured values. Managing uncertainties involves rigorous calibration protocols, statistical modeling to quantify measurement errors, and employing uncertainty propagation techniques to ensure accurate interpretation of sensor data across applications.

Example: A temperature sensor in a controlled environment is calibrated to measure within ±0.5°C accuracy. However, due to slight variations in ambient temperature and sensor aging, the actual recorded temperatures may vary by ±0.2°C from the true values.

Outliers: Outliers in sensor data are aberrant observations that deviate significantly from the expected range of values (Karthick and Pankajavalli 2023). These anomalies can distort statistical analyses and machine learning models, potentially leading to erroneous conclusions or misleading insights. Detecting outliers requires robust statistical techniques such as Z-score analysis, box plots, or clustering algorithms to identify and filter out data points that do not conform to the expected distribution of sensor readings.

Example: In a dataset of heart rate readings from patients, an outlier might be a sudden spike to 180 bpm during a period where most readings are between 60 and 100 bpm. This spike could be due to a temporary irregularity in a patient's heart rhythm.

Missing Values: Missing values in sensor data occur due to transmission failures, sensor malfunctions, or environmental interferences that prevent data from being recorded or transmitted (Karthick and Pankajavalli 2020). These gaps in data can impact the continuity and integrity of time-series analyses and predictive models. Addressing missing values involves data imputation methods such as mean imputation, interpolation techniques, or advanced predictive models to estimate and fill in missing data points while minimizing distortion to the overall dataset.

Example: In a dataset of hourly temperature readings from weather stations, missing values might occur if a sensor malfunctions for a specific hour, resulting in a gap where no temperature data is recorded.

Biases: Biases in sensor data refer to consistent deviations in measurements from the true values, often influenced by calibration errors, environmental conditions, or sensor drift over time. These systematic errors can skew data analysis and decision-making processes if not properly identified and corrected. Mitigating biases requires regular sensor calibration, environmental monitoring, and statistical adjustments to align measured values with known reference standards and minimize systematic errors in sensor outputs.

Example: A pH sensor used in water quality monitoring consistently reads 0.2 units higher than the actual pH value due to calibration drift or contamination on the sensor probe (Table 1.12).

Drifts: Drifts in sensor data occur when sensor readings gradually shift away from their calibrated values over time. This phenomenon is commonly observed in sensors due to aging components, changes in environmental conditions, or prolonged operation without recalibration. Monitoring and correcting drifts involve periodic sensor recalibration, data trend analysis, and adaptive algorithms to adjust for gradual changes in sensor performance and maintain measurement accuracy over extended periods.

Example: A pressure sensor in an industrial process may exhibit drift, where its readings gradually increase by 0.1 bar per month due to wear and tear on internal components, affecting the accuracy of pressure measurements over time.

Stuck-At Faults: Stuck-at faults in sensor data manifest as persistent readings that remain at a single value (e.g., zero or maximum) due to sensor malfunctions, signal transmission errors, or hardware failures. These faults can disrupt data continuity and compromise the reliability of sensor outputs. Detecting and mitigating stuck-at faults requires real-time

TABLE 1.12
Types of Errors in Sensor Data, Healthcare Applications, Properties, Inferences, Pros, Cons, Examples, and Techniques for Handling Errors

Error Type	Healthcare Application	Inference	Example	Techniques for Handling
Uncertainties	Patient monitoring	Requires rigorous calibration and uncertainty modeling	Temperature sensor may record ±0.2°C variation due to sensor aging and environmental factors	Rigorous calibration protocols, uncertainty propagation techniques
Outliers	Health anomaly detection	Distorts statistical analysis and ML models	Heart rate sensor records a spike to 180 bpm during a period of normal readings	Statistical methods (Z-score analysis, clustering), robust filtering
Missing values	Remote patient monitoring	Impacts time-series analyses and predictive models	Hourly temperature readings miss data due to sensor malfunction	Imputation (mean, interpolation), predictive models for estimation
Biases	Medical diagnostics	Skews data analysis and decision-making	pH sensor consistently reads 0.2 units higher due to calibration drift	Calibration, environmental monitoring, statistical adjustments
Drifts	Long-term patient monitoring	Affects long-term data accuracy and reliability	Pressure sensor shows gradual increase in readings due to component wear	Trend analysis, adaptive algorithms, periodic recalibration
Stuck-at faults	Remote health monitoring	Disrupts real-time data continuity and reliability	Wind speed sensor consistently reads 0 m/s due to broken connection	Real-time monitoring, redundant sensor systems, fault detection algorithms
Noise	Wearable health devices	Compromises signal accuracy during capture and processing	Accelerometer records small, rapid fluctuations unrelated to actual vibrations	Signal filtering, noise reduction algorithms, digital signal processing

monitoring, fault detection algorithms, and redundant sensor systems to ensure timely identification and correction of erroneous data outputs.

Example: A wind speed sensor in a weather station continuously shows a reading of 0 m/s, despite varying wind conditions, due to a malfunctioning anemometer or a broken connection in the data transmission line.

Noise: Noise in sensor data refers to unwanted variations or distortions in signal measurements caused by electrical interference, environmental factors, or inherent sensor characteristics. This extraneous noise can obscure true signal patterns and compromise data accuracy during signal capture, transmission, or processing stages. Minimizing noise involves signal filtering techniques, noise reduction algorithms, and signal processing methods to enhance the signal-to-noise ratio and extract meaningful information from sensor data while mitigating the effects of unwanted noise sources.

Example: In an accelerometer dataset measuring vibration levels in machinery, noise might manifest as small, rapid fluctuations in sensor readings unrelated to actual machine vibrations, potentially obscuring meaningful data patterns.

1.11 CONCLUSION

In conclusion, the exploration of sensor data in healthcare underscores its pivotal role in advancing diagnostics, treatment, and patient care. This chapter has highlighted fundamental aspects essential for effectively leveraging sensor data within healthcare environments. It has detailed the criticality of various sensor types, ranging from physiological monitors to environmental sensors, and outlined robust techniques for acquiring and preprocessing data to ensure its reliability and quality. By emphasizing methods such as noise reduction, filtering, normalization, and scaling, the chapter has underscored their significance in preparing sensor data for rigorous analysis.

Moreover, the discussion on feature extraction methods—including time-domain, frequency-domain, and statistical features—has highlighted their importance in deriving meaningful insights from sensor data, particularly in healthcare applications. Additionally, the chapter has examined various types of errors that can affect sensor data, from uncertainties and outliers to biases, drifts, stuck-at faults, and noise. Through practical examples, it has illustrated the impact of these errors and emphasized the necessity of robust error detection and mitigation strategies.

REFERENCES

Ahmad, M.A., M. Al Hemairy, S. Amin, "A New Algorithm for Online Diseases Diagnosis," in *2018 Innovations in Intelligent Systems and Applications (INISTA)*, Thessaloniki, Greece (2018), 1–14.

Akhbarifar, S., H.H.S. Javadi, A.M. Rahmani, M. Hosseinzadeh, "A Secure Remote Health Monitoring Model for Early Disease Diagnosis in Cloud-Based IoT Environment," *Personal and Ubiquitous Computing* 27 (2020), 1–17.

Baig, M.M., H. Gholamhosseini, "Smart Health Monitoring Systems: An Overview of Design and Modeling," *Journal of Medical Systems* 37, no. 2 (2013), 9898. https://doi.org/10.1007/s10916-012-9898-z

Banaee, H., M.U. Ahmed, A. Loutfi, "Data Mining for Wearable Sensors in Health Monitoring Systems: A Review of Recent Trends and Challenges," *Sensors* 13, no. 12 (2013): 17472–17500. https://doi.org/10.3390/s131217472

Chang, R.C.-H., H.-L. Chen, C.-H. Lin, K.-H. Lin, "Design of a Low-Complexity Real-Time Arrhythmia Detection System," *Journal of Signal Processing Systems* 90, no. 1 (2018), 145–156.

Dias, D., J. Paulo Silva Cunha, "Wearable Health Devices-Vital Sign Monitoring, Systems and Technologies," *Sensors* 18, no. 8 (2018), 2414.

Dyskin, A., H. Basarir, J. Doherty, M. Elchalakani, G. Joldes, A. Karrech, B. Lehane, K. Miller, E. Pasternak, I. Shufrin, A. Wittek, "Computational Monitoring in Real Time: Review of Methods and Applications," *Geomechanics, Geophysics, Geo-Energy and Geo-Resources* 4 (2018), 235–271.

Esposito, M., A. Minutolo, R. Megna, M. Forastiere, M. Magliulo, G. De Pietro, "A Smart Mobile, Self-Configuring, Context-Aware Architecture for Personal Health Monitoring," *Engineering Applications of Artificial Intelligence* 67 (2018), 136–156. https://doi.org/10.1016/j.engappai.2017.09.019

Forkan, A.R.M., I. Khalil, "A Clinical Decision-Making Mechanism for Context-Aware and Patient-Specific Remote Monitoring Systems Using the Correlations of Multiple Vital Signs," *Computer Methods and Programs in Biomedicine* 139 (2017), 1–16. https://doi.org/10.1016/j.cmpb.2016.10.018

Hartmann, M., U.S. Hashmi, A. Imran, "Edge Computing in Smart Healthcare Systems: Review, Challenges, and Research Directions," *Transactions on Emerging Telecommunications Technologies* 33, no. 3 (2019), e3710.

Islam, M.S., M.M. Hasan, X. Wang, H.D. Germack, M. Noor-E-Alam, "A Systematic Review on Healthcare Analytics: Application and Theoretical Perspective of Data Mining," *Healthcare* 6, no. 2 (2018), 54. https://doi.org/10.3390/healthcare6020054

Jeon, T., B. Kim, M. Jeon, B.-G. Lee, "Implementation of a Portable Device for Real-Time ECG Signal Analysis," *BioMedical Engineering OnLine* 13, no. 1 (2014), 160. https://doi.org/10.1186/1475-925X-13-160

Joshi, M., H. Ashrafian, L. Aufegger, S. Khan, S. Arora, G. Cooke, A. Darzi, "Wearable Sensors to Improve Detection of Patient Deterioration," *Expert Review of Medical Devices* 16, no. 2 (2018), 145–154.

Kakria, P., N.K. Tripathi, P. Kitipawang, "A Real-Time Health Monitoring System for Remote Cardiac Patients Using Smartphone and Wearable Sensors," *International Journal of Telemedicine and Applications* 2015 (2015), 373474. https://doi.org/10.1155/2015/373474

Karthick, G. S., P. B. Pankajavalli. "A Review on Human Healthcare Internet of Things: A Technical Perspective," *SN Computer Science* 1, no. 4 (2020), 198.

Karthick, G. S., P. B. Pankajavalli. "Chronic Obstructive Pulmonary Disease Prediction Using Internet of Things-Spiro System and Fuzzy-Based Quantum Neural Network Classifier," *Theoretical Computer Science* 941 (2023), 55–76.

Lu, L., J. Zhang, Y. Xie, F. Gao, S. Xu, X. Wu, Z. Ye, "Wearable Health Devices in Health Care: Narrative Systematic Review," *JMIR mHealth and uHealth* 8, no. 11 (2020), e18907.

Malik, N., S.K. Malik, *Using IoT and Semantic Web Technologies for Healthcare and Medical Sector* (John Wiley & Sons, Ltd, 2020), Ch. 5, 91–115. https://doi.org/10.1002/9781119641391.ch5

Mustafa, T., A. Varol, "Review of the Internet of Things for Healthcare Monitoring," in *2020 8th International Symposium on Digital Forensics and Security (ISDFS)*, Beirut, Lebanon (2020), 1–6.

Nubenthan, S., K. Ravichelvan, "A Wireless Continuous Patient Monitoring System for Dengue; Wi-Mon," in *2017 International Conference on Wireless Communications, Signal Processing and Networking (WiSPNET)* (2017), 2201–2205. https://doi.org/10.1109/WiSPNET.2017.8300150

Otoom, M., H. Alshraideh, H.M. Almasaeid, D. Lopez-de Ipina, J. Bravo, "A Real-Time Insulin Injection System," in *Ambient Assisted Living and Active Aging*, eds. C. Nugent, A. Coronato, J. Bravo (Springer International Publishing, 2013), 120–127.

Syed, L., S. Jabeen, S. Manimala, H.A. Elsayed, *Data Science Algorithms and Techniques for Smart Healthcare Using IoT and Big Data Analytics* (Springer International Publishing, 2019), 211–241. https://doi.org/10.1007/978-3-030-03131-2_11

2 Statistical Approximation of Streaming Sensor Data for Enhancing Healthcare Analytics

B. Aadharsh and C. Arunpriya

2.1 INTRODUCTION

"Healthcare providers are increasingly turning to data streaming technologies to monitor patient health in real-time and predict potential health issues before they arise" (Shukla, 2023). The use of low-cost wearable healthcare devices and proactive monitoring of vital physiological data is seen as a solution for the high costs and risks associated with personal healthcare. However, the healthcare data generated from these sensors cannot be manually analyzed for anomalies by clinicians due to its scale. Therefore, automated techniques have to be developed. Statistical approximation of streaming sensor data is an invaluable tool in healthcare. Statistical approximation methods assist in transforming raw sensor data, initially presented as continuous-time analog signals, to achieve filtered and smoothed signals (in the continuous-time domain). Such statistical approximations not only enhance the interpretability of the data but also facilitate timely healthcare interventions.

2.1.1 Practical Example

"Automatic and continuous blood pressure monitoring is important for preventing cardiovascular diseases such as hypertension. The evaluation of medication effects and the diagnosis of clinical hypertension can both benefit from continuous monitoring" (Li, 2023). Monitoring blood pressure (BP) continuously in real-time is a dynamic challenge, especially when dealing with analog measurements that can fluctuate due to various factors. Consider a continuous time – blood pressure monitoring system (CT – BPMS) that captures continuous variations in BP. Interpreting this raw, analog sensor data is inherently challenging due to its infinite sampling rates and frequency bandwidths. Raw analog data also accommodates noises during data measurement, such as:

1. Inaccuracies in BP readings during scenarios where users might move their arms, and,
2. Brief spikes in BP, due to unprecedented increase in heart or breathing rates.

Therefore, mathematical tools are employed to filter out unwanted noise and fluctuations in the data. Statistical approximations act as a smart filter that distinguishes meaningful changes in a stream of sensor data by isolating useful data from transients and environmental noises. This allows us to represent the streams of sensor data concisely and comprehensibly.

2.2 TECHNIQUES FOR STATISTICAL APPROXIMATION

Statistical approximation techniques play a vital role in extracting valuable information from continuous data sequences, contributing significantly to a clearer and more precise understanding of

DOI: 10.1201/9781003486640-2

real-time sensor input. Some commonly used techniques for the statistical approximation of streaming sensor data are as follows:

1. **Moving Averages:** The method of moving averages is applied to smooth out fluctuations and highlight trends and variations in the data. These methods are useful for identifying patterns and reducing noise in the streaming sensor data.
2. **Statistical Indicators:** Statistical indicators include measures of central tendency, variability, and distribution. This incorporates key metrics like mean, median, standard deviation, and percentiles. Aggregating these statistics over fixed time intervals can help in effective screening of streaming data effectively.
3. **Histograms:** Constructing histograms can be beneficial to visualize the distribution of sensor data over time. Histograms help in identifying common values and outliers, providing insights into the data's characteristics.
4. **Clustering:** "Data clustering techniques are descriptive data analysis techniques that can be applied to multivariate data sets to uncover the structure present in the data" (Morissette, 2013). Utilizing clustering algorithms such as k-means can help group similar patterns or behaviors within the streaming sensor data. This approach can be valuable for identifying distinct clusters or anomalies in the data.
5. **Change Detection:** Statistical methods for change detection, like cumulative sum or sequential probability ratio test, can be employed to identify sudden shifts or anomalies in the streaming sensor data.
6. **Time Series Analysis:** Techniques like autoregressive models, moving average models, or machine learning models tailored for time series data can be used to make predictions and detect patterns in the streaming sensor data.
7. **Compression Algorithms:** Using compression techniques like delta encoding or variable-length encoding can reduce the data size while preserving important information, making it easier to store and transmit.
8. **Statistical Tests:** Applying statistical tests to check for correlations, trends, or deviations from expected behavior can be valuable in understanding the streaming sensor data.

In this chapter, the details of a few of the statistical approximation methods discussed above, namely, moving averages, statistical indicators, and clustering, are discussed.

2.3 MOVING AVERAGES

Moving averages can broadly be classified into two major types:

1. Simple Moving Average (SMA) and
2. Exponential Moving Average (EMA)

2.4 SIMPLE MOVING AVERAGE

SMA calculates the average of a set of data points over a specific period, assigning equal weight to each data point in the calculation as shown in equation (2.1).

$$\overline{X} = \frac{\text{Sum of Data Points}}{\text{Number of Data Points in the Period}} \tag{2.1}$$

Let $x_1, x_2, x_3, x_4 \cdots x_n$ be a data sequence with n data points, then the Simple Moving Average (SMA) $\overline{X}$ is given by the equation (2.2),

$$\bar{X} = \frac{x_1 + x_2 + x_3 + x_4 + \cdots + x_n}{n} \tag{2.2}$$

2.4.1 Practical Example

Consider a 3×3 matrix (Figure 2.1), the color of each tile is to be updated with the corresponding SMA (average color) of the current tile and its adjacent tiles, as shown in Figure 2.2.

$$\bar{X} = \frac{\sum(\text{Colors in Current \& Adjacent Blocks})}{\text{Number of Blocks}} \tag{2.3}$$

In equation (2.3), $\bar{X}$ represents the color corresponding to the SMA of colors in the current tile and adjacent tiles.

2.4.2 SMA Blocks 1, 3, 7, 9

Blocks 1, 3, 7, and 9 are red, each with two adjacent blue blocks: (2, 4), (2, 6), (4, 8), and (6, 8).

Substitute the color of blocks 1, 2, 3,..., 9 in the equations given in Figure 2.3a–d to obtain the SMA (average color) of the current tile and its adjacent tiles.

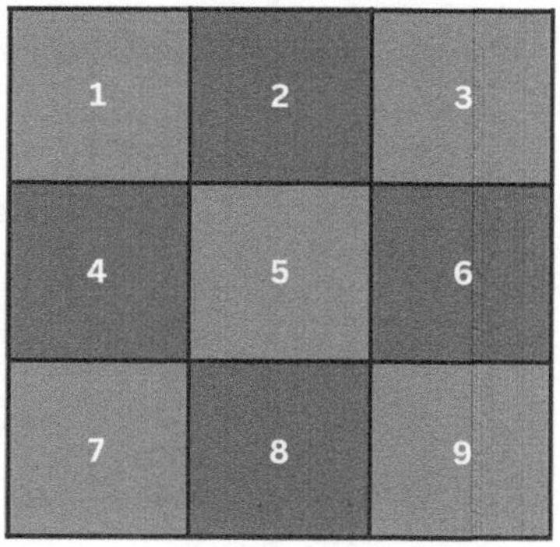

FIGURE 2.1 Original matrix.

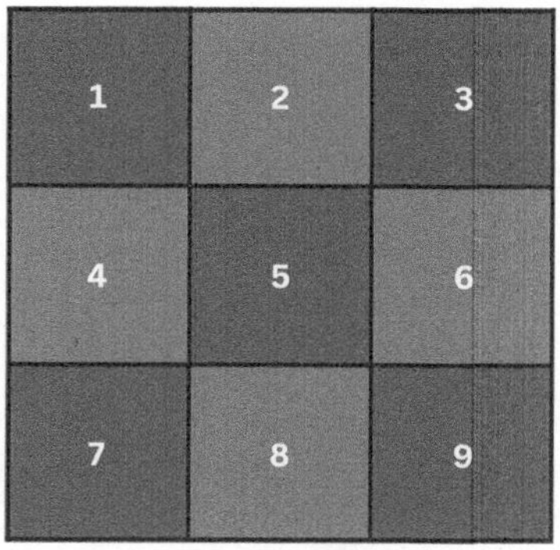

FIGURE 2.2 Post SMA matrix.

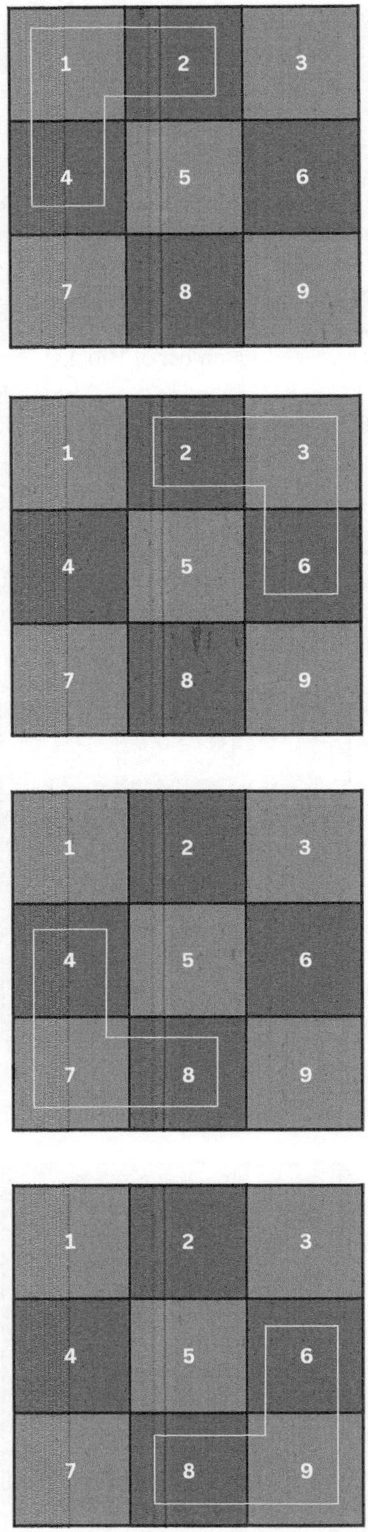

FIGURE 2.3 (a) Evaluating the SMA of tile 1. (b) Evaluating the SMA of tile 3. (c) Evaluating the SMA of tile 7. (d) Evaluating the SMA of tile 9.

$$\text{SMA} = \bar{X} = \text{average}(\text{Current, Adjacent, Adjacent}) = \text{average}(\text{Red, Blue, Blue})$$

Blue dominates Red in the SMA (average) calculation of Red, Blue, Blue due to the equal weighting assigned to each color. With Blue appearing twice and Red appearing once in the calculation, the resultant average leans toward Blue, as shown in equation (2.4).

$$\bar{X} = \text{average}(\text{Red, Blue, Blue}) \approx \text{Cool Shade} \tag{2.4}$$

2.4.3 SMA Block 5

Block 5, colored red, is surrounded by four adjacent blue blocks: 2, 4, 6, and 8. Therefore, the SMA is given in equation (2.5):

$$\begin{aligned}\bar{X} &= \text{average}(\text{Block 2, Block 4, Block 6, Block 8, Block 5}) \\ &= \text{average}(\text{Blue, Blue, Blue, Blue, Red})\end{aligned} \tag{2.5}$$

The blue color appears four times in the list of colors being averaged, while Red appears only once. Thus, the average color would be closer to Blue (cooler than SMA of Blocks 1, 3, 7 and 9) due to its greater frequency in the calculation and is shown by Figure 2.4.

2.4.4 SMA Block 2, 4, 6, 8

Blocks 2, 4, 6, and 8 are Blue in color, with respective adjacent blocks (1, 3, 5), (3, 5, 9), (5, 7, 9), and (1, 5, 7) that are red in color. Therefore, the SMA is given by the equation (2.6)

$$\bar{X} = \text{average}(\text{red, red, red, blue}) = \text{Warm Shade} \tag{2.6}$$

Red, being a warm color, dominates the average due to its greater frequency, while the cooler tone of blue is offset by the three occurrences of red (Figure 2.5).

2.4.5 Advantages

Easy to Evaluate: Simple mathematical models reduce computational loads and time required for statistical approximation and interpretation.

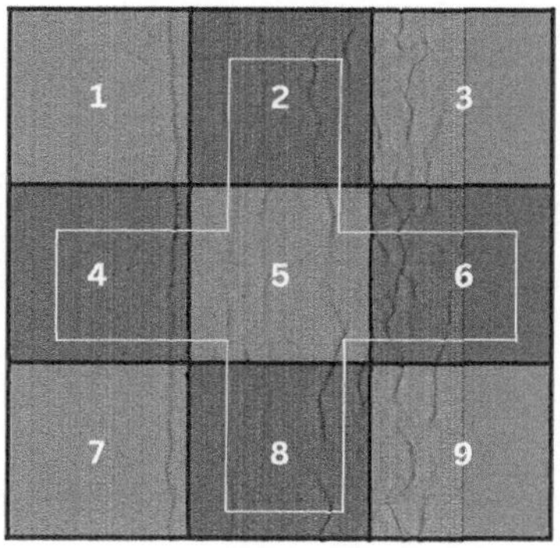

FIGURE 2.4 Evaluation of SMA for Block 5.

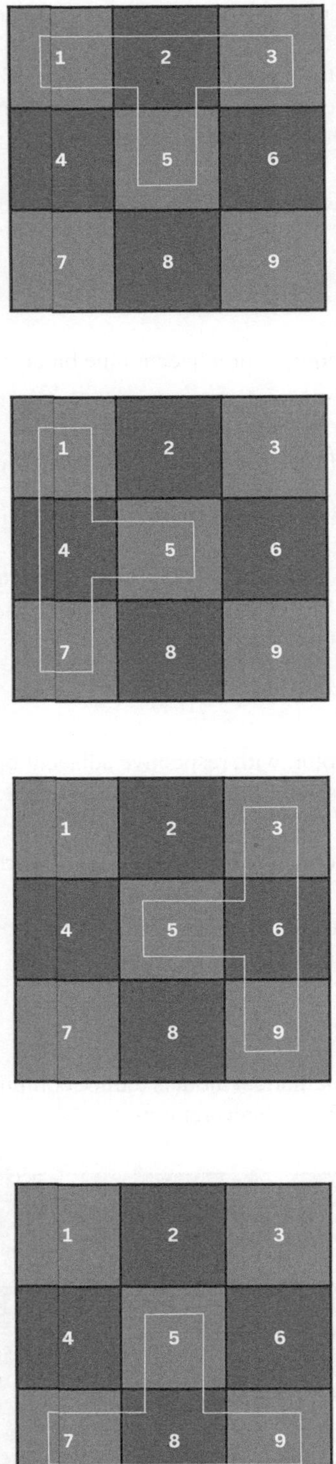

FIGURE 2.5 (a) Evaluation of SMA for Block 2. (b) Evaluation of SMA for Block 4. (c) Evaluation of SMA for Block 6. (d) Evaluation of SMA for Block 8.

2.4.6 Disadvantages

The processed, averaged image is significantly different from the unprocessed, raw data.

2.5 EXPONENTIAL MOVING AVERAGE

EMA acts as a low pass filter by assigning higher weights to recent data, smoothing out fluctuations and emphasizing the trend, providing a refined and responsive analysis. "More weight is assigned to recent data points" (Sarwar and Cantero, 2024), and exponentially decreasing weights to older observations, thereby increasing its responsiveness to changes. EMA, x_t is defined using equation (2.7), where α is the smoothing factor (or the low-pass filter constant).

$$x_t = \alpha x_t + (1-\alpha) x_{t-1} \tag{2.7}$$

2.5.1 Smoothing Factor

Assume an arbitrary value, say 0.2, for the smoothing factor α (i.e., α=0.2). Substituting this value into equation (2.7) results in the equation (2.8).

$$x_t = (0.2) x_t + (0.8) x_{t-1} \tag{2.8}$$

Expanding x_{t-1} in terms of x_{t-2}, equation (2.9) is obtained.

$$x_t = (0.2) x_t + (0.8)\left((0.2) x_{t-1} + (0.8) x_{t-2}\right) \tag{2.9}$$

Simplify equation (2.9) and obtain equation(2.10)

$$x_t = (0.2) x_t + (0.16) x_{t-1} + (0.64) x_{t-2} \tag{2.10}$$

Equation (2.10) can be expanded infinitely, following a similar process to the expansion of equation (2.8) to equation (2.10). This yields the infinite series presented in equation (2.11).

$$x_t = (0.2) x_t + (0.16) x_{t-1} + (0.128) x_{t-2} + \ldots \tag{2.11}$$

Equation (2.11) can be expressed in its shorthand notation, as presented in equation (2.12). Subsequently, the value 0.8 is expressed as (1−0.2), resulting in equation (2.13).

$$x_t = (0.2) \sum_{k=0}^{n} (0.8)^k \cdot x_{t-k} \tag{2.12}$$

$$x_t = (0.2) \sum_{k=0}^{n} (1-0.2)^k \cdot x_{t-k} \tag{2.13}$$

The general EMA expansion, represented by equation (2.14), is derived by generalizing the smoothing factor. In this context, the arbitrary smoothing constant 0.2 is replaced with its general variable notation, α.

$$Y = x_t = (\alpha)\sum_{k=0}^{n}(1-\alpha)^k \cdot x_{t-k} \tag{2.14}$$

2.5.2 Influence of the Smoothing Factor on Graphical Data

The parameter α in the context of EMA serves as a crucial factor in determining the level of smoothness in the resulting output. When α is assigned a value of 0, the EMA produces the smoothest possible curve, effectively minimizing the impact of fluctuations in the input data. For values between 0 and 1 (exclusive), a smoothing effect is maintained, with higher α values leading to a progressively less smooth output. Notably, as α approaches 1, the smoothing effect diminishes, and the resulting EMA output mirrors the raw, unaltered data.

In conditions where $\alpha \rightarrow 0$, The output signal is '0' for any given input signal, i.e. at $\alpha \rightarrow 0$, the system exhibits maximum smoothing effects (Figure 2.6).

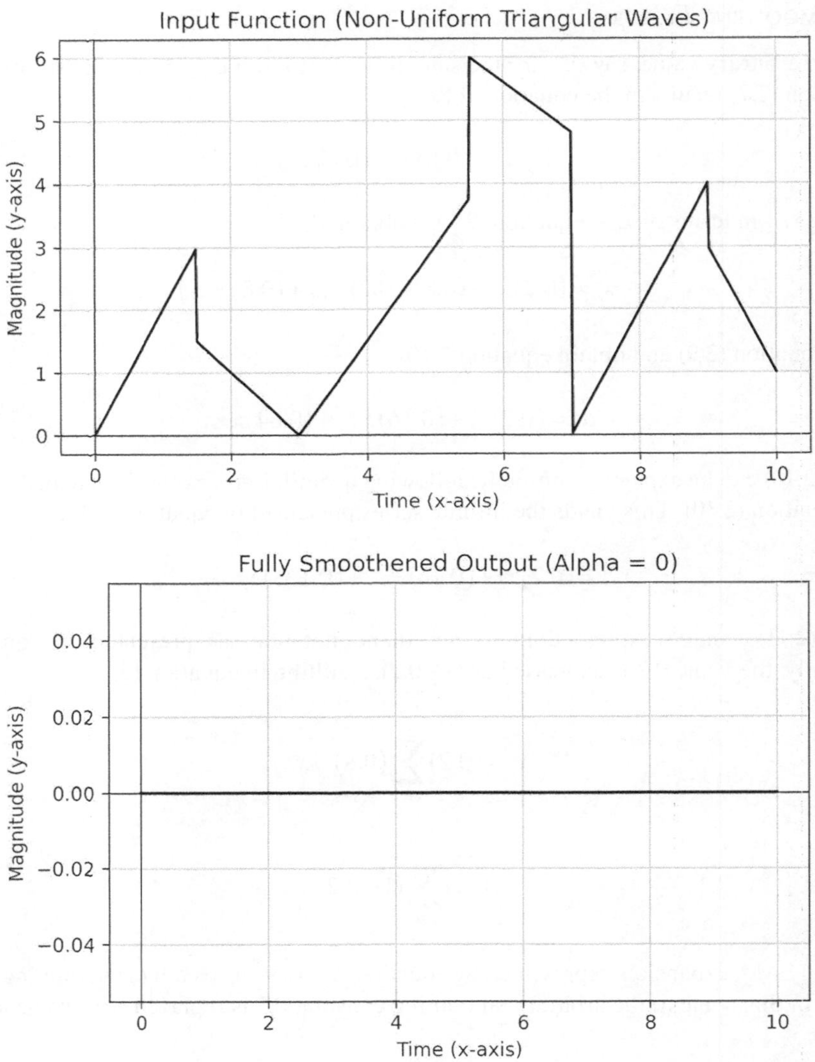

FIGURE 2.6 (a) Input signal. (b) Output signal ($\alpha = 0$). (c) Output signal ($0 > \alpha > 1$). (d) Output signal ($\alpha = 1$). *(Continued)*

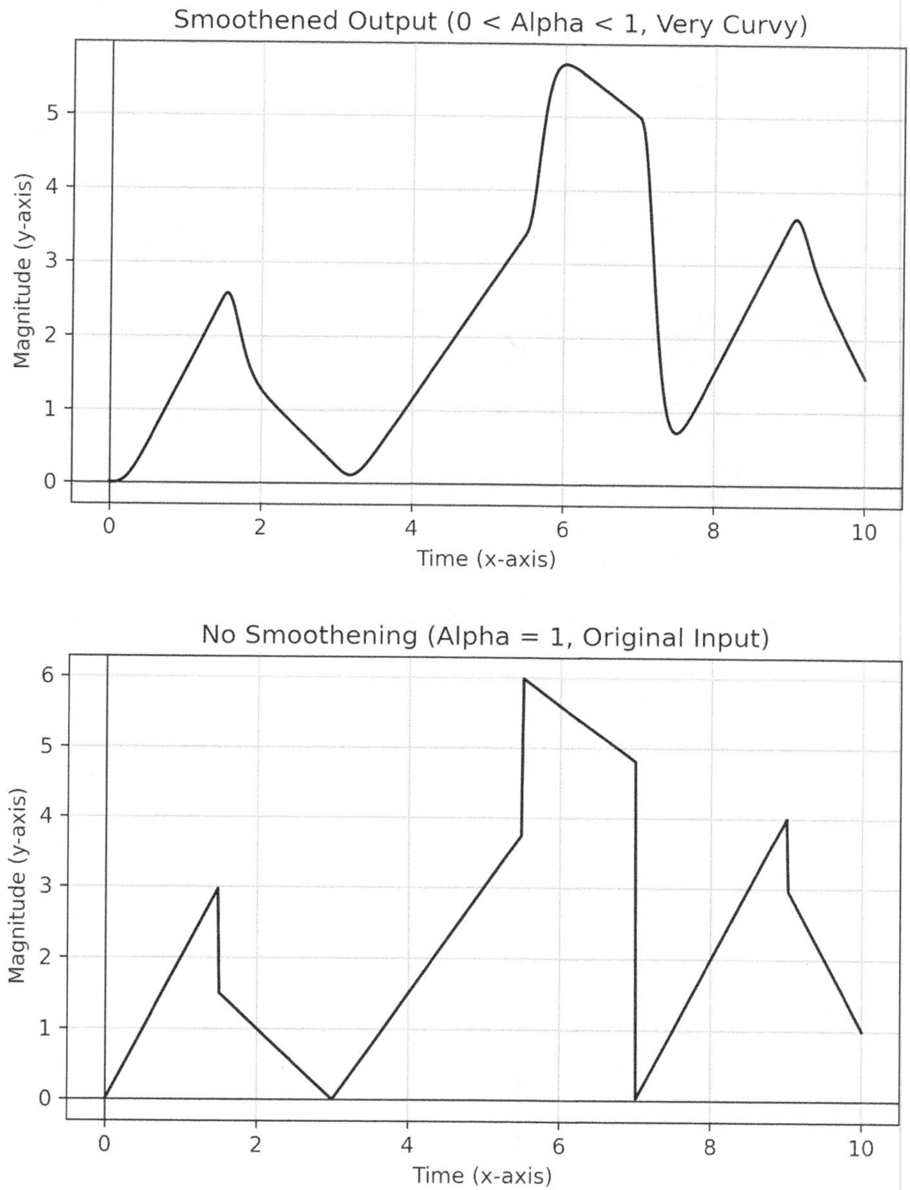

FIGURE 2.6 (*Continued*) (a) Input signal. (b) Output signal (α=0). (c) Output signal (0 > α > 1). (d) Output signal (α = 1).

$$Y = \lim_{\alpha \to 0} \alpha \sum_{k=0}^{n} (1-\alpha)^k \cdot x[n-k] = 0 \tag{2.15}$$

$$Y = 0 \tag{2.16}$$

By examining the weights assigned to the function at various sampling points, it becomes evident that, $\alpha \to 1$, input holds greater significance in influencing the EMA, and the input signal is returned as it is. Meaning that there is no signal smoothing effect as $\alpha \to 1$

$$x_t = \lim_{\alpha \to 1} \alpha \sum_{k=0}^{n} (1-\alpha)^k \cdot x[n-k] = \alpha(x_t) = x_t \tag{2.17}$$

$$x_t = x_t \tag{2.18}$$

Appropriate adjustment of the smoothness parameter 'α' allows for a dynamic balance between responsiveness to recent data and the degree of smoothness desired in the EMA curve.

2.6 CAUSAL, DECAYING EXPONENTIAL FREQUENCY RESPONSE AS LOW PASS FILTER

A low pass filter (LPF) is an analog filter used in signal processing to allow low-frequency components of a signal to pass through while attenuating high-frequency components. It achieves this by selectively allowing signals with frequencies below a certain cutoff frequency to pass through, while attenuating signals with frequencies above the cutoff frequency (Lambda Geeks) (Figure 2.7a–c).

A causal, decaying exponential acts as an LPF as well, as it tends to preserve lower-frequency components of the signal while blocking or attenuating higher-frequency components. This characteristic aligns with the behavior of a practical low-pass filter that allows signals with lower frequencies to pass through relatively unaffected while suppressing higher-frequency components.

2.7 EMA AS A LOW PASS FILTER

Consider that a unit impulse signal is supplied to the EMA Evaluation Algorithm as an input, represented mathematically by the equation (2.19) i.e.,

$$x(t) = \delta(t) \tag{2.19}$$

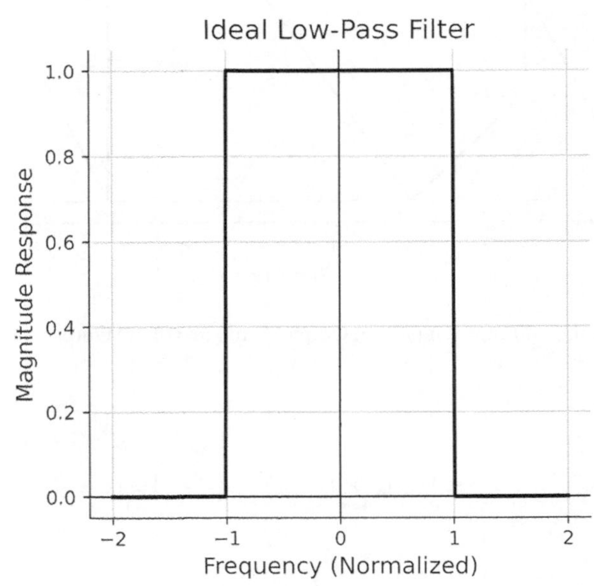

FIGURE 2.7 (a) Ideal low pass filter. (b) Practical low pass filter. (c) Characteristics of practical low pass filter.

(Continued)

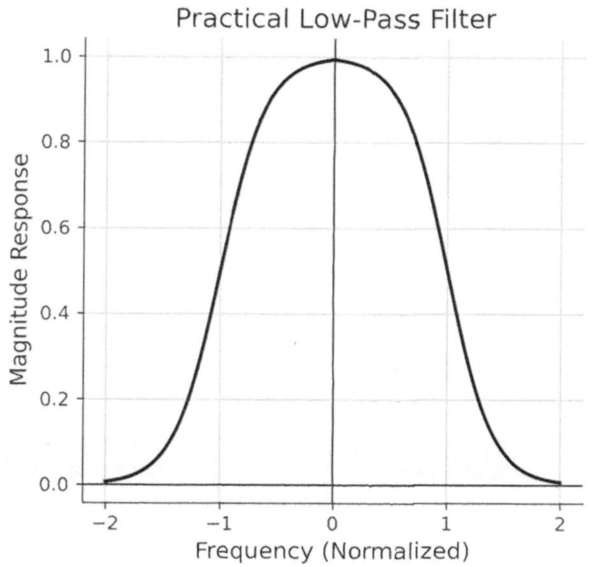

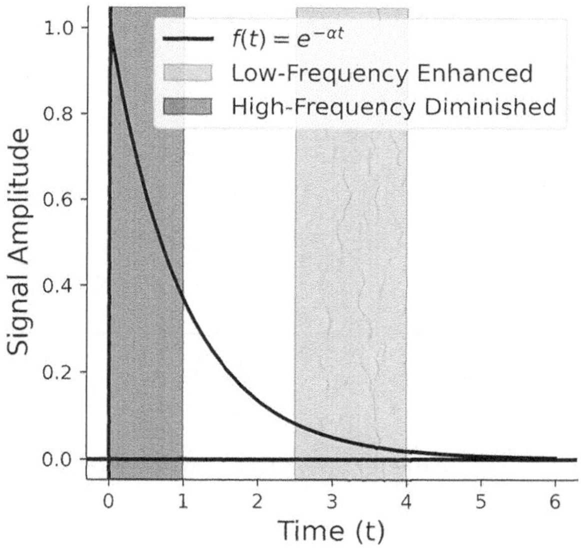

FIGURE 2.7 (*Continued*) (a) Ideal low pass filter. (b) Practical low pass filter. (c) Characteristics of practical low pass filter.

Then its Continuous Time Fourier Transform (CTFT) yields the corresponding frequency response. The frequency response of the unit impulse signal, $x(t) = \delta(t)$ is evaluated, as shown in equation (2.20).

$$X(j\Omega) = \int_{-\infty}^{\infty} x(t)e^{-j\Omega t}dt = \int_{-\infty}^{\infty} \delta(t)e^{-j\Omega t}dt = e^{j\Omega(0)} = 1 \tag{2.20}$$

As evident from equation (2.20) unit impulse in the time domain is equivalent to a constant function of unit magnitude in the frequency domain. It is represented mathematically by the equation (2.21)

$$\delta(t) \Leftrightarrow 1 \tag{2.21}$$

It can then be proven that the frequency domain output for a unit constant input in the frequency domain is a causal, decaying exponential, proof of which exceeds the scope of this chapter (Figure 2.8a and b).

2.7.1 Flow Diagram

The diagram below outlines the steps necessary to demonstrate that an EMA – Evaluator System functions as a LP Filter.

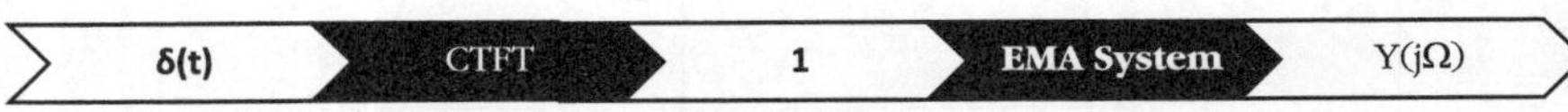

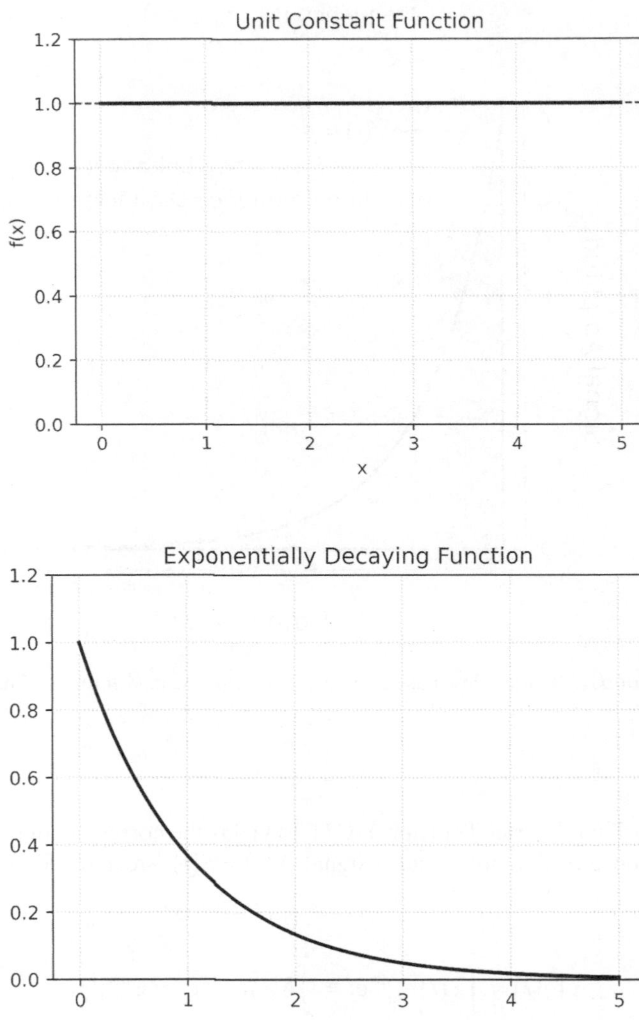

FIGURE 2.8 (a) Constant function. (b) Exponential response.

2.7.2 Advantages of EMA Over SMA

An EMA is better than SMA due to following reasons

1. Sensitivity to recent data
2. Adaptability to trends
3. Reduced lag
4. Smoothing effect
5. Flexibility with time period
6. Weighted influence

2.8 IMPORTANCE OF STATISTICAL INDICATORS

Transitioning beyond their traditional function as timekeeping devices, smartwatches have evolved into essential tools for health monitoring. Smartwatches equipped with health sensors often generate a smoothened curve from the raw data. While this curve encapsulates trends and variations, it can be complex and challenging to interpret for the average user. The continuous fluctuation may not provide a clear understanding of the health metrics, making it difficult for users to extract relevant information promptly. To address this challenge, integrating statistical indicators becomes paramount (Figure 2.9).

Consider the example of heart rate and SpO_2 levels. Rather than presenting users with an intricate curve, the smartwatch can display simplified values like "82 BPM" and "99% SpO_2." This approach transforms the data into easily readable and understandable formats, enabling users to notice trends and take proactive actions regarding their well-being.

2.9 STATISTICAL INDICATORS

Statistical indicators encompass crucial measures such as mean to calculate average values, standard deviation to gauge data variability, and percentile to contextualize the position of a data point

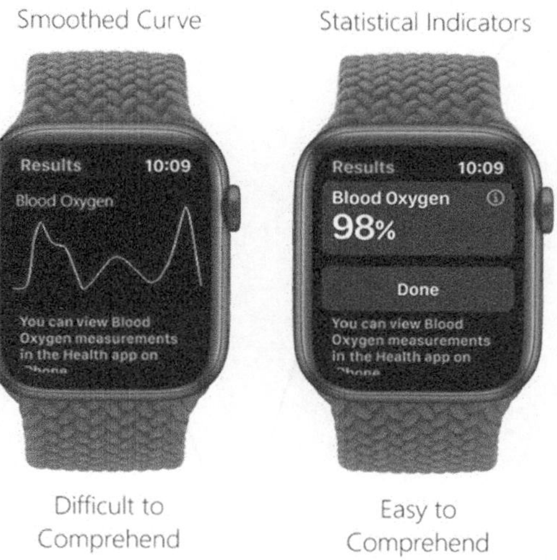

FIGURE 2.9 Importance of statistical indicators.

relative to others. These indicators play a pivotal role in improving the presentation and interpretation of intricate data, whether presented as data sets or parametrized graphs. They provide valuable insights into the central tendency, dispersion, and distribution of data, thereby aiding in the comprehensive analysis and understanding of datasets across various fields.

2.10 MEAN

Mean serves as a vital statistical indicator by offering users a representative value that summarizes their health data. This average provides a baseline for users to gauge the general trend in their metrics, promoting a clearer understanding of their overall health status (Figure 2.10).

Consider that a time period T is divided into N strips of equal thickness, Δt. Then, the mean value of a function $f(t)$ over the period is defined as the average of the heights of all N infinitesimally small strips, each with a thickness of Δt. Mathematically, this representation takes the form:

$$\text{Mean} = \frac{f(0)+f(\Delta t)+f(2\Delta t)+\ldots+f((N-1)\Delta t)}{N} \tag{2.22}$$

$$\text{Mean} = \frac{f(0)+f(\Delta t)+f(2\Delta t)+\ldots+f((N-1)\Delta t)}{\frac{T}{\Delta t}} \tag{2.23}$$

$$\text{Mean} = \frac{\sum_{i=0}^{N-1} f(i(\Delta t))}{T} \Delta t \tag{2.24}$$

As the intervals become infinitesimally small, and the function becomes continuous, the value of Δt approaches 0 for a fixed interval $[0, T]$, and the value of N approaches infinity, effectively transforming the finite discrete sum into a convergent infinite sum (Figure 2.11).

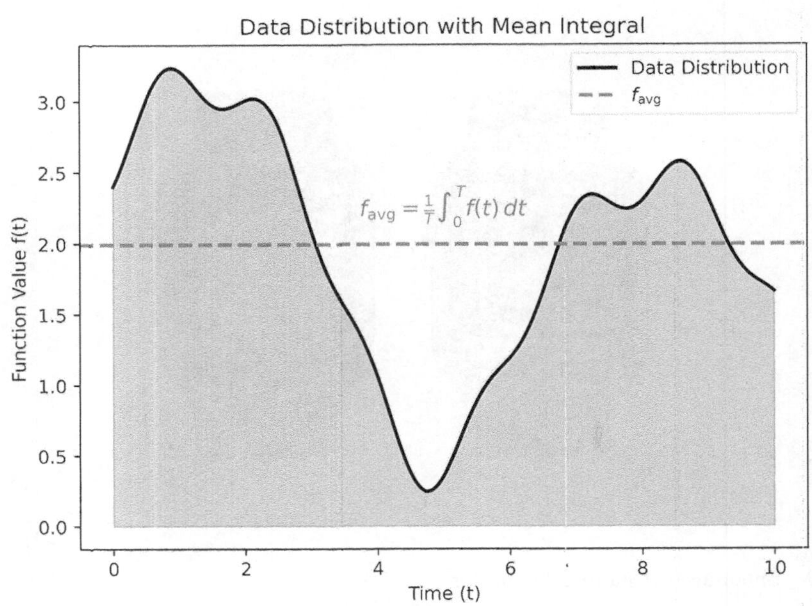

FIGURE 2.10 Time dependent function f(t) & mean of $f(t)$

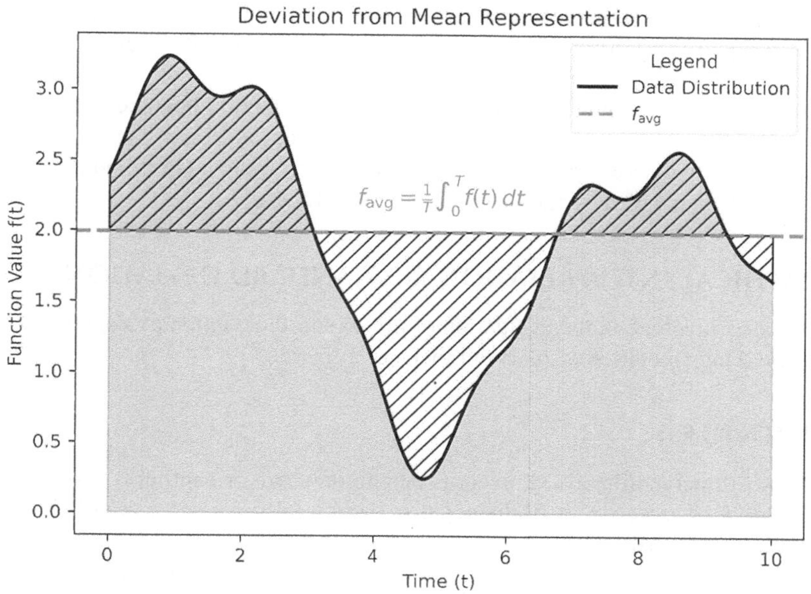

FIGURE 2.11 Evaluation of mean.

$$f(0)+f(\Delta t)+f(2\Delta t)+\ldots+f((N-1)\Delta t).\Delta t = \int_0^T f(t)\,\mathrm{d}t \tag{2.25}$$

$$f(t) = \lim_{\Delta t\to 0} f(t) = \lim_{\Delta t\to 0} \frac{\sum_{i=0}^{N-1} f(i(\Delta t))}{T}\Delta t = \frac{\int_0^T f(t)\,\mathrm{d}t}{T} \tag{2.26}$$

The definite integral,

$$\int_0^T f(t)\,\mathrm{d}t \tag{2.27}$$

of a function $f(t)$ is defined as the area under the curve bounded by the time interval $[0,T]$. Therefore, the mean of a continuous function $f(t)$, averaged over the time interval $[0,T]$, can be interpreted as:

$$f(t) = f_{\text{avg}}(t) = \frac{\int_0^T f(t)\,\mathrm{d}t}{T} = \frac{\text{Area Under the Function}}{T} \tag{2.28}$$

2.11 STANDARD DEVIATION

Standard Deviation complements mean by highlighting the extent of variability in the data. A higher standard deviation suggests more significant deviations from the average, signaling potential irregularities that users should be aware of. This statistical indicator empowers users to discern patterns and variations in their health metrics.

The Standard deviation (σ) of a function, with discrete data points X_i, and mean $\bar{X}$, is defined as the Root Mean Square (RMS) of the deviation of data-points from the mean of the function, refer Table 2.1.

As the intervals become infinitesimally small, and the function becomes continuous, the value of Δt approaches 0 for a fixed interval $[0, T]$, and the value of N approaches infinity, effectively transforming the finite discrete sum into a convergent infinite sum. The standard deviation of such a continuous function is given by the expression—refer Table 2.2.

2.12 GRAPHICAL INTERPRETATION OF STANDARD DEVIATION

The various stages involved in the evaluation of the standard deviation of a signal are graphed, and the mathematical interpretation is analyzed in Table 2.3.

2.13 PERCENTILE

"In statistics, a *K*th percentile, also known as percentile score or centile, is a score below which a given percentage *K* of scores in its frequency distribution falls or a score at or below which a given percentage falls" (Percentile, 2023).

Percentiles are commonly used in health sensor data analysis to provide a contextual understanding of an individual's health metrics in comparison to a larger population. In healthcare analytics, they are used to position the health metric of patients on a scale of 0%–100%, offering insights into where a particular patient's health metric falls within the distribution of values. For instance, being in the 80th percentile for heart rate implies that the user's heart rate is higher than 80% of the population. This contextualizes individual health data, fostering a sense of awareness and encouraging users to strive for optimal well-being.

2.13.1 Example Problem

Consider a dataset with the details about the daily steps taken by individuals in a population. To determine the percentile of a patient who walks 8,500 steps per day, the dataset is as follows:

$$\{5,000, 5,500, 6,000, 6,500, 7,000, 7,500, 8,000, 8,500, 9,000, 9,500, 10,000\}$$

TABLE 2.1
Statistical Formula for Evaluation of Standard Deviation of *N* Data Points

$\sigma = \frac{\sqrt{\sum_{i=0}^{N} (X_i - \bar{X})^2}}{N}$	$(X_i - \bar{X})$: Deviation of data-point X_i from mean $\bar{X}$ of the function N: Number of discrete data-points

TABLE 2.2
Statistical Formula for Evaluation of Standard Deviation of a Function

$\sigma = \sqrt{\frac{\int_0^T (f(t) - f_{avg}(t))^2 dt}{T}}$	$f(t) - f_{avg}(t)$: Deviation of the function's value at a given time instant from the time averaged value T: Time interval over which the function's standard deviation is evaluated

TABLE 2.3
Stages Involved in Deriving and Analyzing the Standard Deviation of Statistical Data

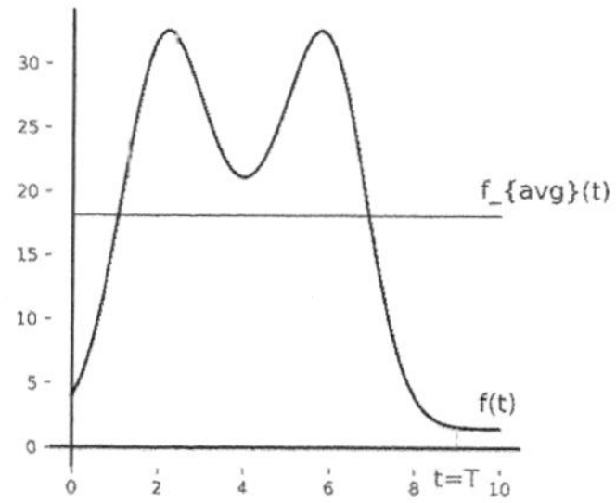 a. Time Varying Input Signal	$f(t)$, $f_{avg}(t)$: Time varying function, Mean of the time varying function
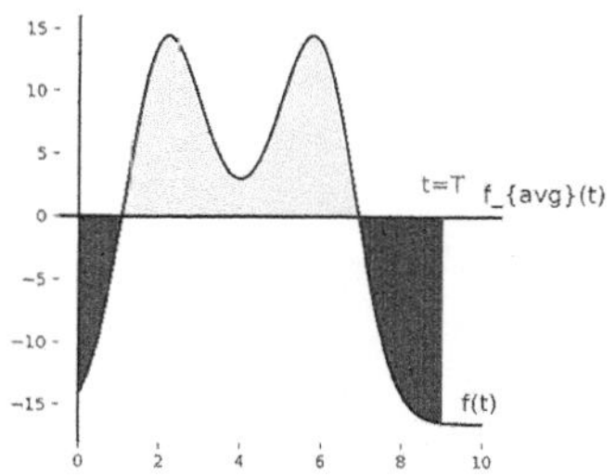 b. Deviation from Mean	$f(t)-f_{avg}(t)$: Deviation of the function's value at a given time instant from the time averaged value Black Region: Negative Deviation from mean, i.e., $f(t)<f_{avg}(t)$ Grey Region: Positive Deviation from mean, i.e., $f(t)>f_{avg}(t)$
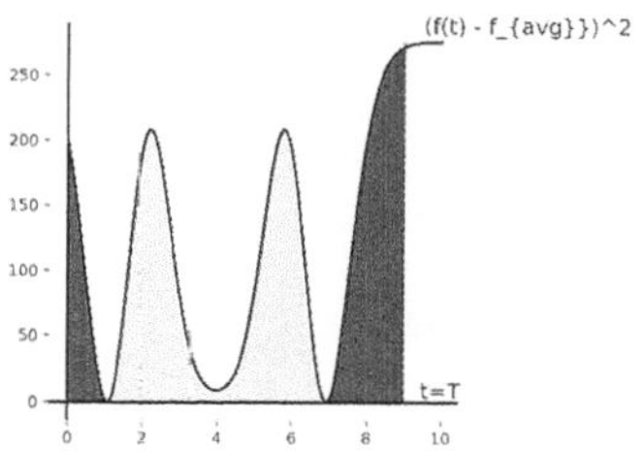 c. – Square of Deviation from Mean	$\left\|f(t)-f_{avg}(t)\right\|^2$: Square of the deviation of the function's value at a given time instant from the time averaged value.
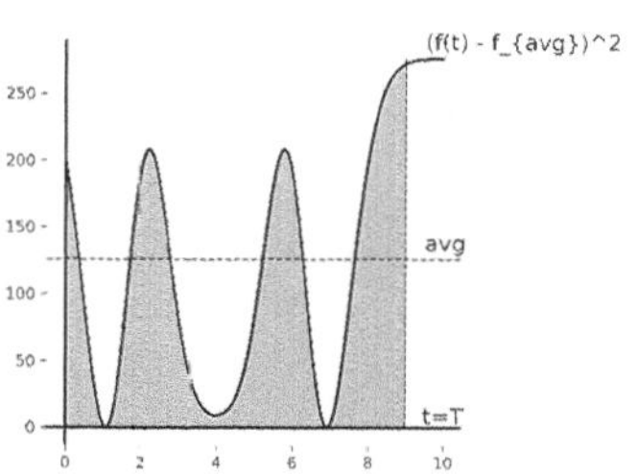 d. Average of square of Standard Deviation	The average of $\left\|f(t)-f_{avg}(t)\right\|^2$ is termed as the variance of the function $f(t)$ in the time interval $[0,T]$, and is equal to the square of standard deviation. $$\text{average}\left(\left\|f(t)-f_{avg}(t)\right\|^2\right)=\frac{\int_0^T \left(f(t)-f_{avg}(t)\right)^2 dt}{T}=\sigma^2=\text{Variance}$$

2.13.2 Percentile Formula

Percentiles are values that help "to understand and interpret data. The Nth percentile of a set of data is the value at which $N\%$ of the data is shown in equation (2.29)." (ep13.revistapasajes.com) (Figure 2.12)

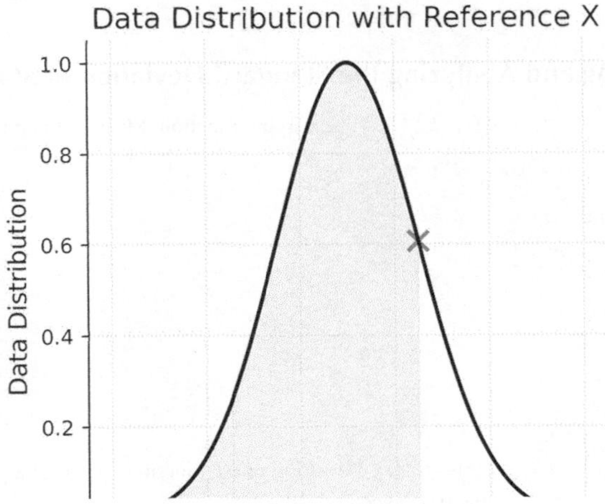

FIGURE 2.12 Percentile.

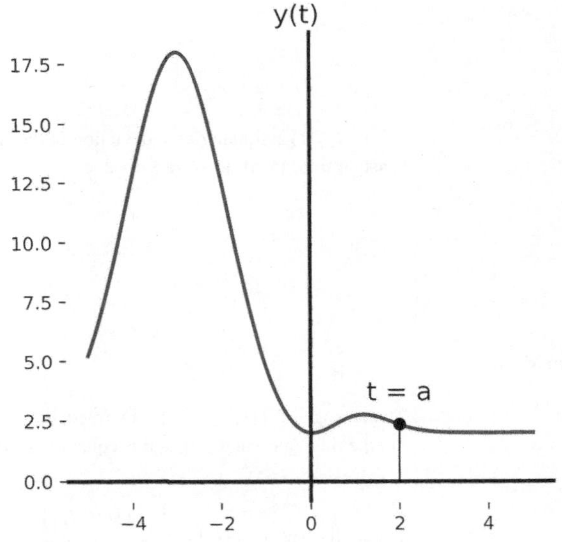

FIGURE 2.13 Percentile of a continuous distribution.

$$\text{Percentile} = \left(\frac{\text{Number of Values Below } X}{\text{Total Number of Values}} \right) \tag{2.29}$$

2.14 PERCENTILE OF A CONTINUOUS DISTRIBUTION

For a continuous distribution $y(t)$, the percentile at a given point $t = a$ is determined using the equation (2.30) (Figure 2.13).

$$\text{Percentile} = \left(\frac{\text{Number of Values Below} X}{\text{Total Number of Values}}\right) = \frac{\int_{-\infty}^{a} f(t)\,\mathrm{d}t}{\int_{-\infty}^{\infty} f(t)\,\mathrm{d}t} \tag{2.30}$$

2.15 PERCENTILE OF A DISCRETE DISTRIBUTION

In a discrete data distribution, there is a finite number of values satisfying the criterion Equal to X. Therefore, a weight of $\frac{1}{2}$ is assigned to the count of values equal to X. This approach ensures equal weightage to values both above and below X. Consequently, half of the count of values equal to X is allocated to the number of values below X, while the remaining half is assigned to the number of values above X, as shown in equation (2.19) (Figure 2.14):

$$\text{Percentile} = \left(\frac{\text{Number of Values Below } X + \frac{1}{2}\text{Number of Values Equal to } X}{\text{Total Number of Values}}\right)100 \tag{2.31}$$

2.15.1 Solution

1. Raw input data is arranged in ascending order

   $\{5{,}000, 5{,}500, 6{,}000, 6{,}500, 7{,}000, 7{,}500, 8{,}000, 8{,}500, 9{,}000, 9{,}500, 10{,}000\}$
2. There are a total of 11 values in the given data set. Out of these, 7 values are below, and 1 value is equal to 8, 500 – reference parameter.

$$\text{Percentile} = \left(\frac{\text{Number of Values Below } X + \frac{1}{2}\text{Number of Values Equal to } X}{\text{Total Number of Values}}\right)100$$

$$= \left(\frac{7 + \frac{1}{2}(1)}{11}\right) \times 100 = 68.18\ \%$$

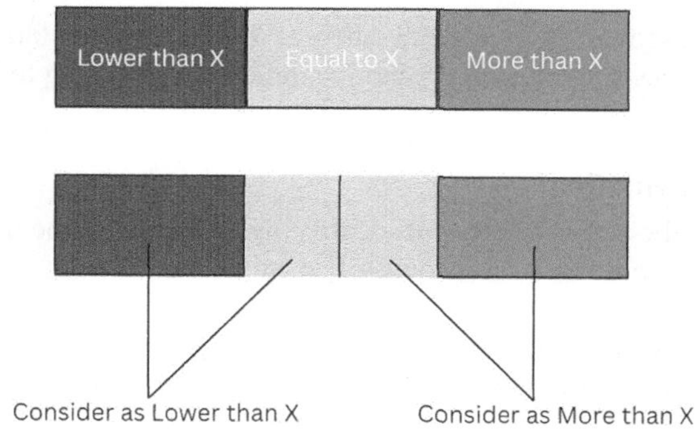

FIGURE 2.14 Percentile of a discrete distribution.

If a patient's score on the pedometer test is in the 68.18th percentile, it indicates that they have walked more steps than 68.18% of the test takers

2.15.2 Observation

Unlike standard reference parameters like mmHg, bpm, BMI, and Complete Blood Cell Counts, percentiles provide a relative measure within a population; being above or below a certain percentile doesn't inherently imply healthiness.

Percentiles provide the relative position of a patient's health metric within a population and do not present as an absolute reference method. In the context of BP, percentiles provide the relative position of a patient's BP within a population and are not an absolute reference method like a standard BP reading in mmHg.

For instance, if the median (50th percentile) blood pressure of a country is 140/90, then all individuals above the 50th percentile will be considered unhealthy. In another population with a median BP of 100/70 mmHg, all individuals with BP below the 50th percentile are considered unhealthy. In summary, being above or below a certain percentile does not inherently imply healthiness or unhealthiness. Rather, it indicates the relative position of an individual's blood pressure within a specific population, and additional factors and individual health assessments are necessary to determine whether someone is considered healthy or unhealthy.

2.16 CLUSTERING

Clustering facilitates the organization and analysis of sensor data by grouping together observations that share common statistical properties. This process aids in the simplification of large datasets, resulting in more comprehensible datasets with fewer data points.

K-means, Hierarchical Clustering, DBSCAN, Mean Shift, OPTICS, Agglomerative Clustering, Spectral Clustering, and Fuzzy C-means are recognized as the most popular clustering algorithms. Among these, *K*-means stands out as a widely adopted technique for segmenting data into distinct clusters. In this chapter, the basic principles of *K*-means clustering method and its importance among other clustering techniques are discussed.

2.17 *K*-MEANS CLUSTERING

In the *K*-means clustering method, data points *(or elements)* are organized into k clusters, where k is a whole number predetermined by the user. An arbitrary set of k elements from the given data set is chosen as centroids *(or reference data points)*. Other data points are then grouped with centroids that are temporally closest to them.

2.17.1 Significance and Applications

K-means clustering is used in various fields such as market segmentation, image compression, anomaly detection, data classification, and genomic data analysis owing to its simplicity, efficiency, and interpretability.

2.17.1.1 Market Segmentation

Market segmentation is the actual process of identifying segments of the market and the process of dividing a broad customer base into sub-groups of consumers consisting of existing and prospective customers.

Market segmentation is the actual process of identifying segments of the market and the process of dividing a broad customer base into sub-groups of consumers consisting of existing and prospective customers. Market segmentation is a consumer-oriented process and can be applied to almost any type of market.

"Market segmentation is the actual process of identifying segments of the market and the process of dividing a broad customer base into sub-groups of consumers consisting of existing and prospective customers. Market segmentation is a consumer-oriented process and can be applied to almost any type of market" (Camilleri, 2018). During this process, prospective buyers are organized into various groups or segments based on demographic, geographic, psychological, and behavioral patterns.

2.17.1.2 Image Compression

"Digital images are composed of pixels, and each pixel represents the color at a single point in the image. By measuring the color of an image at large number of points, digital approximation of the image can be created." "The objective of compression is to reduce redundancy of the image data in order to enable storing or transmitting data with minimal space or bandwidth as much as possible, while keeping the resolution and the visual quality of the reconstructed image as close to the original image" (Samra, 2012). This makes it easier to store, transmit, and display images without sacrificing the image's optical clarity and resolution. One technique used for image compression is color quantization, which reduces the number of colors in an image by grouping similar colors together. When an image has fewer colors, it requires lesser memory to store the color information for each pixel. This results in a smaller file size without sacrificing the image's visual quality.

2.17.1.3 Anomaly Detection

"Anomaly detection describes a class of algorithms that aims at the identification of rare items, events, or observations, which deviate significantly from the majority of the data and do not conform to a well-defined notion of normal behavior" (www.mdpi.com).

2.17.1.4 Genomic Data Analysis

Genomic data analysis is the process of using powerful computational and statistical methods to decode the functional information hidden in DNA sequences. When performed on a spectrum of organisms, genomic data analysis can reveal the differences and similarities between genomic data of different species.

2.18 IMPLEMENTATION OF *K*-MEANS ALGORITHM

K-means clustering is an unsupervised machine learning algorithm that is used to solve the clustering problems in machine learning or data science. It involves four steps: Initialization, Assignment, Updating Centroids, and Iteration. Below, you'll find detailed explanations for each of the four steps mentioned earlier.

2.18.1 Initialization

Initialization involves determining the initial cluster centroids, a critical step that can significantly influence both the convergence of the algorithm and the quality of the resultant clusters. Several methods exist for initializing centroids, and a frequently employed approach involves the random selection of data points from the dataset.

2.18.1.1 Random Selection of Initial Centroids

Randomly select k data points from the dataset to serve as the initial centroids, where k represents the predetermined number of clusters. To illustrate, let's consider a dataset with the following points in a two-dimensional space:

$$(2, 3), (5, 8), (1, 1), (7, 9), (3, 6), (8, 2), (4, 5), (9, 4)$$

TABLE 2.4
Random Selection of Initial Centroids and Clustering at k=3

Input data-set	(2, 3), (5, 8), (1, 1), (7, 9), (3, 6), (8, 2), (4, 5), (9, 4)
Initial Centroids: $k = 3$	(2, 3), (7, 9), (4, 5)

If the objective is to create three clusters $k = 3$, randomly choose three data points as the initial centroids. For example, let's consider the points $(2, 3)$, $(7, 9)$, $(4, 5)$, refer Table 2.4.

2.18.2 Euclidean Distance Metric

Compute the distance between each data point and the initial centroids, then allocate each data point to the centroid to which it is closest. Closeness of two points is determined using *Euclidean Distance Metric.*

The Euclidean distance d between 2 points (x_1, y_1) and (x_2, y_2) in a plane is given by the equation (2.32).

$$d = \sqrt{(y_2 - y_1)^2 + (x_2 - x_1)^2} \tag{2.32}$$

2.18.3 Assignment

Once the starting points (initial centroids) are randomly picked out, the next step is to figure out which cluster each data point should belong to. To do this, measure how close each data point is to these initial centroids.

2.18.3.1 Calculate Distance

For every data point, find out how far it is from each of the initial centroids. The technique often used is Euclidean distance, but other measurements can be used depending on the needs.

2.18.3.2 Assign to Nearest Centroid

Place each data point in the cluster whose centroid is the closest. Proximity is determined by the calculated distance using equation (2.33).

$$\text{Lowest}(d_1, d_2, d_3) \tag{2.33}$$

For example (continuing from the previous steps), consider our data points and the random initial centroids:

Euclidean Distance Metrics

$$0 < 2.8284 < 7.8102$$

Hence, as the point $(2, 3)$ is closest to Centroid A $(2, 3)$, it is assigned to be clustered under Centroid A, refer Table 2.5.

Euclidean Distance Metrics

$$2.2361 < 3.1623 < 5.8310$$

TABLE 2.5
Assigning the Centroid, Clustering under Centroid A

Point $(2, 3)$

Centroid A $(2, 3)$	Centroid B $(7, 9)$	Centroid $(4, 5)$
$\sqrt{(2-2)^2+(3-3)^2}=0$	$\sqrt{(2-7)^2+(3-9)^2}=7.8102$	$\sqrt{(2-4)^2+(3-5)^2}=2.8284$

TABLE 2.6
Assigning the Centroid, Clustering under Centroid B

Point $(5, 8)$

Centroid A $(2,\ 3$	Centroid B $(2,\ 3)$	Centroid $(4, 5)$
$\sqrt{(2-5)^2+(3-8)^2}=5.8310$	$\sqrt{(5-7)^2+(8-9)^2}=2.2361$	$\sqrt{(5-4)^2+(8-5)^2}=3.1623$

TABLE 2.7
Various Data-Points Clustered with Respective Centroids

Centroid A $(2, 3)$	$\{(2, 3),(1, 1)(3, 6)\}$
Centroid B $(7, 9]$	$\{(5, 8),(8, 2),(7, 9),(9, 4)\}$
Centroid C $(4, 5)$	$(4, 5)$

TABLE 2.8
Second Iteration for Evaluation of Centroid

Initial Centroid	Recalculated Centroid
$(2, 3)$	$\left(\frac{2+1+3}{3}, \frac{3+1+6}{3}\right)=(2,\ 3.\ 33)$
$(7, 9)$	$\left(\frac{5+8+7+9}{4}, \frac{8+2+9+4}{4}\right)=(7.25,\ 5.\ 75)$
$(4, 5)$	$(4,\ 5)$

Hence, as the point $(5, 8)$ is closest to Centroid B $(7, 9)$, it is assigned to be clustered under Centroid B, refer Table 2.6.w

Similarly, all the other points in the dataset {(5, 8), (1, 1), (3, 6), (8, 2), (9, 4)} can be clustered under a unique centroid as well. The various data points along with their respective centroids are represented in Table 2.7:

2.18.4 2nd Iteration for Evaluation of Centroid

The new centroid for each cluster is determined by calculating the mean of the data points assigned to that cluster.

So, the updated centroids are: $(2, 3.33)$, $(7.25, 5.75)$, $(4, 5)$, as represented in Table 2.8

The recalculated centroids will be utilized in the subsequent iteration. If there is no significant change in the centroids *(indicative of the convergence condition)*, these centroids become the final centroids for the clusters. If additional iterations are necessary, the assignment and recalculation process is repeated.

2.18.5 Iterations & Condition for Convergence

During each iteration, the algorithm selects centroids from the previous step, assigning data points to the nearest centroid based on the Euclidean distance metric. Following this, centroids are updated by calculating the mean of data points within each cluster. The iterative process persists until convergence, marked by minimal changes in centroids or reaching a predetermined iteration limit. This iterative approach refines clusters, aiming to minimize intra-cluster variance. Known for its simplicity and efficiency, *K*-means is widely applied in diverse fields to reveal patterns and groupings within datasets.

2.18.5.1 Calculate Distance

For every data point, find out how far it is from each of the initial centroids. The method that is used often is Euclidean distance, but other measurements can be used depending on the needs. Refer to equation (2.20).

2.18.5.2 Assign to Nearest Centroid

Place each data point in the cluster whose centroid is the closest. Proximity is determined by the calculated distance. Refer equation (2.21).

$$\text{Lowest}(d_1, d_2, d_3)$$

Euclidean Distance Metrics are applied on Updated Centroids, refer Table 2.9

$$0 < 2.8284 < 5.9266$$

Hence, as the point (2, 3) is closest to Centroid A (2, 3.33), it is assigned to be clustered under Centroid A (Table 2.10).

2.18.5.3 Euclidean Distance Metrics

$3.16 < 3.18 < 5.55$

Hence, as the point $(5, 8)$ is closest to Centroid C $(4, 5)$, it is assigned to be clustered under Centroid C.

Similarly, all points in the dataset can be clustered under a unique centroid, refer Table 2.11.

The points $(1.5, 2)$, $(8, 5)$ and $(4, 6.33)$ are now assigned as the centroids for the next iteration.

TABLE 2.9
Updating with Nearest Centroid

Point $(2, 3)$		
Centroid A $(2, 3.33)$	Centroid B $(7.25, 5.75)$	Centroid $(4, 5)$
$\sqrt{(2-2)^2+(3-3.33)^2}=0.33$	$\sqrt{(2-7.25)^2+(3-5.75)^2}=5.9266$	$\sqrt{(2-4)^2+(3-5)^2}=2.8284$

TABLE 2.10
Updating with Nearest Centroid II

Point $(5, 8)$

Centroid A (2, 3.33)	Centroid B (7.25, 5.75)	Centroid (4, 5)
$\sqrt{(5-2)^2+(8-3.33)^2}=5.55$	$\sqrt{(5-7.25)^2+(8-5.75)^2}=3.18$	$\sqrt{(5-4)^2+(8-5)^2}=3.16$

TABLE 2.11
Updating with Nearest Centroid III

Centroid A (2, 3.33)	$\{(2,3),(1,1)\}$	$\left(\frac{2+1}{2},\frac{3+1}{2}\right)=(1.5,2)$
Centroid B (7.25, 5.75)	$\{(7,9),(8,2),(9,4)\}$	$\left(\frac{7+8+9}{3},\frac{9+2+4}{3}\right)=(8,5)$
Centroid C (4, 5)	$\{(3,6),(4,5),(5,8)\}$	$\left(\frac{3+4+5}{3},\frac{6+5+8}{3}\right)=(4,6.33)$

2.18.6 Condition for Convergence

The dynamic changes in centroid values between successive iterations indicate that the algorithm is still in the process of refining cluster assignments and seeking a stable configuration.

Centroids of Nth Iteration $\neq$ Centroids of $(N+1)$th Iteration

$$\{(2,3.33),(7.25,\ 5.75),(4,\ 5)\}\neq\{(1.5,2),(8,5),(4,6.33)\}$$

Convergence is achieved when the centroids of the clusters undergo minimal changes between successive iterations. This implies that the centroids have stabilized, and the algorithm has effectively identified representative cluster centers. Mathematically, the K-means algorithm is said to converge when:

Centroids of Nth Iteration $=$ Centroids of $(N+1)$th Iteration

2.19 DATA VECTORIZATION

Data vectorization involves expressing data points as vectors within a multidimensional space, and the K-means algorithm is employed to cluster these vectors based on their similarities. "Machine learning algorithms operate in a space of numerical attributes, that is, they expect that a two-dimensional array will be presented at the input, the rows of which are concrete instances, and the columns are attributes or features. Thus, in order to perform machine learning on the text, it is necessary to convert the source documents into vector representations, to which numerical machine learning will subsequently be applied" (Kozhevnikov, 2020).

2.19.1 Multi-Dimensional Vector Encoding

In the process of applying K-means to data vectorization, each data point is initially represented as a vector in a high-dimensional space, with the vector's dimensions corresponding to the features or attributes of the data points. Consider a 2D Data Vectorization Model, parameterized as a function of size and animation.

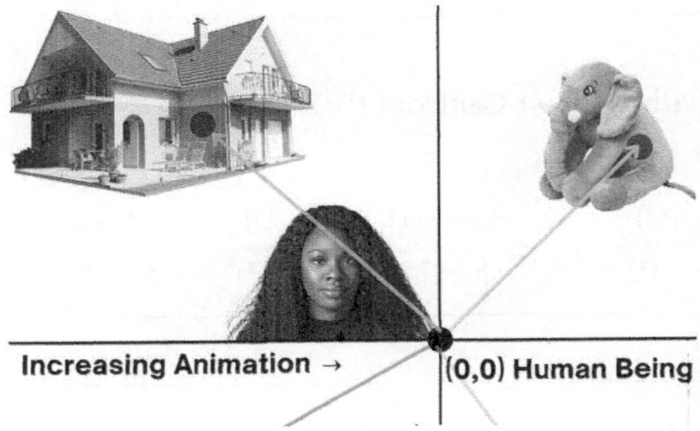

FIGURE 2.15 Graphical (2D) plot of data vectorization.

1. **Origin:** The graph considers an average human being as the point of reference.
2. ***Y*-axis (Vertical):** Represents size relative to a human, with anything larger going above and anything smaller going below.
3. ***X*-axis (Horizontal):** Represents the level of animation or life, with anything more animate than a human going to the right and anything with less life going to the left.

Applying these criteria, objects and creatures can be placed within specific quadrants, creating a visual representation of their characteristics. The following examples further illustrate this classification for a cruise ship, an elephant, an ant, and a microchip within their respective quadrants (Figure 2.15).

1. **Elephant:** Larger than a human (above the y-axis), more animate than a human (to the right of the x-axis), so it's in the 1st quadrant.
2. **Cruise Ship:** Larger than a human (above the y-axis), less animate than a human (to the left of the x-axis), so it's in the 2nd quadrant.
3. **Microchip:** Smaller than a human (below the y-axis), less animate than a human (to the left of the x-axis), so it's in the 3rd quadrant.
4. **Ant:** Smaller than a human (below the y-axis), more animate than a human (to the right of the x-axis), so it's in the 4th quadrant.

In employing 2D multi-dimensional vector encoding techniques, the objects—elephant, microchip, cruise ship, and ant—have been systematically represented as 2D vector coordinates. Each object's unique characteristics, such as size relative to a human and the level of animation or life, are encapsulated in these coordinates. These 2D vector representations now function as raw input datasets for a k-means clustering algorithm.

The k-means algorithm, a popular unsupervised learning method, utilizes these vector coordinates to partition the objects into clusters based on similarities in their feature space. Through an iterative process, the algorithm refines cluster assignments and adjusts cluster centroids, ultimately revealing inherent patterns and relationships among the objects.

It's noteworthy that similar vector encoding techniques can be extended to multidimensional datasets, allowing for a broader range of applications in data analysis, machine learning, and pattern recognition. This approach, leveraging vectorization for diverse types of data, contributes to the systematic exploration and understanding of complex datasets.

2.20 CHALLENGES AND CONSIDERATIONS

While *K*-means is recognized for its robustness, it displays sensitivity to the initial placement of centroids. The attainment of a universal optimum depends on specific sets of initial values and '*k*' values. However, there are instances where the *K*-means clustering algorithm may not converge to the universal optimum, settling instead for a local optimum. Consequently, conducting multiple initializations and evaluations becomes necessary to enhance the reliability of clustering results.

2.21 CONCLUSION

In conclusion, current research focuses on improving the efficiency of clustering algorithms, managing streaming sensor data with various dimensions and types, and integrating domain knowledge and user feedback into statistical approximation methods. These challenges in data analysis and machine learning drive the need for enhanced clustering algorithm efficiency. Future studies should explore autonomously determining the optimal number of clusters in *k*-means clustering, especially for large datasets. Additionally, innovative techniques for handling diverse streaming sensor data and creating a unified framework for statistical approximation and analysis would advance insights, especially in healthcare. Integrating domain knowledge and user feedback into statistical approximation processes could enhance accuracy and interpretability. These research questions highlight the dynamic nature of the field, urging researchers to contribute to evolving data analysis methodologies.

REFERENCES

Camilleri, M. A. (2018). Market segmentation, targeting and positioning. In *Travel Marketing, Tourism Economics and the Airline Product*, ed. Mark Anthony Camilleri (pp. 69–83). Springer, Cham, Switzerland.

Kozhevnikov, V. A., & Pankratova, E. S. (2020). Research of the text data vectorization and classification algorithms of machine learning. *ISJ Theoretical & Applied Science*, 5(85), 574–585.

Li, L., Sheng, S., Liu, Y. Wen, J., Song, C., Chen, Z., Xu, W., Zhang, Z., Fan, W., Chen, C., & Sun, Q. (2023). Automatic and continuous blood pressure monitoring via an optical-fiber-sensor-assisted smartwatch. *PhotoniX*, 4, 21.

Morissette, L., & Chartier, S. (2013). The k-means clustering technique: general considerations and implementation in Mathematica. *Tutorials in Quantitative Methods for Psychology*, 9(1), 15–24.

Percentile. (2023, December 22). In Wikipedia. https://en.wikipedia.org/wiki/Percentile

Samra, H. S. (2012). Image compression techniques. *International Journal of Computers & Technology*, 2(2), 49–52.

Sarwar, M. Z., & Cantero, D. (2024). Probabilistic autoencoder-based bridge damage assessment using train-induced responses. *Mechanical Systems and Signal Processing*, 208, 111046.

Shukla, S. (2023). Real-time monitoring and predictive analytics in healthcare: harnessing the power of data streaming. *International Journal of Computer Applications*, 185(8), 32–37.

3 Sensor Data Analytics for Transformative Healthcare Solutions

A Comprehensive Insights

T. Mathankumar, and S. Vijayarani

3.1 INTRODUCTION

The healthcare analytics domain uses data analysis to enrich both healthcare management and patient care. Emerging developments in the field of IoT, pervasive and wearable devices, mechatronics, and electronics have knowingly augmented the proficiencies of smart sensors and extended the wide variety of applications. The healthcare and medical fields, among others, have been profoundly impacted by these technological developments, providing extensive offerings across various applications. Indeed, smart sensors are progressively proposing innovative results to numerous experiments in healthcare, such as the early discovery of diseases and minimally invasive management and prevention of prevalent conditions like cardiovascular diseases and cancer. Sensor data analytics is vital for gathering and analyzing data from sensor-equipped devices across a wide range of sectors, including healthcare, agriculture, automotive, manufacturing, retail, energy, banking and financial services, oil and gas, logistics, transportation, smart cities, and beyond.

These explanations facilitate on-demand and immediate data analytics, allowing the monitoring of ecological conditions, optimization of asset utilization, and implementation of preventive maintenance measures. In addition, sensor analytics results leverage AI/ML competencies to accurately forecast serious proceedings, develop extremely precise estimates, alleviate long-term threats, and automate procedures through smart guidance. Medical sensors are essential components ensuring the safe functioning of various medical devices across numerous applications. They are incorporated into devices present in intensive care units, hospital wards, general practitioner offices, laboratory equipment, dental practices, and home care products. These sensors are integral to medical devices aiding in the diagnosis, prevention, monitoring, and treatment of diseases or injuries. Additionally, sensors are utilized in devices for cleaning, equipment calibration, and specimen examination.

This chapter provides significant information about sensor data in the healthcare domain. Section 3.2 explores the need for data analytics and its role in the healthcare industry. Section 3.3 deliberates healthcare sensor data analytics and how the sensors are used in healthcare. Section 3.4 discusses the role of IoT in healthcare, IoT data integration challenges, and outcomes. Section 3.5 provides the essential components required for healthcare devices. Section 3.6 discusses the importance and use of artificial intelligence, machine learning, and other algorithms in sensor healthcare analytics. Substantial research challenges are presented in Section 3.7. The successful implementation of sensor data analytics in healthcare is explored in Section 3.8. Future trends in sensor data analytics for healthcare are given in Section 3.9. Section 3.10 concludes the chapter.

DOI: 10.1201/9781003486640-3

3.2 DATA ANALYTICS

In the era of digital transformation, data analytics has emerged as a cornerstone of modern technology, driving innovation and enhancing decision-making processes across various sectors. The size of data generated globally continues to rise exponentially, and the ability to harness and interpret this data has become crucial for businesses, governments, and organizations worldwide. Data analytics is the progression of inspecting, dusting, converting, and exhibiting data to ascertain valued facts, which can inform inferences and assist decision-making. Data analytics encompasses a range of techniques and tools designed to extract meaningful insights, patterns, and trends from raw data that can help organizations make better decisions, solve problems, and gain competitive advantages.

Data analytics comprises a collection of methods and techniques, including data mining, statistical analysis, machine learning, and data visualization. It is used to answer specific questions, uncover hidden patterns, and predict future trends based on historical information. Business industries can gain better perceptions of their operations and services with the help of data analytics, providing them with a deep understanding of customer issues and experiences. Depending on the complexity of the data, it can be moved to cloud data warehouses or data lakes and accessed by business intelligence tools when necessary. By leveraging insights from data, companies can enhance customer experiences, develop relevant digital products, optimize processes, and improve employee productivity.

In industries such as healthcare, finance, retail, and manufacturing, data analytics is revolutionizing traditional practices, leading to more personalized services, improved efficiency, and significant cost savings. In healthcare, for example, data analytics enables predictive modeling and early detection of diseases, ultimately enhancing patient outcomes and reducing healthcare costs. In finance, sophisticated algorithms analyze market trends and consumer behavior, helping institutions manage risks and identify investment opportunities. Retailers leverage data analytics to understand customer preferences, streamline supply chains, and enhance the overall shopping experience. Meanwhile, manufacturers utilize data-driven insights to observe the performance of the equipment, forecast maintenance requirements, and augment manufacturing developments (Kodjin by Edenlab 2023).

3.2.1 Need for Data Analytics

In the present scenario, data analytics has played a vital role due to its capability to fulfill the end user's expectations by providing various services. Figure 3.1 shows the need for data analytics.

Finding Patterns and Trends: By analyzing the data, researchers can find patterns, trends, and connections within the information. Researchers can gain a deeper understanding of the topics they are studying by looking at these patterns.

Testing Hypotheses: Developing and testing hypotheses is a common step in research. Analyzing data gives one the ability to thoroughly assess hypotheses. Researchers can ascertain whether the observed patterns in the data are statistically significant or merely the result of chance by using statistical tests and inferential analysis.

Improving Data Quality: Data cleaning and validation procedures are part of data analysis, which raises the dataset's dependability and quality. Making sure that errors, missing numbers, and outliers are recognized and dealt with guarantees that the research findings appropriately depict the phenomenon under study.

Decision Supporting: Data analysis in applied research helps decision-makers in business, government, and healthcare, among other fields. Research findings are frequently used as the basis for resource allocation, marketing plans, and policy choices.

Finding the Outliers: These features in data may point to mistakes or include important information. Whether it's for product quality control, financial fraud detection, or medical diagnosis, data analysis tools can help to find these unique circumstances.

Revealing Insights: Research data frequently reveal hidden insights that are immediately obvious. These insights can be found through data analysis techniques like text analysis

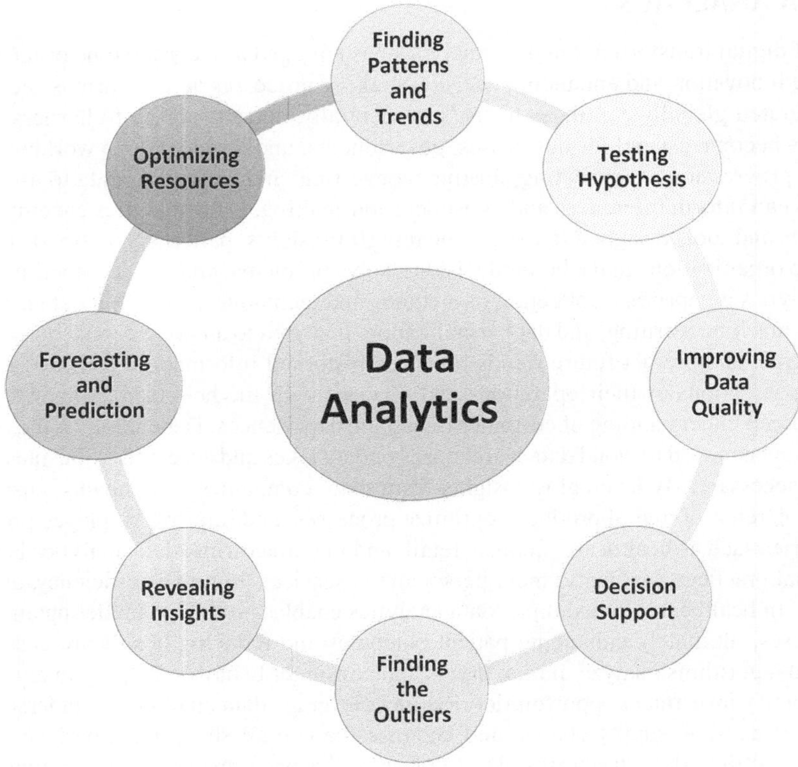

FIGURE 3.1 Need for data analytics.

and clustering. Sentiment analysis of social media data, for instance, can show trends and public opinion on a range of social science topics.

Forecasting and Prediction: Predictive models can be developed during the data analysis. Researchers can create models that predict future trends or outcomes by using previous data. This is useful for predicting stock prices in the finance industry, weather forecasting in meteorology, and the spread of illness in epidemiology.

Optimizing Resources: Allocating resources is a common aspect of research optimization. By pointing out areas where expenditures might be cut or improvements made, data analysis assists researchers and organizations in making the most use of their resources.

3.2.2 Uses of Data Analytics

Data is crucial in today's world as it helps to understand performance, improve processes, and understand (Kodjin by Edenlab 2023) consumers better. Figure 3.2 illustrates the uses of data analytics.

Data in Business: Data is a crucial component for businesses to succeed in today's world. Proper data analytics processes and tools are necessary to access the benefits of the business data. Raw data is also crucial, and it needs to be analyzed to unlock its potential and convert it into useful information for the business. Therefore, data analytics plays a vital role in businesses as it helps in making informed decisions based on the analyzed data.

Data in Healthcare: Data is indispensable in the medical and healthcare industry. Medical devices are designed to handle big data, and doctors use heart and temperature monitoring watches to gather critical information about their patients, which is then stored as data.

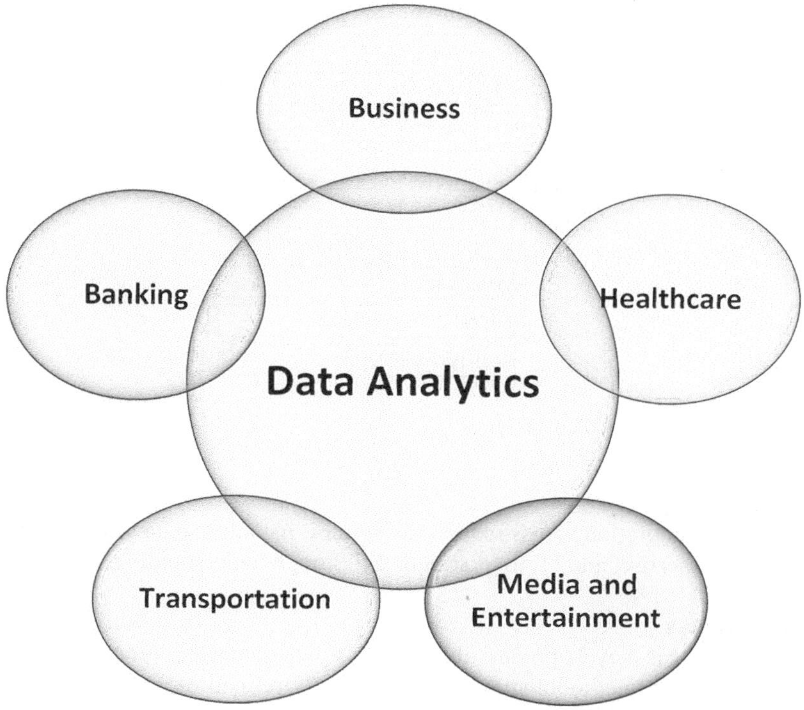

FIGURE 3.2 Uses of data analytics.

Each data record is vital for doctors to monitor their patients' health and prescribe related medicines.

Data in Media and Entertainment: The media and entertainment industry collects, creates, analyzes, markets, and distributes content. Big data helps forecast audience preferences, optimize planning, acquire and retain customers, suggest content, and create new offerings.

Data in Transportation: Data is crucial in the field of transportation. It is necessary for proper communication and synchronization of transport mediums. To analyze the information, data analytics is required. With the potential of data, one can analyze the number of passengers traveling from a source to a destination. This data can be processed in real-time with the help of data analytics for the smooth functioning of transportation.

Data in Banking: Data is crucial in banking as it helps to detect fraudulent activities. Big data helps to identify illegal activities like credit/debit card misuse and improve business efficiency, and customer statistics modification. Public analytics for business can also be carried out effectively using data.

3.2.3 Characteristics of Data Analytics

Figure 3.3 shows the significant characteristics of data analytics.

- **Data-Driven**
  Data analytics uses organized and unstructured data to get insights and make choices.
- **Goal-Oriented**
  It focuses on accomplishing specified objectives or goals, such as boosting operational efficiency, revenue, or customer happiness.

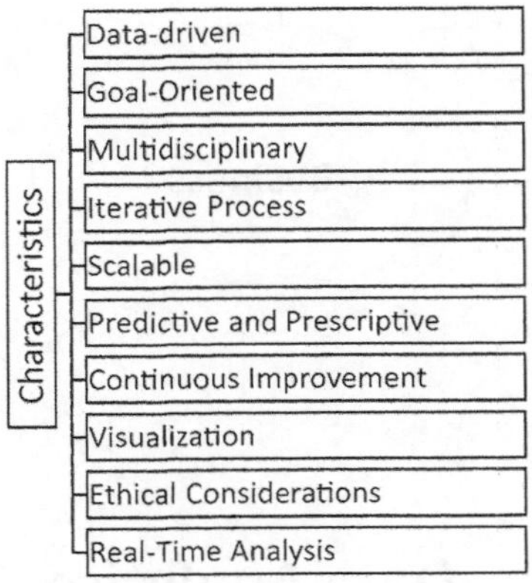

FIGURE 3.3 Characteristics of data analytics.

- **Multidisciplinary**
  It entails collaboration across several disciplines, including data science, business analysis, domain expertise, and IT, to guarantee a thorough understanding and implementation of findings.
- **Iterative Process**
  Data analytics is a cycle process that involves data gathering, processing, analysis, and interpretation, with methodologies being constantly refined depending on new data and insights.
- **Scalable**
  It can manage enormous volumes of data and scale analytical processes to handle larger datasets and increased complexity.
- **Predictive and Prescriptive**
  Predictive and prescriptive analytics are used to estimate future patterns and results based on previous data, as well as to prescribe actions to attain desired outcomes.
- **Continuous Improvement**
  Data analytics encourages continuous learning and improvement of models, algorithms, and analytical methodologies to improve insights' accuracy, efficiency, and relevance.
- **Visualization**
  It uses data visualization tools like charts, graphs, and dashboards to show complicated data in a visually appealing way, making it easier to comprehend and interpret.
- **Ethical Considerations**
  Data analytics follows ethical rules and principles to promote fairness, openness, privacy, and responsible data usage throughout the analytical process.
- **Real-Time Analysis**
  This method allows companies to make rapid choices and adapt swiftly to changing situations by analyzing data as it is created or shortly thereafter.

3.2.4 Process Flow

Data Collection: Collect the information needed to answer the queries. This might include data from a variety of sources, including databases, spreadsheets, APIs, IoT devices, and social media.

Data Cleaning and Preparation: Data cleaning is the process of eliminating or repairing mistakes, inconsistencies, or missing information from data. This phase guarantees that the information is correct and dependable (Banaee et al. 2013).

Data Integration: If necessary, combine data from many sources. This might include combining datasets or linking tables.

Data Transformation: It is the process of converting data into an analytically usable format. This might involve normalization, standardization, or encoding categorical variables.

Exploratory Data Analysis (EDA): This involves summarizing the key features of the data, such as the mean, median, mode, variance, and more.

Data Visualization: Use histograms, scatter plots, box plots, and other visualizations to study data and uncover patterns, trends, or outliers.

Feature Engineering: Develop new features from current data to increase the performance of machine learning systems. This might include transformations, scaling, or the creation of interaction terms (Banaee et al. 2013).

Choosing a Model: Selecting Algorithms: Depending on the nature of the task (classification, regression, clustering, etc.), select appropriate machine learning methods (Banaee et al. 2013)

Split Data: Partition the data into training and testing sets, and occasionally validation sets. Model Training: Execute the selected model(s) on the training data.

Performance Metrics: Use relevant metrics to evaluate the model(s) performance.

Cross-Validation: Cross-validate the model to ensure it is generalizable. Model tuning (if applicable): Tune the model's hyperparameters to increase performance.

Deployment: Once an acceptable model has been trained, it may be used in production to provide predictions or generate insights. This might include connecting the model with current systems or developing APIs for real-time predictions.

Monitoring and Maintenance: Continue to monitor the model's performance in the production environment. To ensure the model remains relevant, it should be updated when new data becomes available and retrained regularly using machine learning methods (Banaee et al. 2013).

The process flow of the data analytics is given in Figure 3.4.

3.2.5 Forms of Data Analytics

The data analytics classification is depicted (Kodjin by Edenlab 2023) in Figure 3.5.

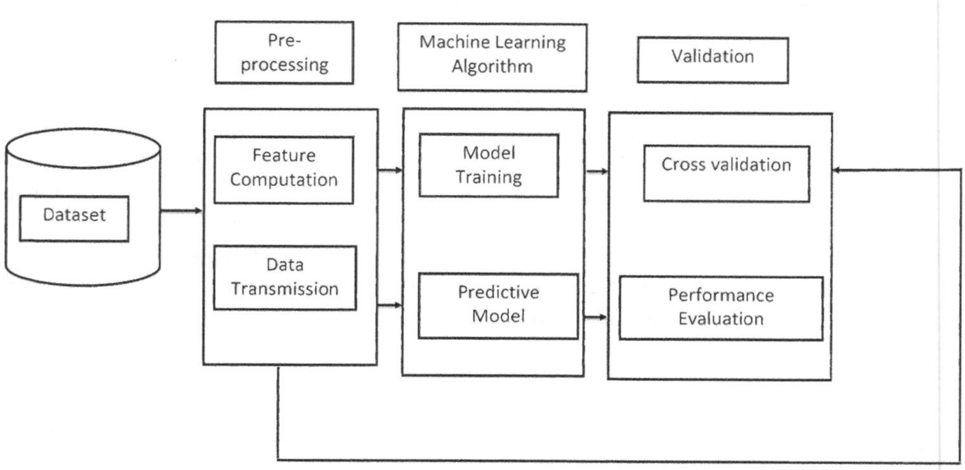

FIGURE 3.4 Data analytics process flow.

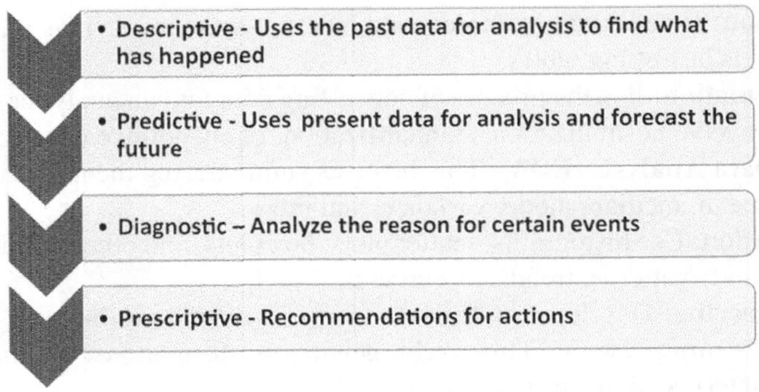

FIGURE 3.5 Forms of data analytics.

3.2.5.1 Descriptive Analytics

Descriptive analytics uses tools like reports, dashboards, and basic statistical measurements to summarize past data and analyze what occurred earlier.

3.2.5.2 Predictive Analytics

Predictive analytics anticipates forthcoming results by utilizing historical facts and statistical techniques, such as machine learning, regression analysis, and predictive modeling.

3.2.5.3 Diagnostic Analytics

Diagnostic analytics studies data to determine why something happened, including techniques such as data mining, drill-down analysis, and correlation analysis.

3.2.5.4 Prescriptive Analytics

Prescriptive analytics makes actionable suggestions based on data analysis, utilizing techniques such as optimization algorithms, simulation, and decision trees.

3.3 HEALTHCARE SENSOR DATA ANALYTICS

Healthcare sensor analytics is the procedure of collecting and using the enormous volume of data from numerous sensors in healthcare settings to gain insights, enhance patient care, and streamline healthcare operations. This entails processing data from wearable devices, implanted sensors, stationary monitors, and ambient sensors to monitor patient health, predict outcomes, adapt therapy, and increase operational efficiency in healthcare settings. Healthcare sensors collect data from individuals, medical equipment, and the environment. These sensors might be wearable, implanted devices, fixed monitors, or mobile apps. This cutting-edge discipline sits at the confluence of healthcare and data analytics, with an emphasis on extracting insights from sensor-generated data. Wearable sensors, fixed monitors, and ambient sensors all capture critical information for improved patient care and healthcare operations. By evaluating this data, healthcare practitioners may acquire real-time insights into patients' health, identify prospective problems, tailor treatment methods, and improve overall facility efficiency. Health data analytics uses advanced statistical and computational approaches to handle an extensive collection of information sources together with electronic health records, public health databases, and wearable devices. Descriptive predictive, and prescriptive analytics are used to improve patient care, operational efficiency, and public health activities. It has a significant impact on clinical decisions, population health, customized care, and research.

3.3.1 Features

- **Monitor Patient Health:** Sensors constantly monitor vital signs, activity levels, glucose levels, and other health data to provide facts on the status of the patient (Harb et al. 2021).
- **Predict and Prevent:** By applying algorithms to sensor data, healthcare professionals may anticipate probable health concerns or difficulties, allowing for preemptive actions to avoid bad conclusions (AumRaj 2023).
- **Personalized Patient Care:** Personalized patient care with tailored treatment plans. Healthcare practitioners can tailor treatment strategies based on specific patient data from sensors. Sensor data enables individualized treatment programs that are suited to each patient's specific needs. For example, diabetic patients' prescription doses can be adjusted depending on real-time glucose observation (AumRaj 2023).
- **Early Detection:** The early detection of health concerns leads to timely interventions and better results. Sensor analytics help identify health problems early, enabling prompt intervention and avoidance of negative consequences (Harb et al. 2021, Goyal and Malviy 2023).
- **Data Fusion:** By combining information from several sensors, a widespread representation of a patient's well-being is made possible, improving the precision and dependability of analytics models
- **Chronic Disease Management:** Continuous monitoring using sensors helps to manage chronic illnesses more proficiently (AumRaj 2023).
- **Improved Operational Efficiency:** By evaluating sensor data, hospitals, and clinics may optimize processes and resource allocations. For example, monitoring equipment utilization to guarantee timely repair or tracking patient flow for more efficient operations.
- **Resource Optimization:** Sensor data may improve operational efficiency by optimizing resource allocation, including hospital beds, staff, and equipment.
- **Workflow Improvement:** Analytic insights can help to simplify operations, reduce waiting times, and improve patient cure.
- **Reducing Readmissions:** Predictive analytics recognize patients who have the chance of readmission and provide preemptive therapy to avoid it.
- **Disease Surveillance:** Detects outbreaks and tracks their spread.
- **Community Health:** Understanding environmental elements through sensor data contributes to better overall community health.
- **Accelerated Research:** Large-scale sensor data can accelerate medical research, leading to breakthrough treatments and cures.
- **New Technologies:** Sensor data are used to generate new medical equipment and technologies.
- **Cost Reduction:** Early action based on sensor data can reduce costs and avert problems.
- **Efficiency in Healthcare Delivery:** Optimizing operations using analytics can result in cost savings for healthcare institutions.
- **Patient Empowerment:** Wearable technologies and applications promote patient empowerment and engagement by allowing them to monitor their health data (Li et al. 2023).
- **Improved Outcomes:** Giving patients real-time health data might encourage them to adjust their behavior and stick to treatment regimens. Overall, healthcare sensor analytics seeks to improve patient outcomes by allowing for early diagnosis of abnormalities, individualized treatment plans, and more efficient healthcare delivery (Li et al. 2023).
- **Data Compliance:** With severe rules such as HIPAA, healthcare sensor analytics ensure the correct management and safeguarding of patient data.
- **Real-Time Monitoring:** Wearable technology and medical sensors, along with healthcare sensor analytics, facilitate uninterrupted, live monitoring of patients' vital signs and physiological characteristics.
- **Remote Monitoring:** Sensor analytics allow for patient monitoring from a distance, eliminating the need for recurrent clinic visits and allowing medical care to be provided outside of conventional healthcare facilities (Li et al. 2023).

3.3.2 Advantages and Disadvantages

3.3.2.1 Advantages

- **Better Patient Outcomes:** Sensor data analytics-enabled early detection and tailored therapies increase patient outcomes and quality of life.
- **Economical Medical Care:** By avoiding complications from untreated health concerns and hospital readmissions, early intervention and remote monitoring help us to save healthcare expenses.
- **Enhanced Productivity:** By automating the tasks, i.e. data collecting, analysis, and decision-making, sensor data analytics optimize healthcare delivery operations, increasing productivity and lowering the burden on medical staff.
- **Patient Empowerment:** Sensor analytics enable patients to actively manage their health and make informed decisions by providing access to their sensor data and actionable insights.

3.3.2.2 Disadvantages

- **Data Privacy Concerns:** The security and confidentiality of patient information are at risk while collecting and evaluating sensitive health data from sensors.
- **Interoperability Challenges:** It can be difficult to guarantee interoperability between various sensor devices and healthcare systems, which might result in problems with data compatibility and integration.
- **Accuracy and Reliability:** The validity and reliability of analytics models and clinical judgments can be impacted by noise, artifacts, and inaccuracies in sensor data.
- **Technical Complexity:** Healthcare companies with limited resources may face difficulties in implementing and maintaining sensor data analytics systems due to the need for specific technical skills and infrastructure.
- **Ethical Considerations:** The proper use of sensor data, informed permission, and the possibility of discrimination or data exploitation can all present ethical challenges.

3.3.3 System Architecture

In healthcare sensor analytics, the processes are conducted by using the steps given below. Figure 3.6 illustrates the system architecture.

Obtaining Data: Patient's heart rates, blood pressure, temperatures, and levels of activity are all measured by sensor equipment. Depending on the needs of the monitoring, this information may be collected constantly or at predetermined intervals (Thakur et al. 2018).

Data Pre-Processing: Before analysis, noise, outliers, and missing values in raw sensor data must be removed. Pre-processing methods are used to clean up and get the data ready for

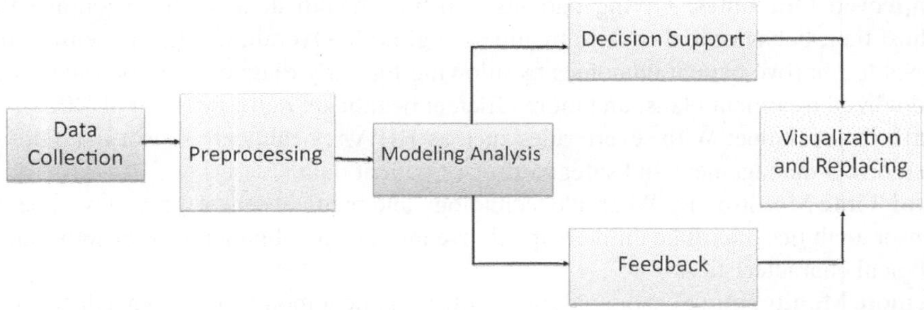

FIGURE 3.6 System architecture.

analysis, including filtering, standardization, and imputation. Feature extraction is the process of taking useful information for analysis out of the pre-processed sensor data by extracting pertinent characteristics. Time-domain analysis, frequency-domain analysis, and statistical metrics that characterize the data are examples of feature extraction techniques (Banaee et al. 2013).

Modeling and Analytics: To extract meaning from the sensor data, analytical methods including statistical analysis, machine learning, and pattern recognition are used. Models are created to forecast health outcomes, spot irregularities, and spot trends that point to certain illnesses (Banaee et al. 2013).

Decision Support: Healthcare practitioners utilize the analytical results to assist in their clinical decision-making. To help with diagnosis, treatment planning, and patient management, decision support systems analyze sensor data and give suggestions, warnings, and visualizations (Banaee et al. 2013).

Feedback and Iteration: To improve models and algorithms, analytics processes take into account input from patients and healthcare experts. Healthcare sensor analytics may be made more accurate and effective through iterative enhancements made possible by continuous monitoring and evaluation of system performance.

Visualization and Reporting: To aid in the understanding and dissemination of results, the sensor data analysis is represented using charts, graphs, and dashboards. To assist physicians, patients, and other stakeholders in healthcare decision-making, reports with critical insights and trends are produced.

3.4 ROLE OF IoT IN HEALTHCARE

3.4.1 Internet of Things

The Internet of Things (IoT) denotes the collection of hardware devices connected to a network. These devices, which can include automobiles, appliances, and various machinery, are equipped with software, sensors, and network connectivity to enable data sharing and gathering. Often termed "smart things," IoT devices encompass a broad spectrum, from simple smart home products like thermostats to wearables such as smartwatches and RFID-enabled clothing, as well as sophisticated industrial and transportation systems. Technology professionals are even visualizing entire "smart cities" built around IoT. These intelligent devices can communicate with one another and with other internet-enabled systems, creating a vast network of interconnected gadgets capable of independent tasks, akin to cell phones and gateways (Harb et al. 2021).

The Internet of Things (IoT) spans numerous sectors, including healthcare, manufacturing, agriculture, and transportation, showcasing its diverse applications. As the proliferation of internet-connected devices grows, IoT influence is set to reshape our world, revolutionizing work, lifestyle, and societal interactions. Within organizational settings, IoT devices monitor a range of metrics from machine performance to energy use, temperature, humidity, and air quality. Utilizing real-time data analysis to detect patterns, trends, and anomalies enables businesses to streamline operations and boost profitability significantly.

3.4.2 IoT Data Integration in Healthcare

3.4.2.1 Challenges

The Internet of Medical Things (IoMT) holds immense potential, but there are many early obstacles to overcome. Research, testing, and licensing are major investments made by health-tech companies before product launch. After effectiveness is established, they create digital ecosystems for smooth data integration. IoT sensor data integration in healthcare, however, is fraught with difficulties.

3.4.2.2 HIPAA Compliance

Due to sensitive data rules, GDPR and HIPAA compliance are essential for IoT healthcare providers. The biggest issues with IoT device integration in healthcare institutions are privacy and data security. HIPAA exclusively safeguards patient health information, termed PHI, requiring consent for its disclosure. PHI encompasses health data combined with personally identifiable information like name and birth date. GDPR also protects healthcare data but necessitates consent for sharing. Compliance involves mindful data transmission and proper storage, discouraging storing all patient data on servers. To ensure anonymity, innovative approaches like generating random IDs are adopted, as advocated by Paul Kressnik of Reha Buddy (Demigos 2020), an Austrian start-up facilitating home rehabilitation.

3.4.2.3 GDPR

The GDPR identifies three categories of personal data that are especially pertinent to the healthcare sector. Health information refers to any information about an individual's state of mind or body, including the kind of care they have gotten (because the patient's condition may be assumed). Genetic information refers to data on a person's genetic composition, including biological sample analysis. Biometric information refers to data on an individual's morphological or behavioral qualities, such as fingerprints, face photos, gait patterns, and more. This information is regarded as personal as biometrics might be used to identify a particular individual. Health, genetic, and biometric data are all considered sensitive data under the GDPR and need to be protected with a higher degree than other categories of personal information (Demigos 2020).

3.4.2.4 Outcomes

Integrating the Internet of Things (IoT) in healthcare has the prospective to greatly improve patient outcomes and operational efficiency. This integration links medical devices, sensors, and healthcare systems via the Internet, enabling real-time data collection, analysis, and sharing. Table 3.1 shows the outcomes of the integration of the IoT in healthcare (Kolodziej and Gonzalez-Velez 2019).

TABLE 3.1
Outcomes – IoT Integration in Healthcare

	Improving Patient Outcomes
Continuous monitoring and real-time alerts	• Fitness trackers and Smartwatches continuously observe vital signs such as blood pressure, oxygen levels, and heart rate • Continuous monitoring allows for early detection of anomalies or critical deviations in a patient's state, enabling timely medical intervention.
Personalized treatment plans	• Devices like continuous glucose monitors (CGMs) for diabetic patients provide detailed insights into blood sugar levels throughout the day. • Healthcare providers can use this data to make effective treatment plans, specifically to the needs of the patients, adjusting medication dosages and dietary recommendations in real-time.
Enhanced chronic disease Management	• IoT platforms that incorporate data from several sensors. Blood pressure monitors, activity trackers, and scales help manage chronic conditions like hypertension, heart disease, and obesity. • IoT enables more effective management of chronic diseases through continuous monitoring and proactive adjustments to treatment plans.
Remote patient monitoring	• IoT-enabled Remote Patient Monitoring (RPM) systems enable patients with conditions like heart failure or COPD to be monitored remotely from their homes. • Patients can receive high-quality care without the need for frequent hospital visits. This enhances both patient comfort and satisfaction while also alleviating the burden on healthcare facilities.

(*Continued*)

TABLE 3.1 (*Continued*)
Outcomes – IoT Integration in Healthcare

	Enhancing Operational Efficiency
Streamlined hospital operations	• IoT-enabled asset tracking systems monitor the location and usage of medical equipment like wheelchairs, ventilators, and defibrillators in real-time. • Efficient tracking and management of medical equipment reduce time wasted searching for devices, leading to more efficient use of resources and improved patient care. • This also helps in better inventory management and reduces operational costs
Improved workflow and staff management	• IoT systems can track the movements and activities of healthcare staff, optimizing workflow and patient assignments. • By analyzing data on staff activities and patient needs, hospitals can improve the allocation of personnel, ensuring that patients receive timely care. • This enhances the overall efficiency of healthcare delivery and reduces wait times
Energy management and cost reduction	• IoT-enabled smart systems control heating, lighting, air conditioning, and ventilation in healthcare facilities based on occupancy and usage patterns. • Efficient energy management leads to significant cost savings and reduces the environmental footprint of healthcare facilities. • These savings can be redirected towards improving patient care services
Predictive maintenance of medical equipment	• IoT sensors monitor the condition and performance of critical medical equipment, predicting when maintenance is required. • Predictive maintenance helps prevent equipment failures, ensuring that devices are always available and functioning correctly when needed. • This reduces downtime, enhances patient safety, and improves the reliability of medical services
Data-driven decision making	• IoT platforms collect and analyze data from diverse sources, offering perceptions of patient care, resource allocation, and operational efficiency. • Data-driven insights enable healthcare administrators to make well-informed decisions regarding staffing, resource distribution, and process enhancements • This leads to better management practices, cost efficiencies, and improved patient outcomes.

3.4.3 Identification of Sensing Technologies

The advancement of semiconductor VLSI technology has resulted in low-power computers, sensors, and intelligent wireless networks, which serve as the foundation for the IoT. IoT provides the capacity to connect things and facilitate communication between them, which necessitates networking and sensing capabilities. Its purpose is to detect, gather, and process data to optimize resource use, which is aided by cloud services. Over the last two decades, networking has become essential for accessing information from anywhere, because of advances in semiconductor and computer technology. This has resulted in the deployment of sensors in a variety of situations, enabling control and monitoring that was previously limited to industrial settings and establishing the framework for IoT and Big Data integration.

Smart Sensors: Smart sensors play a main role in a diversity of disciplines, including environment monitoring, eHealth, and IoT, with applications growing quickly. As the market grows, efficient manufacturing becomes increasingly important in meeting demand, with an emphasis on cost-effectiveness, high production, and quick fabrication cycles. These sensors incorporate processing capabilities to interpret environmental signals before sending data to centralized hubs, creating the foundation of IoT infrastructure. Their adaptability has applications in the scientific, military, civic, and domestic realms, demonstrating their importance in current technology (Li et al. 2023).

Gas Sensors: Gas sensors are essential in chemical sensing because they assess gas concentrations in the surrounding area. They are widely used in environmental monitoring, automotive, and industrial sectors to detect gases in a variety of contexts like as mines and power plants. Their flexibility extends to medical applications such as electronic noses and breath analyzer testing. Gas sensors serve a significant part in a variety of applications, including air quality management and home protection.

3.4.4 Health Monitoring System

An SMS is sent to a doctor's phone or any family member who may be able to help in an emergency by a healthcare monitoring system (HMS), which primarily employs a microcontroller to track and interpret health data. The primary benefit of this system is that it is lightweight, portable, and wireless, making it perfect for carrying around. The ability to continuously and in real-time monitor health issues is another benefit of these systems. Hospitals, home health care, and athlete vitals tracking (heart rate, blood pressure, and body temperature) all employ HMS. Many sensors that are built into the systems are capable of processing all of this data (Paganelli et al. 2022). Figure 3.7 illustrates the Health Monitoring System.

Wearable sensors, FPGA, or microcontrollers are vital in health monitoring. A transmitter captures heartbeat impulses, interprets, and sends data via ZigBee through Wi-Fi. The receiver relays information to a computer for analysis. Microprocessors within the transmitter convert pulse to voltage for display. Wire-free sensors measure temperature, blood pressure, and heart rate attached to the patient. Short-range wireless methods like Bluetooth and ZigBee enable data transmission. The device includes electrodermal activity (EDA) and respiration sensors. Field-programmable gate arrays (FPGAs) with HDL enable post-manufacture programming for versatile applications. An inexpensive analog-to-digital converter aids in system integration. Figure 3.8 illustrates the E-Health Monitoring System Architecture.

Real-time data gathering is achieved by integrating medical and environmental sensors through the Perception layer. While environmental sensors monitor variables that affect patient health, such as oxygen levels and room temperature, medical sensors track vital signs. The API layer has several interfaces that facilitate the storage and retrieval of data using cloud technologies. Through various APIs, it creates patient profiles and retrieves existing medical information. An e-health application

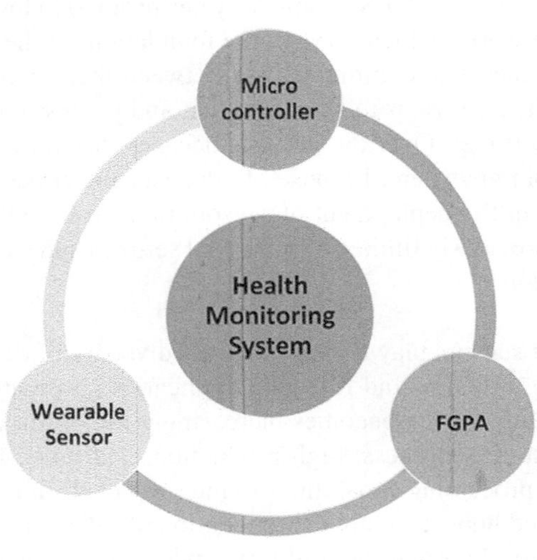

FIGURE 3.7 Health monitoring system.

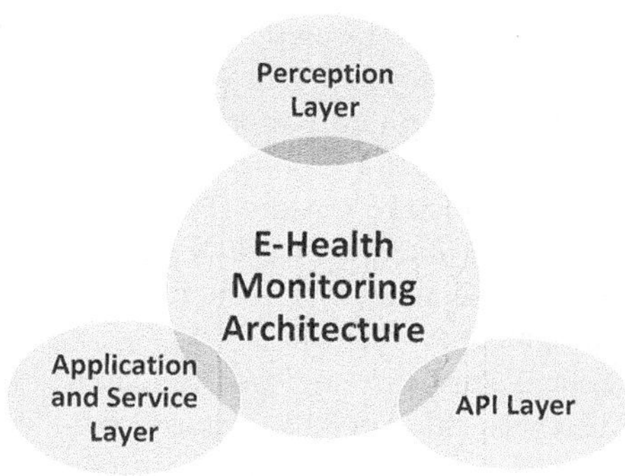

FIGURE 3.8 E-health monitoring architecture.

hosted on the service layer uses data analysis to recommend treatments or medications. When an emergency arises, integrated algorithms analyze data with patient histories and send signals to medical professionals. HMS is a flexible instrument that works well for both homes and hospitals at a reasonable price and has the potential to save lives.

3.5 HEALTHCARE DEVICES

3.5.1 Medical Sensor

The networked healthcare environment is built on sensors. They make it possible to collect data that is trustworthy and give patients and medical professionals vital information on the state of the patient. This is particularly true in medical settings where minimally invasive technology, medical pump equipment, breathing apparatus, and vital sign monitoring gadgets are used. Both the patient and the physician can profit greatly from the integration of these health sensors and wireless communication technologies to monitor the patient's well-being during usual activities. In this example, the wireless sensor network (WSN) related to an essential node in a health facility treats each patient as a node. The real-time extent of health indicators is dependent on the health condition of the patient and the sensors necessary for health monitoring. The suggested healthcare system architecture includes dependable, compact, and low-power medical sensors. To measure the significant five variables, i.e. ECG signals, blood pressure, heart rate, and body temperature, four sensors are required.

3.5.1.1 Types of Medical Sensors

Based on the sensing methods and principles, the significant categories of sensors are biosensors, mechanical sensors, magnetic sensors, thermal sensors, optical sensors, and electrochemical and semiconductor sensors. In the medical domain, some sensors are used specifically for various purposes, including pressure detectors, gas and temperature sensors, flow sensors, acoustic sensors, image sensors, biomedical sensors, magnetic field sensors, and gas sensors. Typically, cameras use image sensors, which might be found in devices like X-ray, optical, and ultrasonic machines. The utilization of sensors in the medical industry is highly dependent on the application. Biomedical sensors detect biological, chemical, or physical processes, and the resulting data is then sent for analysis. These sensors can also be used in systems that handle clinical samples, such as the increasingly popular lab-on-a-chip devices. To collect body and pathology information, biomedical sensors are required. As medical procedures in hospitals and clinics become more expensive, people are increasingly turning to home healthcare services. In various healthcare devices, physical sensors, chemical sensors, biopotential electrodes, biosensors, and bioanalytic sensors are used.

Physical Sensor: A physical sensor might be used to monitor blood flow, blood viscosity, body temperature, blood pressure, bone development velocity, biological magnetic field, and so on. In biomedical applications, there are numerous kinds of physical sensors are used. Gamma-ray-based and X-ray sensors are considered as Radiation sensors. Mechanical sensors include ultrasonic and pressure sensors. Thermal sensors include thermocouples, thermistors, thermopiles, optical fiber devices, P-N junction diodes, and infrared sensors. Magnetic sensors encompass crucial devices for monitoring blood flow and magnetic resonance imaging (MRI) equipment (Singaravel 2019).

Chemical Sensors: A chemical sensor is employed to identify the makeup and strength of bodily fluids, such as pH levels, calcium ions, glucose, and more. Meanwhile, a biosensor is designed to detect enzymes, antigens, antibodies, hormones, DNA, RNA, and microbes. (Singaravel 2019).

Bio Sensor: Biosensors utilize biological components and a suitable platform to identify pathogenic organisms, carcinogenic or mutagenic substances, and toxins, or to capture a biological response. Over recent years, a multitude of biosensor types have emerged, tailored for diverse medical applications. Classification of biosensors is based on both the sensor apparatus and the biological material utilized.

- Electrochemical biosensors operate on enzymatic catalytic reactions that either consume or generate electrons. These enzymes are commonly known as redox enzymes.
- Physical biosensors are categorized into two types: piezoelectric biosensors and thermometric biosensors.
- An optical biosensor utilizes optical measurement principles, employing fiber optics and optoelectronic transducers. Meanwhile, a wearable biosensor is a digital device worn on the human body, integrated into wearable systems like smart watches, smart shirts, and even tattoos, enabling the monitoring of blood glucose, blood pressure, heart rate, and other physiological parameters. (Singaravel 2019)
- A wearable biosensor is digital equipment worn on the body, integrated into systems like smart shirts, smartwatches, and even tattoos, enabling the monitoring of blood pressure, blood glucose, heart rate, and other physiological factors.

3.5.2 Applications of Sensors in Medical Devices

Medical sensors are utilized in an extensive variety of instruments, aiding in both invasive and non-invasive medical procedures.

Diagnostic Devices: *S*ensors are used in various diagnostic instruments, such as blood glucose monitors, electrocardiograms (ECGs), and imaging equipment.

Therapeutic Devices: Medical devices such as pacemakers, insulin pumps, and defibrillators integrate sensors to deliver precise and controlled therapies.

Monitoring Devices: Sensors are essential for monitoring equipment such as vital sign monitors, telemetry devices, and wearable devices to continuously measure patient health data.

Home Health Monitoring: Medical sensors allow medical practitioners to remotely monitor the vital signs of the patients and intervene promptly if needed (TriMedika 2024).

3.5.3 Types of Healthcare Sensors

Wearable Sensors: Wearable sensors include fitness trackers, smart watches, and patches that measure vital indications such as heart rate and activity level.

Implantable Sensors: Implantable sensors are used in various medical equipment to monitor glucose levels, cardiac function, and other parameters. Stationary Monitors: Stationary monitors are used in hospitals to continually monitor patients' vital signs. Environmental Sensors: Monitor air quality, temperature, and humidity in healthcare facilities (Garg et al. 2023).

ECG Sensing: The ECG method uses a unit with five electrodes, they are RL- Right Leg, LL- Left Leg, RA- Right Arm, LA- Left Arm, and V1- Chest) attached to the body to continuously monitor the electrical and muscle activity of the heart. These electrodes detect signals and turn them into electrical signals ranging in amplitude from 1 to 5 mV. A signal conditioning circuit, consisting of an instrumentation amplifier, high-pass filter, low-pass filter (with a cut-off frequency of 150 Hz), gain amplifier, and notch filter, is used to filter and amplify analog signals from ECG electrodes.

Heart Rate and Oxygen Level Monitoring: A finger pulse oximeter monitors both oxygen saturation (SpO2) and heart rate. It is made up of red or infrared LEDs and a photodetector that collects light from the region being measured. This concept is based on the absorption properties of blood hemoglobin when exposed to infrared or red light. Oxygenated hemoglobin absorbs more infrared light whereas Deoxygenated hemoglobin absorbs more red light. By comparing the relative transmittance of infrared and red light, the device calculates absorbance and determines blood oxygenation using pulse oximetry. A microprocessor analyzes the output pulses produced by the pulse oximeter sensor to calculate the heart rate of the patient (Krishnamurthi et al. 2020).

Blood Pressure Monitoring: Blood pressure readings were taken using a Silicon pressure sensor type (ASDX 015PDAA5), which includes an integrated microprocessor with digital interface capabilities. The pressure sensor is connected to a DC motor and a dump valve via an airline, making it easier to gather blood pressure measurements. The integrated microprocessor controls the functioning of the DC motor and dump valve, allowing data gathering. This technology uses pressure fluctuations observed by the sensor in the arm cuff to ensure accuracy. The sensor produces a high voltage output (4.0 Vdc) across the full-scale pressure range, with an accuracy rate of ±2.0%.

Sensing Temperature: The MLX90614, a small and inexpensive non-contact infrared temperature sensor, is made up of two integrated chips: a signal processing chip and an infrared thermopile detector. It provides a 10-bit PWM output signal with a fine precision of 0.14°C, allowing for continuous temperature monitoring. It can be easily interfaced with a microcomputer for streamlined data entry.

Sensor for Medical Ventilators: The use of sensor technology in medical applications enhances patient care by cutting costs, improving outcomes, and monitoring issues through data insights. These sensors monitor not only the equipment but also the patient's internals throughout operations. They satisfy stringent requirements and include robust, compact designs, digital signal processing, low power consumption, and multi-sensor integration. Sensors, which are built into medical equipment like blood pressure monitors and portable ventilators, provide real-time data transfer, supporting patients and professionals in making informed decisions and providing better healthcare.

Medical Pumps: In certain medical settings, such as hemodialysis and infusion therapy, the use of specialist equipment, such as infusion pumps and blood flow monitors, is critical to patient life. These systems include sensors that are meant to maintain a regular flow rate, detect potential obstructions, identify air bubbles in tubing, and correctly measure liquid levels.

Minimally Invasive Equipment: A wide range of medical tools and equipment, from minimally invasive surgical treatments to non-invasive blood pressure monitoring, now prefer less intrusive ways. Sensors for temperature, force, pressure, and other characteristics provide precise and dependable measurements, ensuring that patient monitoring equipment operates properly.

Respiratory Care: Ventilators deliver breathable air into and out of the lungs using either a face mask or an artificial airway (invasive ventilation). Pressure, temperature, location, vibration, and CO_2 detection sensors are utilized to monitor and control the ventilation system as the air moves from the machine to the respiratory system.

Vital Signs Monitoring: Vital signs act as important markers of a patient's overall health. Body pulse rate, temperature, blood pressure, and respiration rate are some of the most commonly measured vital signs. Sensors are at the heart of vital sign monitoring, allowing for continuous tracking and monitoring of these important parameters, resulting in rapid and accurate assessments of a patient's status.

3.5.4 Functions and Uses

The application of data collected from several sensors in healthcare settings to gain insights, boost operational effectiveness, improve patient outcomes, and facilitate improved decision-making is known as healthcare sensor analytics. These sensors can be integrated into wearable technology, medical equipment, or even the environment itself. Here are a few typical applications and roles for sensor analytics in healthcare:

Remote Patient Monitoring: Prime indicators such as blood pressure, heart rate, blood sugar, and oxygen saturation may all be continually tracked by sensors from a distance. Real-time analysis of this data to identify trends or abnormalities enables early intervention and individualized healthcare management (Krishnamurthi et al. 2020).

Fall Prevention and Detection: Alerts to caretakers or medical experts can be sent when a senior or patient at risk falls. This is made possible via sensors. Examination of movement patterns Identifying people who are at risk of falling and putting preventative measures in place can also be aided by movement pattern analysis.

Medicine Adherence: By keeping an eye on wearable medical devices or pill bottle openings, sensors can monitor medicine consumption. Medication compliance and treatment results can be enhanced by using analytics to evaluate adherence levels and warn patients who miss doses.

Chronic Disease Management: Sensors can monitor pertinent physiological indicators and environmental elements for diseases such as diabetes, asthma, or hypertension. Analytics can help manage diseases better by revealing how a condition progresses, pointing out exacerbation triggers, and optimizing treatment plans.

Sleep Monitoring: Wearable sensors can track many aspects of sleep patterns, such as length, intensity, and interruptions. Analytics can assess the effectiveness of sleep and identify sleep abnormalities, allowing for tailored interventions to enhance general health and sleep hygiene.

Infection Control: To stop hospital-acquired infections, environmental sensors can keep an eye on temperature, humidity, air quality, and other variables. Analytics can be used to track adherence to hygiene guidelines, detect high-risk regions for infections, and optimize ventilation systems.

Surgical Safety and Precision: Real-time feedback on tissue temperature, blood flow, and pressure can be obtained during surgeries utilizing sensors built into surgical instruments or wearable technology. Surgeons can improve surgical outcomes, reduce risks, and optimize methods with the use of analytics.

Physical Rehabilitation: During rehabilitation exercises, wearable sensors can monitor muscle activation and movement. Analytics can evaluate development, identify breaks from recommended protocols, and give patients and therapists suggestions for better rehabilitation plans. Health Behavior Monitoring: Data on stress levels, food habits, and physical activity can be recorded via sensors. Analytics is capable of analyzing behavior.

Predictive Analytics and Early Warning Systems: Predictive models can predict unfavorable occurrences like patient deterioration or hospital readmissions by evaluating past data and real-time sensor inputs. Early warning systems have the potential to lower healthcare costs and improve patient safety by alerting healthcare practitioners to take preventive measures.

3.6 ALGORITHMS/TECHNIQUES

Numerous algorithms and methodologies are used in healthcare sensor analytics research to glean insightful information from sensor data. Among the essential formulas and methods.

3.6.1 Machine Learning and Deep Learning

Sensor data is examined using machine learning algorithms to provide predictions or classifications. These algorithms use a variety of methodologies: supervised, unsupervised, and reinforcement learning. Deep learning approaches perform well with sequential sensor data, such as time-series data from wearable sensors. Recurrent neural networks (RNNs) and convolutional neural networks (CNNs) are prevalent choices for this purpose.

3.6.2 Signal Processing

To pre-process sensor data, eliminate noise, and extract pertinent information, signal processing techniques are used. For studying physiological signals like ECG and EEG data, time-domain and frequency-domain analytic techniques like the Fourier transform and wavelet transform are frequently utilized (Banaee et al. 2013).

3.6.3 Pattern Recognition

Pattern recognition techniques are utilized to identify patterns and anomalies in sensor data. Statistical pattern recognition methods, including clustering, classification, and anomaly detection algorithms, are applied to detect abnormal patterns indicative of health conditions or events (Siddiqui et al. 2023).

3.6.4 Feature Selection and Dimensionality Reduction

Feature selection and dimensionality reduction techniques are used to simplify sensor data and enhance algorithm performance. Methods like independent component analysis (ICA), principal component analysis (PCA), and feature ranking algorithms are applied to pinpoint the most pertinent features for analysis.

3.6.5 Probabilistic Modeling

Probabilistic modeling techniques, such as Bayesian networks and hidden Markov models (HMMs), are used to model uncertainty and infer relationships between sensor data and health outcomes. These models enable probabilistic reasoning and decision-making based on sensor observations.

3.6.6 Semantic Interoperability

Semantic interoperability techniques utilize ontologies and semantic models to standardize the representation and interpretation of sensor data. Semantic technologies enable data integration and interoperability across heterogeneous healthcare systems and facilitate semantic reasoning for decision support.

3.6.7 Streaming Analytics

Streaming analytics techniques process sensor data in real time, enabling timely detection and response to health events. Stream processing platforms and algorithms, such as Apache Kafka and Spark Streaming, analyze continuous streams of sensor data and trigger alerts or actions based on predefined rules or thresholds.

3.7 RESEARCH CHALLENGES

Sensor data analytics in healthcare presents unique opportunities to enhance patient care, improve diagnostics, and optimize treatment plans. However, it also faces several specific challenges that need to be addressed to fully realize its potential. These challenges include data quality and integration, privacy and security concerns, real-time processing, and the need for advanced analytical techniques.

3.7.1 Data Quality and Integration

Heterogeneity of Data: Sensor data in healthcare comes from heterogeneous sources, such as wearable devices, electronic health records (EHRs), and medical instruments, and. These data sources often differ in format, scale, and frequency, making integration complex.

Data Accuracy and Reliability: Ensuring the accuracy and reliability of sensor data is critical. Sensors can produce noisy, incomplete, or erroneous data due to device malfunctions, user errors, or environmental factors.

Standardization: The lack of standardized protocols and formats for sensor data can hinder the seamless integration and interoperability of different systems and devices (Shaik et al. 2023).

3.7.2 Privacy and Security Concerns

Data Sensitivity: Healthcare data is extremely sensitive, and any breach can lead to significant consequences for patient privacy and trust. Implementing strong security measures to safeguard sensor data against unauthorized access is critical (Kolodziej and Gonzalez-Velez 2019).

Regulatory Compliance: US regulations HIPAA (Health Insurance Portability and Accountability Act), and European regulations GDPR (General Data Protection Regulation) require stringent data handling and protection protocols, which can be challenging to implement consistently across all sensor data sources (Shaik et al. 2023).

3.7.3 Real-Time Processing

Latency and Response Time: Many healthcare applications demand near-real-time or real-time data processing to provide timely interventions, such as monitoring critical patients or managing chronic conditions. Ensuring low latency and quick response times is essential.

Computational Resources: Significant computational resources are required for processing large volumes of real-time sensor data. Balancing the need for high-performance with cost-effective solutions can be challenging.

3.7.4 Advanced Analytical Techniques

Complexity of Data: Healthcare sensor data is often complex, involving time-series data, multi-dimensional measurements, and dynamic changes. Developing advanced analytical techniques to accurately interpret this data is essential.

AI and Machine Learning Integration: Leveraging AI and machine learning to analyze sensor data can provide powerful insights but also requires specialized expertise and computational resources. Training models with high accuracy and generalizability in the healthcare context remains a challenge.

Clinical Validation: Any analytical models or algorithms developed from sensor data must be clinically validated to ensure their reliability and efficacy in real-world healthcare settings. This process can be time-consuming and resource-intensive.

3.7.5 Scalability and Deployment

Scalability of Solutions: Developing scalable solutions that can handle the increasing volume and variety of sensor data is crucial. Ensuring that analytics platforms can grow with the expanding data landscape in healthcare requires ongoing innovation and investment.

Integration into Clinical Workflows: For sensor data analytics to be effective, it must be seamlessly integrated into existing clinical workflows. This involves ensuring that healthcare professionals can easily access and utilize the insights generated from sensor data without disrupting their routine practices.

3.7.6 User Adoption and Training

Ease of Use: The tools and platforms used for sensor data analytics should be user-friendly and accessible to healthcare professionals who may not have advanced technical expertise.

Training and Education: Providing adequate training and education to healthcare providers on the use and interpretation of sensor data analytics is essential for widespread adoption and effective use. Addressing these issues is essential for maximizing the benefits of sensor data analytics in healthcare. By overcoming these hurdles, healthcare providers can progress patient outcomes, enhance operational efficacy, and pave the way for innovative medical solutions

Data Integration and Fusion: Integrating data from various sensors and sources while ensuring accuracy and consistency is a significant challenge. Fusion techniques must be developed to combine heterogeneous data types effectively (Goyal and Malviy 2023, Thakur et al. 2018).

Real-Time Processing: Processing sensor data in real-time is crucial for timely decision-making in healthcare. Developing algorithms and systems capable of controlling enormous sizes of data with minimal latency is a task, especially in resource-constrained environments.

Security and Privacy: Securing the security and integrity of patient data received by sensors is critical. Developing resilient encryption algorithms and access control systems that protect sensitive healthcare data from unwanted access and potential cyber hazards is a daunting task.

Interoperability: Achieving interoperability among different sensor devices and healthcare systems is essential for seamless data exchange and integration. Developing standardized protocols.

Scalability: To handle the increasing amount of sensor data produced in healthcare settings, healthcare sensor analytics systems need to be scalable. It is difficult to design scalable algorithms and structures that can manage growing data loads without sacrificing performance.

3.8 SUCCESSFUL IMPLEMENTATIONS OF SENSOR DATA ANALYTICS IN HEALTHCARE

Sensor data analytics has been increasingly integrated into healthcare settings with significant success, transforming patient care, improving outcomes, and optimizing operational efficiency. Here are detailed examples of successful implementations:

3.8.1 Remote Patient Monitoring (RPM)

Example: The Veterans Health Administration (VHA) has implemented an extensive remote patient monitoring program that uses sensors to track the health status of veterans with prolonged illnesses such as diabetes, hypertension, and heart disease (Kolodziej and Gonzalez-Velez 2019).

Impact: The VHA can detect early signs of complications, allowing for timely interventions based on the continuous observation of the vital signs, i.e. glucose levels and blood pressure. This program has led to reduced hospital admissions and improved management of chronic diseases.

3.8.2 Wearable Health Devices

Example: The Apple Watch, equipped with advanced sensors, has been used in studies to detect atrial fibrillation (AFib), a common but often undiagnosed heart condition.

Impact: By analyzing heart rate data collected from the watch, users can be alerted to irregular heart rhythms. In collaboration with healthcare providers, this data can facilitate early diagnosis and treatment, potentially preventing strokes and other complications associated with AFib.

3.8.3 Predictive Analytics in Intensive Care Units (ICUs)

Example: The University of Pennsylvania Health System implemented a predictive analytics system called "Penn Signals" in their ICUs.

Impact: By analyzing real-time data from patient monitors (e.g., heart rate, oxygen levels) using machine learning algorithms, the system predicts patient deterioration. This allows for proactive interventions, such as adjusting treatment plans or allocating resources more effectively, which has been shown to reduce mortality rates in ICU patients.

3.8.4 Smart Inhalers for Asthma Management

Example: Propeller Health's smart inhalers use sensors to track medication usage and environmental factors that may trigger asthma symptoms.

Impact: Data collected by the inhalers is examined to offer tailored perceptions and reminders to patients, improving medication adherence and helping patients identify and avoid triggers. Studies have shown that this approach reduces asthma-related emergency visits and hospitalizations.

3.8.5 Post-Surgical Recovery Monitoring

Example: Scripps Health in San Diego implemented a monitoring system using wearable sensors to track the recovery of patients after heart surgery.

Impact: Sensors measure metrics such as heart rate, activity levels, and sleep patterns. The data is analyzed to identify deviations from expected recovery patterns, enabling early intervention if complications arise. This approach has improved recovery outcomes and reduced the length of hospital stays.

3.8.6 Diabetes Management with Continuous Glucose Monitors (CGMs)

Example: Dexcom's CGM systems continuously monitor glucose levels in diabetic patients, providing real-time data and trend analysis.

Impact: The analyzed data helps patients and physicians to make well-versed decisions about diet, exercise, and insulin administration. This real-time monitoring has been revealed to improve glycemic control, diminish the frequency of hypoglycemic episodes, and enhance the overall quality of life for diabetic patients.

3.8.7 Sepsis Detection and Management

Example: The Mayo Clinic developed a sepsis detection system using sensor data analytics to monitor patients' vital signs and laboratory results.

Impact: The system uses machine learning algorithms to identify early signs of sepsis, a life-threatening condition. Early detection allows for prompt treatment, which has significantly reduced sepsis-related mortality and improved patient outcomes.

3.8.8 Fall Detection and Prevention in Elderly Care

Example: Philips Lifeline's fall detection system uses wearable sensors to monitor movements and detect falls among elderly patients.

Impact: When a fall is detected, the system automatically alerts caregivers or emergency services. This rapid response capability has reduced the time to treatment after a fall, mitigating the severity of injuries and improving overall safety for elderly individuals living independently.

3.8.9 Future Trends in Sensor Data Analytics for Healthcare

As sensor data analytics continues to evolve, several emerging trends and potential advancements promise to further transform healthcare. These innovations are expected to enhance patient care, improve operational efficiency, and foster new medical discoveries. Here are some of the key future trends and potential advancements (Kolodziej and Gonzalez-Velez 2019). Table 3.2 presents the future trends in sensor data analytics.

TABLE 3.2
Future Trends in Sensor Data Analytics

Technology	Future Trends	Benefits and Advancements
Integration of artificial intelligence and machine learning	Advanced predictive analytics	• Early detection of diseases • Patient deterioration • Personalized treatment plans
	Improved diagnostic accuracy	• Highly accurate diagnoses • Reducing the likelihood of human error • Enabling earlier intervention
	Automated insights and recommendations	• Automatic analysis of sensor data • Provide actionable insights and recommendations to healthcare providers

(*Continued*)

TABLE 3.2 (*Continued*)
Future Trends in Sensor Data Analytics

Technology	Future Trends	Benefits and Advancements
Enhanced wearable technology	More comprehensive monitoring	• Monitoring not just vital signs but also other physiological parameters such as hydration levels, stress indicators, and sleep quality
	Greater comfort and usability	• More comfortable, user-friendly, and unobtrusive • Encouraging higher adoption rates among patients
IoT-enabled smart healthcare systems	Interconnected medical devices	• Medical devices communicate seamlessly, providing a comprehensive view of patient health
	Smart hospital infrastructure	• Automated systems for patient monitoring, resource management, and operational optimization
Telehealth and remote patient monitoring (RPM) expansion	Wider adoption of telehealth	• More comprehensive remote monitoring and virtual care, especially in rural and underserved areas
	Integration with home health devices	• Enabling continuous monitoring of chronic conditions and reducing the need for in-person visits
Advanced-data integration and interoperability	Unified health records	• Providing a holistic view of patient health across different healthcare providers and systems
	Real-time data sharing	• Facilitating timely and coordinated care
Precision medicine and personalized healthcare	Tailored treatment plans	• Treatments and interventions are tailored to the individual based on their unique physiological data and genetic profile
	Dynamic Adjustments	• Real-time adjustments to treatment plans based on the patient's ongoing response, optimizing therapeutic outcomes
Enhanced patient engagement and self-management	Patient empowerment	• User-friendly apps and devices are used by the patients to take a more dynamic role in handling their health
	Behavioral interventions	• Enable personalized behavioral interventions, guiding patients towards healthier lifestyles and better adherence to treatment plans
Advanced genomic and bioinformatics integration	Genomic data analysis	• Enable more precise risk assessments and personalized healthcare strategies based on an individual's genetic predisposition
	Bioinformatics tools	• Analyze complex biological data in conjunction with sensor data, leading to new insights into disease mechanisms and potential treatments
Blockchain for data security and privacy	Secure data sharing	• Blockchain technology will be used to ensure secure and transparent sharing of sensor data • Protecting patient privacy and enhancing trust in data management systems
	Immutable health records	• Blockchain can create immutable health records • Ensuring data integrity and reducing the risk of tampering or data breaches
Nanotechnology and micro-sensors	Implantable sensors	• Development of tiny, implantable sensors that can continuously monitor health parameters from within the body, providing unprecedented levels of data accuracy
	Non-invasive monitoring	• Micro-sensors will enable non-invasive monitoring techniques, reducing discomfort and risk associated with traditional monitoring methods
Augmented reality (AR) and virtual reality (VR)	Enhanced training and simulation	• To create realistic training simulations for healthcare professionals, improving skills and preparedness
	Patient rehabilitation	• Developed for patient rehabilitation, using real-time sensor data to provide interactive and personalized therapy sessions.

3.9 CONCLUSION

The transformative potential of sensor data analytics in healthcare is vast, as evidenced by the detailed exploration in this chapter. From enhancing patient outcomes through continuous monitoring and real-time alerts to optimizing operational efficiency via predictive maintenance and workflow improvements, sensor data analytics is reshaping the healthcare landscape. The integration of IoT devices and the application of AI and machine learning algorithms further amplify these benefits, enabling more personalized and precise medical care. However, the journey is not without challenges; problems associated with data integration, security, and privacy must be addressed to fully harness the power of sensor data. Successful implementations, such as remote patient monitoring systems and wearable health devices, illustrate the practical benefits and improved health outcomes achievable through sensor data analytics. Looking ahead, advancements in technology promise even greater integration and sophistication, with future trends pointing toward more interconnected, AI-driven, and patient-centered healthcare solutions. By addressing the current challenges and embracing these future trends, the healthcare industry can continue to innovate, ultimately leading to more efficient, effective, and personalized care for patients. This chapter underscores the critical role of sensor data analytics in driving these advancements and shaping the future of healthcare.

REFERENCES

AumRaj. *Healthcare Sensor Types and Cloud-Based IoT System*. 1 Jun, 2023. https://www.linkedin.com/pulse/healthcare-sensor-types-cloud-based-iot-system-aumraj-design-system.

Hadi Banaee, Mobyen Uddin Ahmed, and Amy Loutfi. Data mining for wearable sensors in health monitoring systems – A review of recent trends and challenges. 2013 Dec 17: 13(12); 17472–17500. https://doi.org/10.3390/s131217472.

Demigos. IoT sensor data integration in healthcare: Challenges and solutions. 3 November, 2020. https://demigos.com/blog-post/iot-sensor-data-integration-in-healthcare-challenges-and-solutions.

Mayank Garg, Arpana Parihar, and Md. Saifur Rahman. Advanced and personalized healthcare through integrated wearable sensors. 7th December 2023. https://doi.org/10.1039/D3MA00657.

Priyanshi Goyal, and Rishabha Malviy. Challenges and opportunities of big data analytics in healthcare. 17 August 2023. https://doi.org/10.1002/hcs2.66.

Hassan Harb, Abbass Nasser, Ali Mansour, Eduardo Motta Cruz, and Isabel de La Torre Diez. A sensor-based data analytics for patient monitoring in connected healthcare applications. *IEEE Sensors Journal*, 2021: 21(2); 974–984. https://doi.org/10.1109/JSEN.2020. 2977352.

Kodjin by Edenlab. *Data Analytics in Healthcare: Challenges and Uses*. 23 March, 2023. https://kodjin.com/blog/data-analytics-in-healthcare-challenges-and-solutions.

Joanna Kolodziej, and Horacio Gonzalez-velez (eds). Medical Data Processing and analysis for remote health and activities monitoring. *LNCs*, 2019: 11400; 186–220, 2019. https://doi.org/10.1007/978-3-030-1627 2-6_7.

Rajalakshmi Krishnamurthi, Adarsh Kumar, Dhanalekshmi Gopinathan, Anand Nayyar, and Basit Qureshi. An overview of IoT sensor data processing, fusion and analysis techniques. *Sensors*, 2020: 20; 6076. https://doi.org/10.3390/s20216076.

Chunyan Li, Jiaji Wang, Shuihua Wang, and Yudong Zhang. A review of IoT applications in healthcare. 6 November 2023. https://doi.org/10.1016/j.neucom.2023.127017.

Antonio Iyda Paganelli, Abel Gonz´alezMond´ejar, Abner Cardoso da Silva, Greis Silva-Calpa, Mateus F. Teixeira, Felipe Carvalho, Alberto Raposo, Markus Endler. Real-time data analysis in health monitoring systems: A comprehensive systematic literature review. *Journal of Biomedical Informatics*, 2022; 127: 104009.

Thanveer Shaik, Xiaohui Tao, Lin Li, Haoran Xie, and Juan D. A survey of multimodal information fusion for smart healthcare: Mapping the journey from data to wisdom. 23 September. 2023. https://doi.org/10.1016/j.inffus.2023.102040

Eram Fatima Siddiqui, Tasneem Ahmed, and Sandeep Kumar Nayak. A decision tree approach for enhancing real-time response in exigent healthcare units using edge computing. 14 December 2023. https://doi.org/10.1016/j.measen.2023.100979.

Akshaya Singaravel. NPI Engineer at Viant Medical. Clinical & Manufacturing Aspects of Medical Devices by Professor Folarin Erogbogbo. December 2019. https://www.linkedin.com/pulse/types-sensors-medical-devices-akshaya-singaravel/.

Saurabh Singh Thakur, Shabbir Syed Abdul, Hsiano Yean (Shannon) Chiu, Ram Babu Roy, Po-Yu Huang, Shwetambara Malwade, Aldilas Achmad Nursetyo, and Yu Chuan (Jack) Li. Artificial intelligence based prediction of clinical events among hemodialysis patients using non-contact sensor data. *Sensors,* 2018; 18: 2833. https://doi.org/10.3390/S18092833.

TriMedika Redefining care. Rev. 06. March 26, 2024. https://trimedika.com/sensors-medical-technology-healthcare-industry.

4 Healthcare Sensor Data Analysis for Real-Time Anomaly Detection

A Comprehensive Insights

G. S. Karthick and C. Sivamathi

4.1 INTRODUCTION

Healthcare is undergoing a transformative shift driven by the proliferation of sensor technologies. These sensors, embedded in diverse devices and environments, generate a deluge of data, offering unprecedented opportunities for improving patient care and outcomes. This section introduces the landscape of healthcare sensor data, its sources, and the critical role of real-time anomaly detection in leveraging this data effectively.

The sources of healthcare sensor data are remarkably diverse. Wearable devices, such as smartwatches and fitness trackers, continuously monitor physiological parameters like heart rate, activity levels, and sleep patterns (Aboudi and Benhlima, 2018, Azzalini et al., 2021, Alfian et al., 2018). Implantable sensors, including pacemakers and insulin pumps, provide even more intimate and continuous data streams, offering invaluable insights into internal bodily functions (Aboudi and Benhlima, 2018). Environmental sensors, deployed in homes or hospitals, monitor ambient conditions like temperature, humidity, and air quality, influencing patient comfort and safety (Azzalini et al., 2021). This multifaceted data ecosystem presents both immense potential and significant analytical challenges.

Real-time anomaly detection is paramount because timely identification of deviations from normal physiological patterns can be life-saving. An anomaly in a patient's heart rate, for example, could indicate a cardiac event requiring immediate intervention (Alfian et al., 2018). Similarly, detecting anomalies in sensor readings from a medical implant can prevent device malfunction and avert serious health consequences (Ali et al., 2019). The ability to detect these anomalies in real-time is crucial for optimizing treatment strategies, improving patient safety, and reducing healthcare costs. However, harnessing the power of this data presents significant challenges. The sheer volume, velocity, and variety of data generated by these sensors create a "big data" problem (Al-amri et al., 2021, Ashfaq et al., 2022).

Efficiently processing these high-volume, high-velocity data streams in real-time requires sophisticated algorithms and robust infrastructure. Furthermore, the need for data privacy and security adds another layer of complexity to the process. This book section provides a comprehensive guide to navigating these challenges. We will explore data acquisition methods, preprocessing techniques, anomaly detection algorithms, real-time implementation strategies, and address critical challenges associated with this rapidly evolving field. The section will conclude by highlighting future research directions and the potential impact of real-time anomaly detection on improving healthcare outcomes.

DOI: 10.1201/9781003486640-4

4.2 DATA ACQUISITION AND PREPROCESSING TECHNIQUES

Efficient and reliable data acquisition is the cornerstone of any successful real-time anomaly detection system. This section explores the methods employed to acquire healthcare sensor data and the subsequent preprocessing techniques necessary to prepare this data for analysis. Data acquisition in healthcare relies heavily on various wireless communication protocols. Bluetooth Low Energy (BLE) is frequently used for its low power consumption and suitability for wearable sensors (Bruno et al., 2015). Wi-Fi, while offering higher bandwidth, may be less energy-efficient for always-on monitoring (Chamberlain et al., 2020). Low-Power Wide-Area Networks (LPWAN) protocols, such as LoRaWAN, are well-suited for applications requiring long-range communication with low power consumption, particularly in remote patient monitoring scenarios (Chatterjee & Ahmed, 2022). The choice of communication protocol depends heavily on the specific application's requirements, balancing factors such as range, power consumption, bandwidth, and cost. The wireless communication protocols outlined in Table 4.1 are crucial for determining the range, power consumption, bandwidth, latency, and suitability of technologies like Bluetooth Low Energy (BLE), Wi-Fi, LoRaWAN, Zigbee, and other LPWAN protocols.

Data transmission strategies also play a vital role. Data can be transmitted directly from the sensor to a central server, or it can be routed through intermediate devices (e.g., smartphones, gateways) for aggregation and preprocessing before transmission to the cloud. The choice of transmission strategy impacts latency, bandwidth requirements, and data security. Consideration of data compression techniques can further optimize data transmission, reducing the volume of data sent over the network. The data preprocessing techniques highlighted in Table 4.2 play a key role in enhancing the quality of healthcare sensor data.

Preprocessing plays a crucial role in enhancing the accuracy and efficiency of anomaly detection algorithms. Raw sensor data is often noisy and incomplete, necessitating careful cleaning and transformation. Noise reduction techniques, such as filtering, smooth out random fluctuations in the data (Dwivedi et al., 2021). Outlier removal identifies and eliminates data points that deviate significantly from the expected values (Gudovskiy et al., 2021). Missing data imputation techniques fill in gaps in the data using various methods, such as linear interpolation or more sophisticated model-based approaches (Kaur & Mann, 2018). The choice of preprocessing techniques should be guided by the characteristics of the sensor data and the specific anomaly detection algorithm to be used. The impact of these preprocessing steps on the accuracy and computational efficiency of the subsequent analysis must be carefully considered.

TABLE 4.1
Wireless Communication Protocols for Healthcare Sensor Data

Protocol	Range	Power Consumption	Bandwidth	Latency	Suitability
Bluetooth low energy (BLE)	Short	Low	Low	Low	Wearable sensors
Wi-Fi	Medium	Medium	High	Medium	High-bandwidth applications
LoRaWAN	Long	Very Low	Low	High	Remote patient monitoring
Zigbee	Short-Medium	Low	Low-Medium	Low	Home healthcare networks
Other LPWAN protocols (Sigfox, NB-IoT)	Varies	Very Low	Low	High	Long-range, low-power applications

TABLE 4.2
Data Preprocessing Techniques for Healthcare Sensor Data

Technique	Description	Advantages	Disadvantages
Noise reduction (Filtering)	Removes random fluctuations in the data using methods like moving averages or Kalman filters.	Improves signal-to-noise ratio, enhances accuracy of anomaly detection.	Can introduce bias if not carefully implemented.
Outlier removal	Identifies and eliminates data points significantly deviating from expected values.	Improves accuracy of anomaly detection, reduces impact of erroneous measurements.	Can remove legitimate but unusual data points.
Missing data imputation	Fills gaps in the data using methods like linear interpolation or model-based imputation.	Ensures complete datasets for analysis.	Can introduce bias if the imputation method is inappropriate.
Data transformation	Converts data into a more suitable format for analysis (e.g., normalization, standardization).	Improves algorithm performance, enhances comparability of different features.	Can obscure important information if not carefully implemented.

4.3 ANOMALY DETECTION ALGORITHMS FOR HEALTHCARE DATA

This section provides a comprehensive overview of anomaly detection algorithms applicable to healthcare sensor data, emphasizing their suitability for real-time applications. We will examine both unsupervised and supervised methods, highlighting their strengths and weaknesses in this specific context.

Unsupervised anomaly detection methods are particularly useful when labeled data is scarce or unavailable. Principal Component Analysis (PCA) is a well-established technique for dimensionality reduction and anomaly detection by identifying principal components and flagging data points deviating significantly from the principal subspace (Khaledian et al., 2021). Isolation Forest works by isolating anomalies based on their relative isolation in a random tree structure (Kim et al., 2022). *K*-means clustering groups data points into clusters, identifying anomalies as points far from any cluster center (Krishnamurthi et al., 2020). One-class SVM models the normal data distribution and identifies anomalies as points falling outside this model (Kumar & Singh, 2018). Autoencoders, neural networks trained to reconstruct input data, detect anomalies as data points that the autoencoder struggles to reconstruct accurately (Lakshmi et al., 2021, Li et al., 2017). Conditional normalizing flows offer a more sophisticated approach by modeling the probability distribution of normal data and identifying anomalies as low-probability data points (Mehnaz & Bertino, 2020). The anomaly detection algorithms discussed in Table 4.3 are commonly used for identifying abnormal patterns in healthcare sensor data.

Supervised methods, in contrast, require labeled data for training. Support Vector Machines (SVM) are effective classifiers that can be trained to distinguish between normal and anomalous data points (Moallemi et al., 2022). Gaussian distribution-based methods assume that normal data follows a Gaussian distribution and identify anomalies as points deviating significantly from this distribution. Multilayer Perceptrons (MLP) and Long Short-Term Memory (LSTM) networks are powerful deep learning models capable of learning complex patterns in time-series data (Sunny et al., 2022). LSTMs are particularly well-suited for handling temporal dependencies in healthcare data.

The choice of algorithm depends on several factors, including the availability of labeled data, the nature of the data, the desired computational complexity, and the specific application requirements. A critical evaluation of each algorithm's strengths and weaknesses in the context of healthcare data is essential for selecting the most suitable approach (Tripathi et al., 2020). The trade-offs between accuracy, computational cost, and real-time performance must be carefully considered.

TABLE 4.3
Anomaly Detection Algorithms for Healthcare Sensor Data

Algorithm	Type	Description	Advantages	Disadvantages
Principal component analysis (PCA)	Unsupervised	Dimensionality reduction; identifies principal components and flags data points deviating significantly from the principal subspace.	Simple, computationally efficient.	Assumes linear relationships, sensitive to outliers.
Isolation forest	Unsupervised	Isolates anomalies based on their relative isolation in a random tree structure.	Effective for high-dimensional data, handles outliers well.	Performance can degrade with very high-dimensional data.
K-means clustering	Unsupervised	Groups data points into clusters; identifies anomalies as points far from any cluster center.	Simple, relatively fast.	Sensitive to initial cluster centers, struggles with non-spherical clusters.
Support vector machine (SVM)	Supervised	Trains a classifier to distinguish between normal and anomalous data points.	Effective for high-dimensional data, versatile.	Can be computationally expensive for large datasets, requires labeled data.
Long short-term memory (LSTM)	Supervised	Recurrent neural network suitable for handling temporal dependencies in time-series data.	Captures temporal patterns effectively.	Computationally expensive, requires significant labeled data.
DeepAnT	Supervised	Uses a convolutional neural network (CNN) for prediction and an anomaly detector module for tagging anomalies.	Effective in detecting a wide range of anomalies, including contextual discords in data.	Requires careful parameter tuning.
Conditional normalizing flows	Unsupervised	Models the probability distribution of normal data and identifies anomalies as low-probability data points.	Computationally and memory efficient, high accuracy.	Requires careful model selection and training.

4.3.1 Unsupervised Anomaly Detection Algorithms

Unsupervised anomaly detection algorithms are particularly valuable in healthcare settings where labeled data—data explicitly marked as normal or anomalous—is often scarce, expensive to obtain, or simply unavailable. These algorithms learn patterns directly from the data itself without relying on pre-defined labels. This makes them adaptable to situations where the characteristics of anomalies are not fully understood or where the types of anomalies are highly variable.

4.3.1.1 Principal Component Analysis (PCA)

Principal Component Analysis (PCA) is a widely used dimensionality reduction technique that identifies the principal components, which represent the directions of maximum variance in the data. Anomalies often exhibit significant deviations from these principal components, making PCA a useful tool for anomaly detection.

The PCA algorithm involves several key steps: first, the covariance matrix of the data is computed. This matrix quantifies the relationships between different variables in the dataset. Next, the eigenvectors (principal components) of the covariance matrix are calculated. These eigenvectors represent the directions of maximum variance in the data. The data is then projected onto the subspace spanned by the principal components, effectively reducing the dimensionality of the data while preserving most of the variance. Finally, data points with large reconstruction errors—the distances between the original data points and their projections onto the principal subspace—are flagged as potential anomalies.

PCA's computational efficiency is a significant advantage, making it suitable for real-time applications. However, PCA's reliance on the assumption of linear relationships in the data and its sensitivity to outliers are significant limitations. In healthcare sensor data, where non-linear relationships and outliers are common, the performance of PCA might be compromised. Furthermore, the interpretation of the results can be challenging, especially in high-dimensional datasets.

4.3.1.2 Isolation Forest

Isolation Forest is an ensemble-based anomaly detection algorithm that operates on the principle of isolating anomalies by randomly partitioning the data. The core idea is that anomalies, being inherently different from normal data points, are typically located at the periphery of the data distribution and thus require fewer partitions to be isolated.

The algorithm constructs multiple isolation trees, each randomly partitioning the data using a process similar to recursive partitioning. Anomalies are identified based on their average path length in these trees; anomalies tend to have shorter path lengths because they are isolated more quickly. Isolation Forest is particularly effective for high-dimensional data and shows relative robustness to outliers. However, its performance can degrade when dealing with extremely high-dimensional data, a situation that is not uncommon in healthcare sensor data. The effectiveness of Isolation Forest also depends on the appropriate selection of the number of trees and the sub-sampling size used in the algorithm.

4.3.1.3 *K*-Means Clustering

K-means clustering is a partitioning-based clustering algorithm that aims to group data points into k clusters based on their proximity to cluster centroids [2]. In anomaly detection, data points that are distant from any cluster centroid or belong to small, sparsely populated clusters are identified as potential anomalies.

The algorithm iteratively updates the cluster centroids until convergence. The process begins by randomly initializing k centroids. Then, each data point is assigned to the nearest centroid. The centroids are then recalculated as the mean of the data points assigned to each cluster. This process of assignment and centroid recalculation continues until the centroids no longer change significantly. While computationally efficient for relatively low-dimensional data, K-means has limitations. It is sensitive to the initial placement of cluster centroids, and it struggles with non-spherical clusters or clusters of varying densities. The algorithm also requires the specification of the number of clusters (k) beforehand, which can be challenging to determine without prior knowledge of the data. In the context of healthcare sensor data, determining the optimal number of clusters can be particularly difficult due to the complex and often non-linear relationships between data points.

4.3.1.4 One-Class Support Vector Machine (One-Class SVM)

One-class SVM is a supervised machine learning algorithm that models the distribution of normal data points and identifies anomalies as points that fall outside this learned model. This makes it particularly useful in situations where only normal data is available for training, a common scenario in healthcare where obtaining sufficient anomalous data for training a traditional two-class SVM can be difficult.

The algorithm aims to find a hyperplane that maximizes the margin between the origin and the data points, effectively defining a boundary around the normal data. Data points located outside this boundary are classified as anomalies. One-class SVM is effective for high-dimensional data, a characteristic often found in healthcare sensor datasets. However, it requires careful parameter tuning to achieve optimal performance. The choice of kernel function also significantly influences the algorithm's performance and its ability to capture complex non-linear relationships in the data.

4.3.1.5 Autoencoders

Autoencoders are neural networks designed to learn compressed representations of input data. They consist of an encoder that compresses the input data into a lower-dimensional representation (latent space) and a decoder that reconstructs the original data from this compressed representation. Anomalies are often characterized by large reconstruction errors; that is, the difference between the original data and the data reconstructed by the autoencoder is significantly larger for anomalies than for normal data points.

Autoencoders are particularly powerful for non-linear data, making them well-suited for many healthcare applications where complex, non-linear relationships between variables are common. However, they require careful design of the network architecture and careful parameter tuning for optimal performance. The choice of activation functions, the number of layers, and the size of the latent space can all significantly affect the autoencoder's ability to accurately reconstruct normal data and identify anomalies. Deep autoencoders, with multiple layers, can capture more complex patterns in the data than shallow autoencoders, but this comes at the cost of increased computational complexity.

4.3.1.6 Conditional Normalizing Flows

Conditional normalizing flows represent a more sophisticated approach to unsupervised anomaly detection by explicitly modeling the probability distribution of the normal data. They utilize a series of invertible transformations to map a simple probability distribution (e.g., a standard Gaussian distribution) to a complex, high-dimensional distribution that closely approximates the distribution of the normal data. Anomalies are then identified as data points with low probability under this learned distribution.

The key advantage of conditional normalizing flows is their computational efficiency and their ability to achieve high accuracy in anomaly detection. However, they require careful selection of the model architecture and its hyperparameters, and the training process can be computationally intensive. The choice of the base distribution, the types of transformations used, and the number of transformations all affect the model's ability to accurately capture the distribution of normal data and identify anomalies. Despite these challenges, conditional normalizing flows offer a promising approach for real-time anomaly detection in healthcare due to their high accuracy and relatively low computational cost.

4.3.2 Supervised Anomaly Detection Algorithms

Supervised anomaly detection algorithms require labeled data for training, allowing them to learn a more precise boundary between normal and anomalous data points. While this can lead to higher accuracy compared to unsupervised methods, obtaining sufficient labeled data in healthcare can be a significant challenge due to the relatively low frequency of anomalous events and the associated costs of labeling.

4.3.2.1 Support Vector Machines (SVMs)

Support Vector Machines (SVMs) are powerful and versatile classifiers that can be effectively trained to distinguish between normal and anomalous data points. The algorithm's core objective is to find an optimal hyperplane that maximizes the margin between the two classes (normal and anomalous). This hyperplane acts as a decision boundary, classifying new data points based on their position relative to this boundary.

Various kernel functions can be employed with SVMs to handle non-linear relationships in the data, extending their applicability beyond linearly separable data. The choice of kernel function significantly influences the algorithm's performance and is often determined through experimentation and validation. SVMs are particularly effective for high-dimensional data, a characteristic frequently encountered in healthcare sensor datasets. However, they can be computationally expensive for very large datasets, and they require careful parameter tuning to achieve optimal performance. The availability of sufficient labeled data is also crucial for training an accurate and reliable SVM model.

4.3.2.2 Gaussian Distribution-Based Methods

Gaussian distribution-based methods assume that normal data follows a Gaussian (normal) distribution. Anomalies are identified as data points that deviate significantly from this distribution. The algorithm involves estimating the parameters of the Gaussian distribution—the mean and covariance matrix—using the normal data points.

Anomaly scores are then calculated for each data point based on its Mahalanobis distance from the estimated mean. The Mahalanobis distance takes into account the covariance structure of the data, providing a more robust measure of distance than the Euclidean distance. Data points with high Mahalanobis distances are classified as anomalies. These methods are computationally efficient, but their reliance on the assumption of normality can be a significant limitation. Real-world healthcare sensor data may not always conform to a Gaussian distribution, and violating this assumption can lead to inaccurate anomaly detection. The performance of these methods can also be affected by the presence of outliers in the training data.

4.3.2.3 Multilayer Perceptrons (MLPs) and Long Short-Term Memory (LSTM) Networks

Multilayer Perceptrons (MLPs) and Long Short-Term Memory (LSTM) networks are powerful deep learning models capable of learning complex, non-linear patterns in time-series data. MLPs are feedforward neural networks that can model intricate relationships between input features and the anomaly label. LSTMs, a type of recurrent neural network (RNN), are particularly well-suited for time-series data because they can capture temporal dependencies and long-range patterns in sequential data.

Both MLPs and LSTMs are capable of achieving high accuracy in detecting complex anomalies in healthcare sensor data. However, they require substantial labeled data for training, and their computational cost can be significant, especially for deep networks with many layers and parameters. The training process can also be computationally intensive, requiring substantial computing resources and time. Furthermore, deep learning models can be difficult to interpret, making it challenging to understand the reasons behind their anomaly detection decisions. This lack of interpretability can limit their applicability in certain healthcare settings where transparency and explainability are crucial.

4.3.2.4 DeepAnT

DeepAnT is a deep learning-based approach specifically designed for unsupervised anomaly detection in time-series data. It is particularly well-suited for handling data with periodic seasonality; a characteristic often present in healthcare sensor data. DeepAnT consists of two main modules: a time predictor module and an anomaly detector module.

The time predictor module, implemented using a convolutional neural network (CNN), is trained to predict the next time stamp in the time series. The anomaly detector module then compares the predicted value with the actual value. A significant difference between the predicted and actual values indicates a potential anomaly. DeepAnT is designed to be trained on unlabeled data, making it suitable for scenarios where labeled data is scarce or unavailable. However, similar to other deep learning models, DeepAnT can be computationally intensive and may require careful parameter tuning to achieve optimal performance. The model's interpretability can also be a limitation, hindering the understanding of the reasons behind its anomaly detection decisions.

4.4 ALGORITHM SELECTION AND IMPLEMENTATION CONSIDERATIONS

The selection of an appropriate anomaly detection algorithm for a given healthcare application is not a straightforward process. Several factors must be carefully considered to ensure the chosen algorithm is both effective and suitable for the specific context. These factors include the characteristics of the data, the availability of labeled data, the real-time requirements of the application, and the importance of interpretability.

Data Characteristics: The dimensionality, linearity, and distribution of the data significantly influence the choice of algorithm. High-dimensional data may benefit from algorithms like Isolation Forest or One-class SVM, which are relatively robust to the curse of dimensionality. Data exhibiting clear clusters might be well-suited for *K*-means clustering. Non-linear data often requires algorithms that can capture complex, non-linear relationships, such as autoencoders or deep learning models. The presence of significant noise or outliers might necessitate the use of robust algorithms or preprocessing techniques to mitigate their impact.

Data Availability: The availability of labeled data is a critical factor in determining whether unsupervised or supervised methods are appropriate. When labeled data is scarce or unavailable, unsupervised methods are the only viable option. However, supervised methods often achieve higher accuracy when sufficient labeled data is available. The cost and effort required to obtain labeled data must be weighed against the potential improvement in accuracy.

Real-Time Requirements: For real-time applications, the computational complexity and latency of the chosen algorithm are crucial considerations. Simpler algorithms like PCA or K-means are generally faster than deep learning models like LSTMs or autoencoders. The acceptable latency for anomaly detection will depend on the specific application; for life-critical applications, very low latency is essential. In these situations, simpler algorithms may be preferred even if their accuracy is slightly lower.

Interpretability: In many healthcare applications, understanding the reasons behind an anomaly detection decision is vital for clinical decision-making and building trust. Simpler algorithms are often more interpretable than complex deep learning models. If interpretability is a high priority, simpler methods might be preferred, even if they sacrifice some accuracy.

Implementation Considerations: Beyond algorithm selection, several implementation considerations are crucial for building a robust and effective anomaly detection system. These include data preprocessing, parameter tuning, model evaluation, and scalability.

Data Preprocessing: Thorough data preprocessing is essential to improve the performance of anomaly detection algorithms. This involves steps such as noise reduction, outlier removal, missing data imputation, and data transformation. The specific preprocessing steps should be tailored to the characteristics of the data and the chosen algorithm.

Parameter Tuning: Most anomaly detection algorithms have hyperparameters that must be carefully tuned to optimize their performance. This often involves experimentation and validation on representative datasets using techniques like cross-validation. The optimal hyperparameter settings will depend on the specific dataset and the application requirements.

Model Evaluation: Appropriate metrics, such as precision, recall, F1-score, area under the receiver operating characteristic curve (AUC), and others, should be used to evaluate the performance of the chosen algorithm. The choice of evaluation metric depends on the specific application and the relative importance of different types of errors (false positives vs. false negatives).

Scalability: For large healthcare datasets, scalability is crucial. Distributed computing frameworks can be used to parallelize computations and handle high data volumes. The chosen architecture should be designed to handle the expected data volume and velocity in a timely manner.

TABLE 4.4
Architectural Models for Real-Time Anomaly Detection in Healthcare

Architecture	Description	Advantages	Disadvantages
Cloud-based	Data processed in a central cloud server.	Scalable, centralized data storage.	Potential latency due to data transmission delays.
Edge computing	Data processed closer to the source (e.g., on wearable devices or gateways).	Low latency, reduced bandwidth requirements.	Limited computational resources at the edge.
Fog computing	Hybrid approach combining cloud and edge computing.	Balances latency, scalability, and resource constraints.	Increased complexity in system design and management.
Hybrid	Combination of cloud, edge, and other approaches tailored to specific application needs.	Optimized for specific application requirements, leveraging strengths of different approaches.	Increased complexity in system design and management. Requires careful planning and integration of diverse technologies and expertise.

4.5 ARCHITECTURAL MODELS FOR REAL-TIME ANOMALY DETECTION IN HEALTHCARE

Implementing real-time anomaly detection systems for healthcare requires careful consideration of architectural design and technological choices. This section examines different architectural models and their implications for system performance and scalability.

Cloud-based solutions offer scalability and centralized data storage but may introduce latency due to data transmission delays. Edge computing frameworks, by processing data closer to the source, reduce latency but may require more sophisticated resource management at the edge devices. Fog computing, a hybrid approach that combines cloud and edge computing, attempts to strike a balance between these two extremes. The choice of architecture involves a trade-off between latency, scalability, cost, and data security.

Specific technologies play a crucial role in enabling real-time processing. Apache Kafka, a distributed streaming platform, enables high-throughput, low-latency data ingestion and processing. MongoDB, a NoSQL database, offers flexible and scalable data storage, suitable for handling the diverse and potentially unstructured nature of healthcare data. Other technologies, such as message queues and real-time databases, can be employed to optimize data flow and minimize latency. The selection of specific technologies should be guided by the application's requirements, considering factors such as data volume, velocity, and the desired level of fault tolerance. The integration of these technologies within the chosen architectural framework is crucial for building a robust and efficient real-time anomaly detection system. The architectural models detailed in Table 4.4 provide frameworks for deploying real-time anomaly detection systems in healthcare.

4.6 ADDRESSING CHALLENGES IN REAL-TIME ANOMALY DETECTION

Real-time anomaly detection in healthcare faces several significant challenges, primarily related to the characteristics of the data itself and the complexities of the healthcare environment. This section addresses these challenges, providing strategies for mitigating their impact.

The 4 Vs of big data—volume, velocity, variety, and veracity—pose significant hurdles. The sheer volume of data generated by numerous sensors requires efficient storage and processing capabilities. The high velocity of data necessitates real-time processing techniques to ensure timely detection of anomalies. The variety of data sources and formats necessitates algorithms capable of handling diverse data types. The veracity, or trustworthiness, of the data requires robust data quality control mechanisms to ensure accuracy and reliability. Addressing these challenges requires careful planning and selection of appropriate technologies and algorithms.

Imbalanced datasets, where one class (e.g., anomalies) is significantly underrepresented compared to another, pose a challenge for many anomaly detection algorithms. Techniques like oversampling, undersampling, and cost-sensitive learning can help mitigate this issue. Concept drift, where the statistical properties of the data change over time, necessitates adaptive algorithms capable of adjusting to evolving patterns (Karthick & Pankajavalli, 2020). Data privacy and security are paramount in healthcare, requiring robust mechanisms to protect patient data throughout the entire data lifecycle (Karthick, 2023). Encryption, anonymization, and access control are crucial for ensuring compliance with regulations and maintaining patient trust.

4.7 CASE STUDIES AND APPLICATIONS

This section presents several real-world case studies demonstrating the successful application of real-time anomaly detection in various healthcare settings. These examples illustrate the practical value and potential impact of the techniques discussed in previous sections.

Patient monitoring for chronic diseases is a prime application area (Pankajavalli & Karthick, 2022a, b). Real-time monitoring of vital signs, such as heart rate and blood glucose levels, allows for early detection of critical events and timely intervention, preventing hospitalizations and improving patient outcomes. Early warning systems for critical events, such as cardiac arrest or hypoglycemia, rely on real-time anomaly detection to trigger alerts and facilitate rapid response. Anomaly detection in medical wireless sensor networks (MWSNs) is crucial for ensuring the reliability and accuracy of data collected from multiple sensors deployed on a patient. The use of smart thermometers for infectious disease surveillance demonstrates the potential of real-time data analysis for public health applications. These examples illustrate the broad applicability and significant benefits of real-time anomaly detection across various healthcare settings (Pankajavalli et al., 2021). Further examples can include applications in structural health monitoring of medical equipment, predictive maintenance of medical devices, and fraud detection in healthcare claims processing. Each of these applications requires tailored algorithms and implementation strategies, highlighting the adaptability and versatility of real-time anomaly detection in healthcare.

4.8 FUTURE DIRECTIONS AND RESEARCH TRENDS

The field of real-time anomaly detection in healthcare is rapidly evolving, with several promising trends emerging (Karthick & Pankajavalli, 2023). This section explores these future directions and research opportunities. Advanced machine learning techniques, particularly deep learning, hold immense potential for improving the accuracy and efficiency of anomaly detection. Deep learning models, such as convolutional neural networks (CNNs) and recurrent neural networks (RNNs), can learn complex patterns in high-dimensional data and adapt to evolving data distributions. Federated learning, a privacy-preserving approach that allows for collaborative model training without sharing raw data, is gaining traction in healthcare. This approach is particularly relevant in the context of patient data privacy and security. The integration of artificial intelligence (AI) for improved anomaly detection and interpretation is another significant trend. AI can assist in automating anomaly detection, providing insights into the causes of anomalies, and guiding clinical decision-making (Pankajavalli & Karthick, 2022a, b).

Explainable AI (XAI) is crucial for enhancing trust and transparency in AI-driven healthcare systems. XAI techniques aim to make the decision-making process of AI models more understandable and interpretable, facilitating clinical acceptance and improving accountability. The development of more robust and adaptive algorithms capable of handling concept drift, imbalanced datasets, and high-dimensional data remains a crucial research area. The integration of sensor data from multiple sources and modalities, as well as the development of standardized data formats and interoperability protocols, will further enhance the capabilities of real-time anomaly detection systems. Addressing ethical considerations, such as algorithmic bias and data privacy, is also essential for responsible development and deployment of these systems.

4.9 CONCLUSION

This section summarizes the key findings and insights presented throughout this book section, emphasizing the importance of real-time anomaly detection in healthcare. The integration of sensor technologies in healthcare has ushered in an era of data-rich opportunities to improve patient care and outcomes. However, effectively harnessing this data requires sophisticated techniques for real-time anomaly detection. This section has provided a comprehensive overview of the methods, challenges, and future directions in this rapidly evolving field.

We have explored various data acquisition methods, including wireless communication protocols and data transmission strategies. We have examined a wide range of anomaly detection algorithms, including both unsupervised and supervised methods, highlighting their strengths and weaknesses in the context of healthcare data. We have discussed real-time implementation strategies and architectural considerations, including cloud-based, edge computing, and fog computing approaches. We have addressed key challenges, such as the 4 Vs of big data, imbalanced datasets, concept drift, and data privacy. We have presented real-world case studies illustrating the practical applications of real-time anomaly detection in diverse healthcare settings. Finally, we have explored emerging trends and future research directions, including the potential of advanced machine learning techniques, federated learning, AI integration, and XAI.

Real-time anomaly detection holds immense potential for improving patient outcomes, optimizing treatment strategies, and reducing healthcare costs. However, realizing this potential requires continued research and development efforts to address the challenges associated with data volume, velocity, variety, and veracity, as well as ensuring data privacy and security. The ethical considerations related to algorithmic bias and data privacy must be carefully addressed to ensure responsible development and deployment of these systems. The future of healthcare is inextricably linked to the advancement of real-time anomaly detection technologies, promising a more efficient, effective, and patient-centric approach to healthcare delivery.

REFERENCES

Aboudi, N. E., and Benhlima, L. 2018. Big data management for healthcare systems: architecture, requirements, and implementation. https://doi.org/10.1155/2018/4059018

Al-amri, R., Murugesan, R. K., Man, M., Fareed, A., Al-Sharafi, M. A., and Alkahtani, A. A. 2021. A review of machine learning and deep learning techniques for anomaly detection in IoT data. https://doi.org/10.3390/app11125320

Alfian, G., Syafrudin, M., Ijaz, M., Syaekhoni, M. A., Fitriyani, N. L., and Rhee, J. 2018. A personalized healthcare monitoring system for diabetic patients by utilizing BLE-based sensors and real-time data processing. https://doi.org/10.3390/s18072183

Ali, A. S., Cot, C., Heidarinejad, M., and Stephens, B. T. 2019. Elemental: an open-source wireless hardware and software platform for building energy and indoor environmental monitoring and control. https://doi.org/10.3390/s19184017

Ashfaq, Z., Mumtaz, R., Rafay, A., Zaidi, S. M. H., Saleem, H., Mumtaz, S., Shahid, A., Poorter, E. D., and Moerman, I. 2022. Embedded AI-based Digi-Healthcare. https://doi.org/10.3390/app12010519

Azzalini, D., Bonali, L., and Amigoni, F. 2021. A minimally supervised approach based on variational autoencoders for anomaly detection in autonomous robots. https://doi.org/10.1109/lra.2021.3062597

Bruno, B., Mastrogiovanni, F., and Sgorbissa, A. 2015. Wearable inertial sensors: applications, challenges, and public test benches. *IEEE Robotics & Automation Magazine*. https://doi.org/10.1109/MRA.2015.2448279

Chamberlain, S. D., Singh, I., Ariza, C., Daitch, A., Philips, P., and Dalziel, B. D. 2020. Real-time detection of COVID-19 epicenters within the United States using a network of smart thermometers. https://doi.org/10.1101/2020.04.06.20039909

Chatterjee, A., and Ahmed, B. S. 2022. IoT anomaly detection methods and applications: a survey. https://doi.org/10.1016/j.iot.2022.100568

Dwivedi, R. K., Kumar, R., and Buyya, R. 2021. Gaussian distribution-based machine learning scheme for anomaly detection in healthcare sensor cloud. *International Journal of Cloud Applications and Computing*. https://doi.org/10.4018/ijcac.2021010103

Gudovskiy, D. A., Ishizaka, S., and Kozuka, K. 2021. CFLOW-AD: real-time unsupervised anomaly detection with localization via conditional normalizing flows. In *IEEE Workshop/Winter Conference on Applications of Computer Vision*. https://doi.org/10.1109/WACV51458.2022.00188

Karthick, G. S. 2023. Energy-aware reliable medium access control protocol for energy-efficient and reliable data communication in wireless sensor networks. *SN Computer Science, 4*(5), 449. https://doi.org/10.1007/s42979-023-01525-4

Karthick, G. S., and Pankajavalli, P. B. 2020. A review on human healthcare Internet of Things: a technical perspective. *SN Computer Science, 1*(4), 198. https://doi.org/10.1007/s42979-020-00402-5

Karthick, G. S., and Pankajavalli, P. B. 2023. Chronic obstructive pulmonary disease prediction using Internet of things-spiro system and fuzzy-based quantum neural network classifier. *Theoretical Computer Science, 941*, 55–76. https://doi.org/10.1016/j.tcs.2022.08.021

Kaur, J., and Mann, K. S. 2018. AI based healthcare platform for real time. *Predictive and Prescriptive Analytics using Reactive Programming*. https://doi.org/10.1088/1742-6596/933/1/012010

Khaledian, E., Pandey, S., Kundu, P., and Srivastava, A. 2021. Real-time synchrophasor data anomaly detection and classification using *isolation forest, KMeans, and LoOP*. *IEEE Transactions on Smart Grid*. https://doi.org/10.1109/TSG.2020.3046602

Kim, D., Park, C., Cho, S., and Lee, S. 2022. FAPM: fast adaptive patch memory for real-time industrial anomaly detection. In *IEEE International Conference on Acoustics, Speech, and Signal Processing*. https://doi.org/10.1109/ICASSP49357.2023.10096400

Krishnamurthi, R., Kumar, A., Gopinathan, D., Nayyar, A., and Qureshi, B. 2020. An Overview of IoT sensor data processing, fusion, and analysis techniques. https://doi.org/10.3390/s20216076

Kumar, S., and Singh, M. 2018. Big data analytics for healthcare industry: impact, applications, and tools. https://doi.org/10.26599/bdma.2018.9020031

Lakshmi, G. J., Ghonge, M. M., and Obaid, A. J. 2021. Cloud based IoT smart healthcare system for remote patient monitoring. https://doi.org/10.4108/eai.15-7-2021.170296

Li, J., Liu, L., Fong, S., Wong, R., Mohammed, S., Fiaidhi, J., Sung, Y., and Wong, K. K. L. 2017. Adaptive swarm balancing algorithms for rare-event prediction in imbalanced healthcare data. *PLoS ONE*. https://doi.org/10.1371/journal.pone.0180830

Mehnaz, S., and Bertino, E. 2020. Privacy-preserving real-time anomaly detection using edge computing. *IEEE International Conference on Data Engineering*. https://doi.org/10.1109/ICDE48307.2020.00047

Moallemi, A., Burrello, A., Brunelli, D., and Benini, L. 2022. Exploring scalable, distributed real-time anomaly detection for bridge health monitoring. *IEEE Internet of Things Journal*. https://doi.org/10.1109/JIOT.2022.3157532

Pankajavalli, P. B., and Karthick, G. S. 2022a. Efficient data flow graph modeling using free Poisson law for fault-tolerant routing in Internet of Things. In *Computer Networks and Inventive Communication Technologies: Proceedings of Fifth ICCNCT 2022* (pp. 475–487). Singapore: Springer Nature Singapore. https://doi.org/10.1007/978-981-16-8662-1_49

Pankajavalli, P. B., and Karthick, G. S. 2022b. An independent constructive multi-class classification algorithm for predicting the risk level of stress using multi-modal data. *Arabian Journal for Science and Engineering, 47*(8), 10547–10562. https://doi.org/10.1007/s13369-022-07037-7

Pankajavalli, P. B., Karthick, G. S., and Sakthivel, R. 2021. An efficient machine learning framework for stress prediction via sensor integrated keyboard data. *IEEE Access, 9*, 95023–95035. https://doi.org/10.1109/ACCESS.2021.3095648

Sunny, J. S., Patro, C. P. K., Karnani, K., Pingle, S., Lin, F., Anekoji, M., Jones, L. D., Kesari, S., and Ashili S. 2022. Anomaly detection framework for wearables data: a perspective review on data concepts, data analysis algorithms and prospects. In *Italian National Conference on Sensors*. https://doi.org/10.3390/s22030756

Tripathi, G., Ahad, M. A., and Paiva, S. 2020. SMS: a secure healthcare model for smart cities. *Electronics*. https://doi.org/10.339

5 Basic Concepts and Principles of Healthcare Sensor Data Analytics

Mani Deepak Choudhry, M. Sundarrajan, S. Jeevanandham, and Akshya Jothi

5.1 INTRODUCTION

Sensor technologies have revolutionized healthcare by helping in the continuous and non-invasive monitoring of patient health parameters. Such sensors may be wearable, implantable, or remote monitoring systems, and the data generated associated with such a device **are** of tremendous potential in the improvement of patient care and clinical decision-making. However, realizing this potential requires understanding the basis and principles underlying healthcare sensor data analytics. This chapter involves extensive research of these foundational elements to help researchers, practitioners, and healthcare professionals develop important insights that will enable them to navigate the complexities of sensor data analytics in healthcare settings (Burk and Miner 2020).

First, it is important to understand how, in modern healthcare, the utilization of real-time physiological signals and activity levels, along with environmental factors, allows for the monitoring of health status, disease progression, and treatment effectiveness. Sensor data enables the early detection of abnormalities and trends, allowing timely interventions and preventive measures. So, a proper understanding of the roots of healthcare sensor data analytics provides a gateway for dealing with this wealth of information, which can be used for bettering the general state of health and healthcare delivery (Wang et al. 2018).

Data acquisition plays a very vital role in healthcare sensor data analytics methods and technologies. In this chapter, we shall discuss different sensor modalities, including wearable sensors, medical devices, and IoT platforms, in evaluating their capabilities, limitations, and deployment considerations. Similarly, it will study the preprocessing steps for data, which contain filtering, noise reduction, and feature extraction, to improve the quality and utility of sensor data for further analysis (Kotov 2015). Therein, we then introduce the principles of data-driven decision-making in healthcare sensor data analytics. Emphasis is given to assess the quality of data, feature selection, and model validation, and ensuring that an analytical framework is robust enough to derive actionable insights from sensor data. In this regard, in ensuring that their findings are not only reliable but also valid, researchers and practitioners should ensure that findings from sensor data analytics are relevant and applicable within the clinical setting. These principles will ensure that the collected data is valid and reliable, which will increase the acceptability and application of findings in clinical practice (Haque et al. 2014, Demchenko et al. 2014). However, several ethical considerations and regulatory requirements demand more attentive handling: privacy protection, data security, and informed consent (Baheti and Gill 2011).

Healthcare is a data-heavy field, and as a result, traditional electronic medical records (EMR)-based software is inadequate (Zhang et al. 2015, 2017. Also, the capture systems in healthcare have advanced due to their engagement in social networks, which is significantly influenced by health status. Furthermore, the pervasive presence of health data in capture is a consequence of patients tracking their health on social media, an increase in cyber-physical systems (CPS), and the

DOI: 10.1201/9781003486640-5

general participation of patients in monitoring their health (Tawalbeh et al. 2016). Consequently, big data and the field of computational intelligence offer the development of cutting-edge health systems. Therefore, the current hospital informatics systems may not be adept at carrying out the required data analysis. Big data in the present circumstance exists in varied forms and rapidly arises from diverse platforms (Wang et al. 2017). The analytics system should be capable of consolidating all the data and delivering the physicians' insights in real-time, as there is an imperative need to take prompt action in the event of a medical emergency.

This chapter provides an overview of the regulatory frameworks governing data collection, storage, and analysis in healthcare, including standards such as HIPAA and GDPR. The ethical and legal landscape positions stakeholders in such a manner that it allows them to be able to advocate for the ethical provision and usage of sensor data in a way that is in keeping with preserving patients' privacy and confidentiality. This chapter is also organized around some of the major ethical issues of concern regarding private health information while ensuring safe and ethical management of data.

5.2 PRINCIPLES OF HEALTHCARE ANALYTICS

Healthcare analytics can be regarded as the process that entails the collection and management of healthcare data for information and decisions to be gained to guide healthcare industries (Suganthi et al. 2021, Kumar and Singh 2019). Some of the key principles include:

- **Quality Data:** The basic and reliable source of data is healthcare analytics. The reason lies in ensuring that data is free from errors, is complete, and that it is consistent, hence ensuring meaningful insights.
- **Privacy and Security:** Sensitive information is often an element of healthcare data. The maintenance of privacy and the conformity to regulated standards like HIPAA (Health Insurance Portability and Accountability Act) is necessary because this sensitive data is associated with human beings.
- **Interoperability:** In healthcare, one of the most common silos occurs with healthcare data, which is found across a number of systems and formats. This means that data must be able to be exchanged seamlessly from different sources with proper integration for complete analysis. In other words, interoperability.
- **Predictive Modeling, Machine Learning, and Natural Language Processing:** Cutting-edge analytical methodologies play a crucial role in healthcare data, enabling the discovery of valuable patterns, trends, and correlations.
- **Clinical and Operational Insights:** Healthcare analytics aims to analyze the clinical and operational aspects of healthcare delivery. It supports optimizing workflows to improve patient outcomes and operational efficiency.
- **Evidence-Based Decision Making:** Making decisions based on evidence for healthcare analytics means using actual evidence instead of intuition or anecdotal evidence. This helps healthcare organizations develop effective strategies for resource allocation and implementing interventions.
- **Continuous Improvement:** Healthcare analytics is a developing process in which the analytics models are evaluated at intervals and the methodologies are refined to improve the insights and adapt to the changing landscape of healthcare.
- **Patient-Centric Approach:** Healthcare analytics aims to improve the quality of care and outcomes for patients. Hence, this means coming to grips with the preferences and needs of patients, along with their behavior, in providing effective care.
- **Ethical Considerations:** Healthcare analytics has to consider some ethical issues, like fairness, transparency, and accountability. It's crucial to avoid bias, use data responsibly, and make sure that everyone involved receives the final answers in a fair and ethical manner.

- **Collaboration and Stakeholder Engagement:** Healthcare analytics has to be an idea that fosters collaboration from the healthcare providers, researchers, policymakers, and patients who act as stakeholders. The stakeholders are engaged in a planned way to ensure there is alignment with organizational objectives, promoting innovation, and knowledge sharing.

5.3 METHODOLOGIES & TECHNIQUES

In the healthcare industry, data goes beyond the scope of healthcare systems and health brokers, clinical investigators, online networking, and government agencies; it encompasses multiple data sources, which produce different types and massive amounts of data (Belle et al. 2015). Traditional software and hardware, as well as storage approaches and tools, are not able to handle this large data. Data analytics involves examining data to recognize trends and patterns to acquire valuable insights.

In the healthcare industry, big data and analytics play crucial roles in early disease detection, personalized treatment options, operational efficiencies, and fraud prevention. The sharing of diverse health data repositories is vital for evidence-based decision-making. Analyzing large, diverse, and high-velocity data is crucial for obtaining valuable insights. Genomic analysis, patient profiling, and advanced analytics are transforming healthcare practices. Figure 5.1 is an illustration which involves elaboration on the general framework of big data architecture in healthcare.

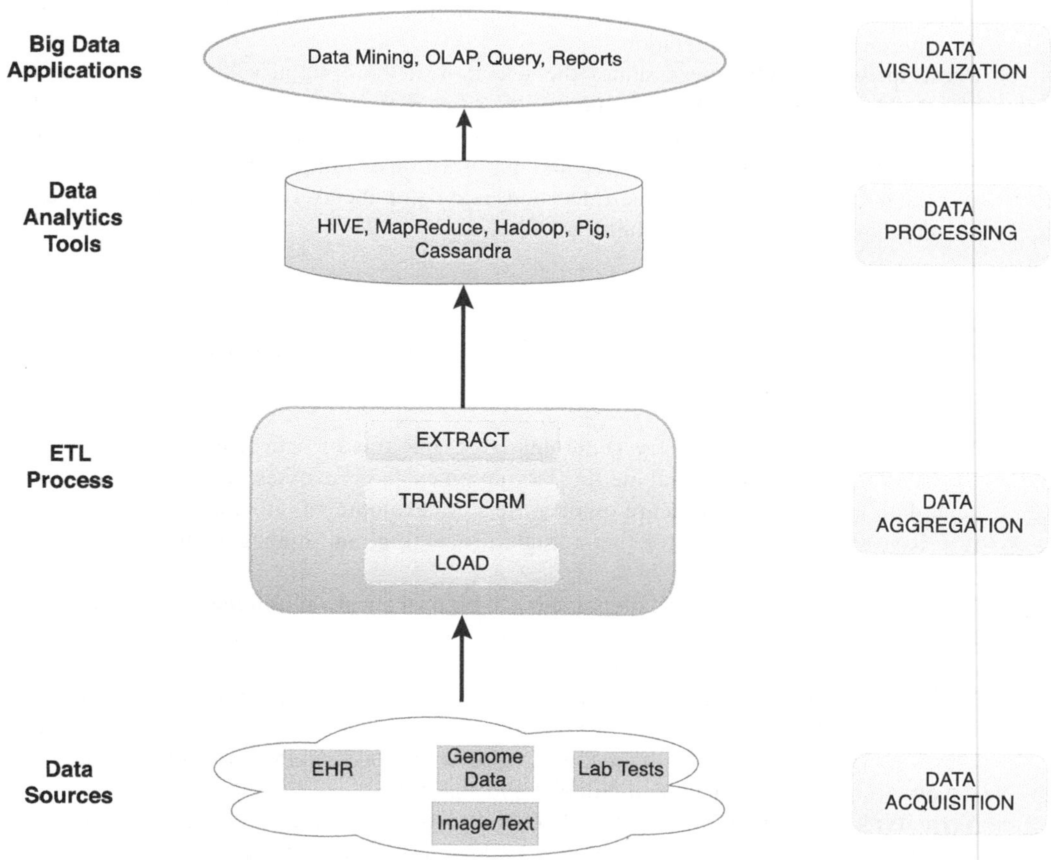

FIGURE 5.1 Framework of big data in healthcare analytics.

5.3.1 Data Analytics

Healthcare data analytics uses sophisticated analytical techniques to extract actionable insights from datasets that are diverse and, therefore, rich, starting from the vast areas of healthcare. Clinical, administrative, and operational data in healthcare organizations identify patterns, trends, and correlations that reflect **enhancements** in the delivery of care to patients, operational efficiencies, and resource management. Data analytics gives the direction to healthcare providers to predict and improve decision-making skills while monitoring in real time, which results in the optimization of workflows, cost reduction, and patient outcome improvement. Healthcare analytics applies machine learning and natural language processing techniques to the effort to implement personalized medicine, risk stratification, early intervention, and population health management. Considering patients and privacy and ethical standards, healthcare analytics becomes the catalyst of change toward transformative improvement in the quality, accessibility, and affordability of healthcare services. There exist three levels of analytics with increasing complexity and value, which are given below (Raghupathi and Raghupathi 2014, Mehta and Pandit 2018):

- **Descriptive Analytics** involves using statistical tools such as tables and graphs to describe current or past events. This can help medical practitioners study and understand patients' past behavioral patterns using operational data, which can be useful in solving current problems.
- **Predictive Analysis** empowers individuals to anticipate future events based on historical data, leveraging statistical techniques such as machine learning, simulation, and data exploration for data interpretation.
- **Prescriptive Analytics** necessitates the selection of the optimal solution from a range of possible alternatives related to the given issues. Real-time data is analyzed alongside historical data by utilizing artificial intelligence, data mining, and machine learning techniques. Through the use of simulation and optimization techniques, practitioners can forecast the potential outcomes of their decisions and equip themselves to effectively manage any outcome, be it a success or failure.

5.3.2 Characteristics of Big Data

Major characteristics of big data include the four Vs, which include (Wan and Alagar 2016, Ward et al. 2014):

- **Volume:** The medical industry generates large amounts of data from various sources like EHRs, LIMSs, and social media. Technologies and processes deliver insights from such data to enhance healthcare quality. Recent developments in storage and architecture have made it possible for the storage, processing, and management of large data volumes.
- **Velocity:** Medical data generation is subject to high frequency requirements, and that calls for specific processing methods. Batch processing, stream processing, and real-time processing have been used to manage data in healthcare.
- **Variety:** The variety of healthcare data comes from different types of sources. About 80% is unstructured (images, signals, text), while 20% is structured (e.g., temperature, blood pressure). Highly efficient techniques are required to transform the unstructured data into structured form for efficient manipulation and analysis.
- **Veracity:** The accuracy in the data collected directly affects the value yielded through it. Reliable, trustworthy, and verifiable data promise error-free data analysis for healthcare services to offer more reliable services.

5.4 HEALTHCARE ANALYTICS FRAMEWORK

As depicted in Figure 5.1 the following section describes the framework in as detailed manner:

5.4.1 Data Aggregation

Healthcare data aggregation is the process of collecting raw data from different sources and organizing it into a standard format. This organized data can then be analyzed, processed, and stored in a data warehouse using methods like data extraction, transformation, and loading (Ullah et al. 2021)

5.4.2 Data Extraction

Heterogeneous, voluminous medical data is sourced from medical records, surveys, and clinical trials, not to mention administrative records. They are further classified as structured data, such as data with predefined formats allowing for easy management, and unstructured data with image, text, or signal requirements for processing (Wijnen et al. 2016). These formats include EHRs, images, genomic data, and clinical text, often represented in text/ASCII, XML, JSON, or DICOM image formats. Medical images usually have PACS that allow interaction via DICOM standards for communication of the workstation.

5.4.3 Data Transformation

After collecting the raw data, we process it to extract relevant insights. This involves filtering out unnecessary information and cleaning the data by normalizing it, reducing noise, and managing missing values. Once transformed, the data conforms to a standard format suitable for in-depth analysis (Poniszewska-Marańda et al. 2023).

5.4.4 Data Loading

Healthcare systems have their own ways of organizing medical data in databases. After the data is organized, it can be analyzed further and stored in different types of databases for future use. These databases could be SQL relational databases, NoSQL databases, or a combination of these (Dash et al. 2019).

5.4.5 Data Processing

In healthcare, batch and stream processing methods for data processing are applied. The method of batch processing is when data is analyzed from pre-existing or previously collected and stored data, not being given immediate response considerations. On the other hand, stream processing handles real-time data that calls for instant responses. Stream processing applies data-mining methods such as clustering and classification for the rapid extraction of information from noisy, continuously changing data. The Hadoop Distributed File System (HDFS) ensures that large data volumes are efficiently stored and retrieved across multiple nodes, thereby ensuring fault tolerance. MapReduce breaks down the process into two nodes: a map phase for data segmentation and a reduce phase for aggregation. Data storage tools other than Hadoop include HBase, Hive, Cassandra, and relational databases, with Apache Zookeeper ensuring reliability among applications and Apache Mahout for machine learning (Dash et al. 2019).

5.4.6 Data Visualization

- **Visualization in Data Analytics** (Ko and Chang 2017)**:** The visual representation of data enables data analytics to get insights. Before visualization, data is preprocessed through cleansing, evaluation, and data-mining algorithms.

- **Applications in Healthcare:** Data analytics in healthcare has given rise to many applications, such as querying, reporting, OLAP, and data mining.
- **Predictive Reports and Proactive Messages:** Predictive analytics generate summaries of reports or messages that can be used for forecasting or to inform of activities that will be carried out.
- **Visualization of Patient Health Records** (Stadler et al. 2016)**:** Data visualization tools help to visualize the records of a patient, which are easier to interpret and take informed decisions with the use of healthcare providers.
- **Real-Time Alerts:** Analytics systems in healthcare enable real-time alerts over critical health events or anomalies to quickly respond.
- **Dashboards for Monitoring:** Dashboards give a complete picture of daily health status and are significantly useful for the monitoring and managing of the patients on an everyday basis.

5.4.7 Data Analytics Tools

Data analytics tools are increasingly important in healthcare for developing the most effective strategic approach to analyzing large amounts of data. This is aimed at improving patient health, enhancing operational efficiency, and optimizing costs. One of the main challenges in healthcare systems is figuring out how to efficiently use the large amounts of data that are generated every day. Healthcare systems need access to appropriate and effective tools to ensure that this data is used optimally. Figure 5.2 illustrates the data analytics tools that are employed in healthcare (Kumar and Singh 2019, Mehta and Pandit 2018).

At the core of healthcare, **data integration tools** play a part in bringing together data from diverse systems into one unified set that is analyzable (Bergamaschi et al. 2018). Attunity, for instance, emerges as an effective integration tool enabling health data aggregation across major databases, cloud platforms, and Hadoop in real-time. Its support for the Health Level 7 (HL7) messaging standard makes it integrate with health systems, while real-time integration capabilities will enhance efficiency in the organization. Informatica offers advanced multi-cloud and hybrid data integration solutions, wherein data integration takes place seamlessly across datasets. This builds a platform for efficiencies in managing patients and cost optimization leading to better outcomes. Information Builder is particularly efficient in the measuring and aggregation of big health data; this guarantees always having the right information at the right time during development and deploying healthcare services.

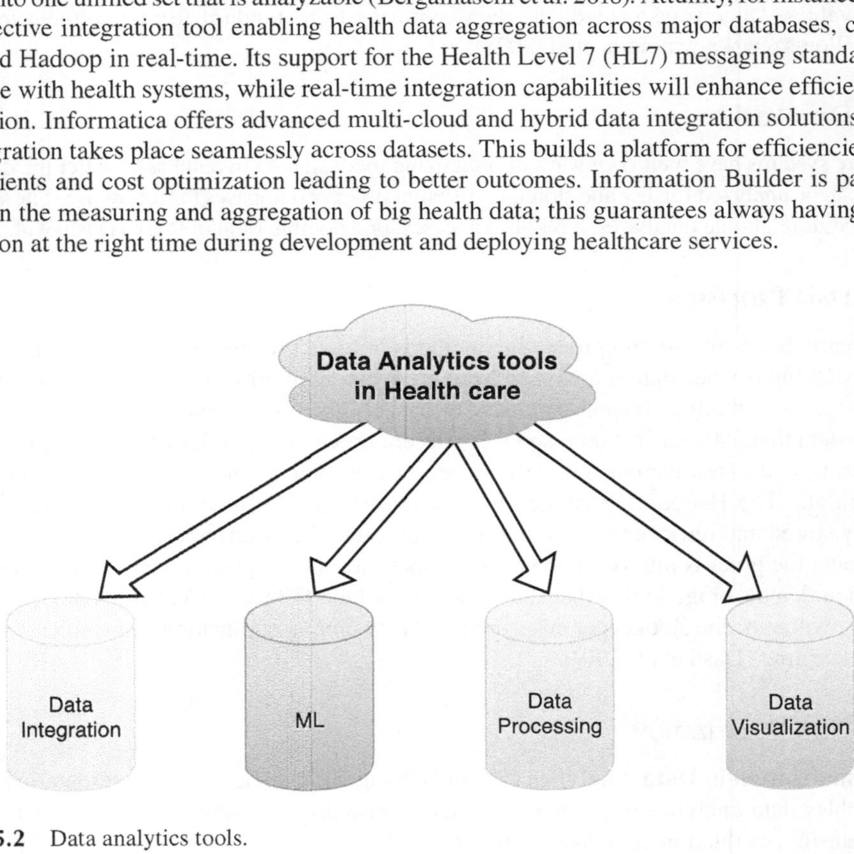

FIGURE 5.2 Data analytics tools.

Searching and Processing Tools are highly crucial for large volumes of unstructured healthcare data. Lucene indexing can quickly locate large blocks of unstructured text as they seamlessly integrate with Hadoop, providing distributed text management. Google Dremel, on the other hand, offers interactive query processing for large datasets and provides better speed and efficiency during data retrieval.

Machine Learning Tools are vital in converting large datasets of information into actionable insights relevant to the healthcare context for well-informed decision-making in clinical settings (Jayatilake and Ganegoda 2021). Apache Mahout presents a set of scalable machine-learning algorithms directed at classification, clustering, and collaborative filtering. Skytree provides accurate predictive analytics models to operate on large data sets for high precision without downsampling. Apache SAMOA allows us to instantiate and run distributed streaming machine learning algorithms in real time. BigML provides a scalable, open-source framework for more advanced workflows of machine learning inside the company or externally, along with reducing costs and increasing reliability with data analysis and decision support.

Real-Time and Streaming Data Processing Tools are indispensable to handle the rapid influx of data from IoT devices and medical sensors in smart healthcare systems. Apache Storm takes on stream computing and real-time data processing through its fault-tolerant framework, providing important real-time analytics and ML applications. SQL Stream Blaze provides a platform of high-throughput streaming analytics that can further enhance real-time threat detection and data wrangling. Apache Flink enables efficient processing of both bounded and unbounded data streams, supporting both batch and stream processing with fault tolerance.

Visual Data Analytical Tools play a crucial role in healthcare to enable the presentation of such information so that one can see patterns, trends, or even data that would be useful in making an informed decision. Tableau aggregates raw datasets into structured data for real-time decision support, aiding in diagnosis and treatment planning, and speeding up treatment decisions. QlikView creates electronic medical records integrated with data from various sources that have in-memory analysis to keep up with safety metrics as well as ensure regulatory compliance. These tools help healthcare professionals find visualization methods to improve patient care and public health policy.

5.4.8 Data Analytics Methodologies

Big data in healthcare is the massive dataset generated from a collection of healthcare data sources, which includes structured and unstructured data. Examples include scan images, health records from electronic health records (EHRs), biomedical signals (ECG, EEG, etc.), and prescriptions written manually. Since healthcare data are multidimensional and dynamic, traditional techniques and technologies are not adequate to manage them. Big data analytics techniques are needed to analyze such diverse data with effective decision-making techniques (Suganthi et al. 2021, Kumar and Singh 2019, Raghupathi and Raghupathi 2014, Mehta and Pandit 2018, Wijnen et al. 2016, Poniszewska-Marańda et al. 2023, Dash et al. 2019). Figure 5.3 illustrates various big data analytics techniques utilized in the healthcare sector, some of which are elaborated below.

Machine Learning (ML): Diagnosis, classification, and predictive modeling from medical imaging data (X-rays, MRIs), risk assessment for patient outcomes (e.g., readmission risk, mortality prediction), and personalized treatment recommendations based on patient characteristics and medical histories. Predictive maintenance for medical equipment to minimize downtime and improve operational efficiency. Fraud detection and prevention in healthcare insurance claims.

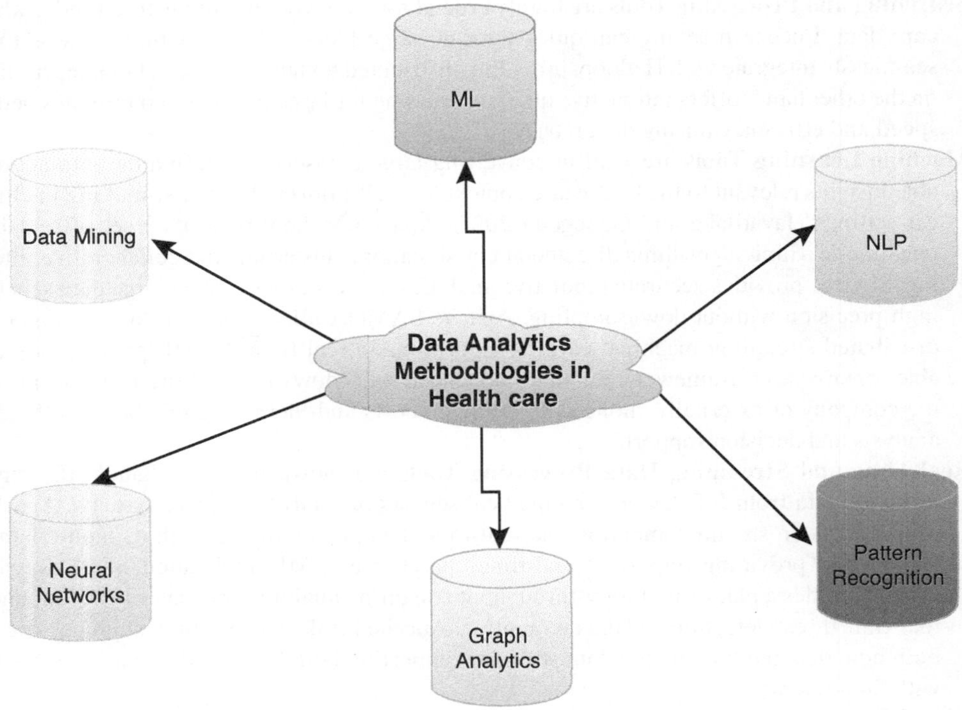

FIGURE 5.3 Methodologies of data analytics in health care.

- **Neural Networks:** Medical image analysis for abnormality detection like tumors or fractures using convolutional neural networks (CNNs). Time-series forecasting for vital signs and early detection of deteriorating health using recurrent neural networks (RNNs). NLP tasks, such as clinical text mining, extracting information from electronic health records (EHRs), using RNNs or transformer-based models like BERT. Molecular structure analysis and drug discovery, through deep learning techniques. Predicting patient outcomes based on holistic information from clinical, genomic, and environmental data sets by using deep neural networks.
- **Pattern Recognition:** Identifying disease patterns and trends from large-scale population health data. Patient vital signs pattern recognition for early detection of sepsis or other critical health conditions. Pattern recognition in genomic data toward the identification of genetic predispositions to some diseases. Automated interpretation of medical test results (e.g., blood tests, electrocardiograms) for diagnosis and monitoring of health conditions.
- **Data Mining:** EHR records of patient characteristics, treatments, and outcomes. Clustering of patients in similar clinical profiles for personalized medicine and targeted interventions. Identifying hidden patterns or trends in the claims data of healthcare to optimize billing and reimbursement processes. Analyzing medication usage patterns and adverse drug reactions to improve medication safety. Early detection of disease outbreaks and public health concerns through the analysis of social media and online health forums.
- **NLP:** Extracting structured information from unstructured clinical notes, radiology reports, and discharge summaries. Automatic coding and classification of medical diagnoses and procedures from free-text clinical narratives. Sentiment analysis on feedback or social media posts to measure patient satisfaction and indicate areas for

improvement. Summarizing medical literature and research articles on evidence-based decision-making. Chatbots or virtual assistants for patient engagement, scheduling appointments, and answering medical queries.

- **Graph Analytics:** Analyzing healthcare networks, including referral patterns and care pathways. Identification of referral patterns and care pathways among healthcare providers. Healthcare fraud and abuse by analyzing networks of patients, providers, and insurance claims. Disease transmission dynamics analysis and disease outbreak prediction by utilizing population health data. Evaluation of healthcare quality and performance by analyzing networks of hospitals and healthcare providers. Identify key opinion leaders and influencers in medical research and clinical practice through social network analysis.

5.5 CHALLENGES

Extensive data analysis has vastly bolstered the healthcare sector by augmenting operational efficiency, diminishing healthcare expenses, advancing drug exploration, providing top-notch healthcare services, enabling individualized patient care, ensuring efficacious treatments, and yielding enhanced clinical results. Although, unquestionably, big data presents several challenges, it is worthy of attention. These challenges collectively represent the multifaceted landscape of data analytics in healthcare and underscore the complexity involved in harnessing data to drive meaningful improvements in patient care and healthcare operations. Table 5.1 summarizes the challenges with possible solutions:

5.5.1 Healthcare Data Security and Privacy

The shift to digital health and patient data digitization has become a fast-growing revolution globally. The transformational shift is supported by, among other things, aging populations, technological advances, and evidence-based medicine, which provide formidable opportunities for health care delivery and management improvement. In the meantime, the push to digitize big data analytics in health care presents several challenges, particularly regarding data security and privacy. Healthcare organizations should adopt a comprehensive approach proactively to address such a concern and to fully exploit the potential inherent in big data analytics in health care. (Bommareddy et al. 2022) further identifies the fact that digitization of healthcare data has been done quickly and, with better patient care and decision-making, the benefits are many. The following section discusses the

TABLE 5.1
Challenges and Strategies in Healthcare Analytics

Challenges	Issues Related to the Challenges	Possible Strategies
Data quality	• Accuracy • Completeness • Reliability	• Data validation checks • Data cleansing • Data governance policy implementation
Data integration	• Multiple source • Different formats	• Interoperability standard development • API for Data Exchange
Privacy & security	• Patient data loss	• Robust Encryption • Security Assessment
Scalability	• Performance degradation while managing the large volume of data	• Cloud-based solutions • Scalable database architectures • Optimize data processing algorithms

potential privacy and security risks, including data breaches and cyber-attacks, together with the major regulatory frameworks, including HIPAA. The authors explained and discussed the technology, including encryption and access controls, and the best practices for data protection. They also pointed out challenges, including data complexity and the evolving cyber threat, and gave pointers on future research works, in which there is a critical need for continued improvement in both technologies and security policies. (Keshta and Odeh 2021) addresses the major security and privacy concerns associated with electronic health records (EHRs). It outlines challenges such as unauthorized access, data breaches, and the need for robust encryption methods to protect sensitive patient information. (Newaz et al. 2021) explores various security and privacy issues prevalent in modern healthcare systems, detailing common attacks and corresponding defenses. The paper highlights the importance of multi-layered security approaches to safeguard healthcare data from emerging cyber threats. (May and Denecke 2022) a scoping review examines the security and privacy concerns related to healthcare conversational agents, such as chatbots. It discusses potential risks, including data breaches and unauthorized data access, and suggests strategies to enhance the security and privacy of these systems. (Rawat et al. 2022) investigates the issue of organ trafficking facilitated through the dark web and the associated data security and privacy concerns in healthcare systems. It emphasizes the need for advanced machine learning techniques to enhance security and prevent illicit activities within healthcare networks. The following are the various encryption strategies and compliance standards involved in making the healthcare data more secure:

5.5.2 Encryption Methods

Encryption is the primary technology used to protect healthcare data. It scrambles readable data into illegible data to ensure that only individuals with authority can access it.

- **Symmetric Encryption:** Symmetric encryption applies the same key to encryption and decryption functions. This method is effective and efficient when used to encrypt large amounts of data. However, it requires safe key management practices to deter the possibility of illegal access.
- **Asymmetric Encryption:** Asymmetric encryption, also known as public key encryption, makes use of two keys: one that is used for encryption (public key) and another for decryption (private key). This method provides a secure process for transmitting data over the internet and ensures that the intended receiver is capable of decrypting the data.
- **Encryption in Transit and at Rest:** In Transit: If data is being transmitted to other networks, the encryption of data while in transfer across networks will help safeguard it from being intercepted. Some of the technologies include transport layer security. At Rest: This refers to the encryption of data stored on the devices and servers, which safeguards it from illegal access. Encryption technologies typically used include full disk encryption and database encryption.
- **Access Control Mechanisms:** Robust access control mechanisms need to be in place to ensure that sensitive healthcare data is only accessed by the authorized personnel.
- **Role-Based Access Control (RBAC):** RBAC only allows access to the system by the authorized personnel of the organization based on roles assigned to them. It, therefore, restricts the employees from accessing any information they would wish for if not in line with their job functions.
- **Attribute-Based Access Control (ABAC):** ABAC allows access based on the attributes of a user, resource, and environment. It is more granular compared to RBAC and allows more complex and fine-grained access policies to be implemented.
- **Multi-Factor Authentication (MFA):** MFA will provide an additional security layer that requires the user to give more than one verification factor, such as a password, fingerprint, or security token, to access. This method greatly minimizes the risk of illegal access due to stolen or forged user credentials.

5.6 CONCLUSION

The integration of healthcare sensor data analytics into clinical practice presents several challenges, including ensuring data accuracy and reliability, integrating data from multiple sensors, and addressing privacy and security concerns. Robust data validation methods, advanced data fusion techniques, and compliance with regulatory standards such as HIPAA and GDPR are essential to mitigate these issues. Strategic decisions regarding the adoption of AI and machine learning technologies, establishing clear data governance protocols, and standardizing data formats are crucial for overcoming these challenges. Effective implementation of sensor data analytics enables continuous patient monitoring, supports personalized and proactive care, optimizes resource allocation, and contributes to clinical research, ultimately improving patient outcomes and healthcare efficiency. Looking ahead, the role of sensor data analytics in healthcare is poised to expand significantly. Advances in sensor technology, AI, and ML will enhance data quality and predictive capabilities, enabling more precise and tailored healthcare solutions. Ethical considerations and regulatory compliance will remain critical, requiring collaborative efforts between policymakers, healthcare leaders, and stakeholders to create balanced frameworks that promote innovation while protecting patient rights. The potential for global health improvement through affordable sensor devices and telemedicine is immense, offering improved access to healthcare in underserved regions. By addressing current challenges and focusing on informed decision-making, the healthcare industry can harness sensor data analytics to deliver better, more personalized care, paving the way for a more efficient, effective, and equitable healthcare system.

REFERENCES

Baheti, R., & Gill, H. (2011). Cyber-physical systems, *Impact Control Technol.*, *12*, 161–166.

Belle, A., Thiagarajan, R., Soroushmehr, S. M. R., Navidi, F., Beard, D. A., & Najarian, K. (2015). Big data analytics in healthcare. *Biomedical Res. Int.*, *2015*, 16. https://dx. doi.org/10.1155/2015/370194

Bergamaschi, S., Beneventano, D., Mandreoli, F., Martoglia, R., Guerra, F., Orsini, M., ... & Magnotta, L. (2018). From data integration to big data integration. In: *A Comprehensive Guide through the Italian Database Research over the Last 25 Years*, ed. Sergio Flesca et al. (pp. 43–59).

Bommareddy, S., Khan, J. A., & Anand, R. (2022). A review on healthcare data privacy and security. In: *Networking Technologies in Smart Healthcare*, eds, Pooja Singh et al. (pp. 165–187).

Burk, S., & Miner, G. D. (2020). *It's All Analytics!: The Foundations of Al, Big Data and Data Science Landscape for Professionals in Healthcare, Business, and Government*. Productivity Press, USA.

Dash, S., Shakyawar, S. K., Sharma, M., & Kaushik, S. (2019). Big data in healthcare: Management, analysis and future prospects. *J. Big Data*, *6*(1), 1–25.

Demchenko, Y., De Laat, C., & Membrey, P. (2014). Defining architecture components of the big data ecosystem. In: *Proceedings of International Conference Collaboration Technoloies and Systems (CTS)* (pp. 104–112), Pennsylvania, USA.

Haque, S. A., Aziz, S. M., & Rahman, M. (2014). Review of cyber-physical system in healthcare. *Int. J. Distrib. Sensor Netw.*, *10*(4), 217415.

Jayatilake, S. M. D. A. C., & Ganegoda, G. U. (2021). Involvement of machine learning tools in healthcare decision making. *J. Healthcare Eng.*, *2021*, 1–20.

Keshta, I., & Odeh, A. (2021). Security and privacy of electronic health records: Concerns and challenges. *Egypt. Inform. J.*, *22*(2), 177–183.

Ko, I., & Chang, H. (2017). Interactive visualization of healthcare data using tableau. *Healthc. Inform. Res.*, *23*(4), 349.

Kotov, A. (2015). Social media analytics for healthcare. Healthcare Data Anal., *1*, 309–340.

Kumar, S., & Singh, M. (2019). Big data analytics for healthcare industry: Impact, applications, and tools. *IEEE*, *2*(1), 48–57.

May, R., & Denecke, K. (2022). Security, privacy, and healthcare-related conversational agents: A scoping review. *Inform. Health Social Care*, *47*(2), 194–210.

Mehta, N., & Pandit, A. (2018). Concurrence of big data analytics and healthcare: A systematic review. *Int. J. Med. Inform.*, *114*, 57–65.

Newaz, A. I., Sikder, A. K., Rahman, M. A., & Uluagac, A. S. (2021). A survey on security and privacy issues in modern healthcare systems: Attacks and defenses. *ACM Trans.Comput. Healthc.*, *2*(3), 1–44.

Poniszewska-Marańda, A., Vynogradnyk, E., & Marańda, W. (2023). Medical data transformations in healthcare systems with the use of natural language processing algorithms. *Appl. Sci.*, *13*(2), 682.

Raghupathi, W., & Raghupathi, V. (2014). Big data analytics in healthcare: Promise and potential. *Health Inform. Sci. Syst.*, *2*, 1–10.

Rawat, R., Garg, B., Mahor, V., Telang, S., Pachlasiya, K., & Chouhan, M. (2022). Organ trafficking on the dark web—The data security and privacy concern in healthcare systems. In: *Internet of Healthcare Things: Machine Learning for Security and Privacy* (pp. 189–216). John Wiley & Sons, USA.

Stadler, J. G., Donlon, K., Siewert, J. D., Franken, T., & Lewis, N. E. (2016). Improving the efficiency and ease of healthcare analysis through use of data visualization dashboards *Big Data*, *4*(2), 129–135.

Suganthi, S., Gupta, V., Sisaudia, V., & Poongodi, T. (2021). Data analytics in healthcare systems–principles, challenges, and applications. In: *Machine Learning and Analytics in Healthcare Systems* (pp. 1–22), CRC Press, England.

Tawalbeh, L. A., Mehmood R., Benkhlifa E., & Song H. (2016). Mobile cloud computing model and big data analysis for healthcare applications. *IEEE Access*, ***4***, 6171–6180.

Ullah, A., Azeem, M., Ashraf, H., Alaboudi, A. A., Humayun, M., & Jhanjhi, N. Z. (2021). Secure healthcare data aggregation and transmission in IoT—A survey. *IEEE Access*, *9*, 16849–16865.

Wan, K., & Alagar, V. (2016). Characteristics and classification of big data in health care sector. In: *2016 12th International Conference on Natural Computation, Fuzzy Systems and Knowledge Discovery (ICNC-FSKD)*, Chengdu, China (pp. 1439–1446). IEEE.

Wang, C., Li, F., Wang, L., Li, F., Wang, L., Zhou, W., Zhu, B., Zhang, X., Ding, L., He, Z., Song, P., & Jin, C. (2017). The impact of population aging on medical expenses: A big data study based on the life table. *BioSci. Trends,* ***11***(6), 619–631.

Wang, Y., Kung, L., & Byrd, T. A. (2018). Big data analytics: Understanding its capabilities and potential benefits for healthcare organizations. *Technol. Forecast. Soc. Change*, *126*, 3–13.

Ward, M. J., Marsolo, K. A., & Froehle, C. M. (2014). Applications of business analytics in healthcare. *Bus. Horiz.*, *57*, 571–582.

Wijnen, B. F. M., Van Mastrigt, G. A. P. G., Redekop, W. K., Majoie, H. J. M., De Kinderen, R. J. A., & Evers, S. M. A. A. (2016). How to prepare a systematic review of economic evaluations for informing evidence-based healthcare decisions: Data extraction, risk of bias, and transferability (part 3/3). *Expert Rev. Pharmacoecon. Outcomes Res.*, *16*(6), 723–732.

Zhang, Y., Qiu, M., Tsai, C. W., Hassan, M. M., & Alamri A. (2015). Health-CPS: Healthcare cyber-physical system assisted by cloud and big data. *IEEE Syst. J.*, ***11***(1), 88–95. https://doi.org/10.1109/jsyst.2015.2460747

6 Design and Development of Physiotherapy Robot to Aid Medical Practitioners for Human Upper-Limb Rehabilitation

Mukul Kumar Gupta, Sowrabh S, Varnita Verma, and Roushan Kumar

6.1 INTRODUCTION

The broad consensus is that exoskeletons are a type of technology that extends, complements, replaces, or enhances human function and capability, or strengthens the human limb where it is worn. In contrast to other robots, an exoskeleton's operator is a human who must make decisions and perform duties while wearing an exoskeleton. Exoskeletons enhance both the capabilities of human force and machine intelligence by integrating them. Exoskeleton robots, therapeutic robots, assistive robots, and prosthetic robots are the four primary categories of rehabilitation robotics (Park et al. 2018). Robotic exoskeletons are utilized as augmentation tools to enhance the body's physical performance. Humans can use exoskeletons, mechanical devices, to enhance their strength and endurance. For sections like the lower extremity and upper extremities, the numerous rehabilitation robotics patient groups include adults and pediatric patients (Bronzino 2000). Gait treatment and limb mobility are two examples of the various applications of rehabilitation robotics that are employed by end users like hospitals and rehabilitation facilities.

Stroke is a leading cause of long-term disability worldwide, with over 17 million persons experiencing a stroke each year (Feigin et al. 2015). This neurological condition occurs when the blood supply to the brain is interrupted, leading to a lack of oxygen and nutrients to brain tissue. As a result, brain cells can be damaged or perish, which can cause a range of physical and cognitive impairments. Stroke can have a profound impact on an individual's ability to conduct activities of daily living, and it can significantly affect their quality of life. In addition to the physical and cognitive impairments associated with stroke, there can also be psychological and emotional effects. Depression and anxiety are common among stroke survivors, and these conditions can have a significant influence on recovery and quality of life. Addressing the psychological needs of stroke survivors is therefore an essential component of comprehensive stroke care (Gupta et al. 2019, Kumar, et al. 2022). Upper limb function is often affected following a stroke, with impairments including paralysis, spasticity, and decreased range of motion. These impairments can limit an individual's ability to carry out daily activities, such as dressing, grooming, and dining (Park et al. 2018, Solomon and Baptiste 2005). Upper limb rehabilitation is therefore an essential component of stroke recovery, as it seeks to improve upper limb function and promote independence (Pollock et al. 2014).

DOI: 10.1201/9781003486640-6

6.1.1 Upper Limb Rehabilitation for Stroke Survivors

Upper limb rehabilitation can take many forms, including exercise-based interventions, neuromuscular electrical stimulation, and constraint-induced movement therapy. These interventions seek to promote motor recovery, reduce spasticity, and improve range of motion. In recent years, there has been a growing interest in the use of technology to assist upper limb rehabilitation, including robotics and virtual reality (Kumar et al. 2018, Das et al. 2024). These technologies offer a potentially effective and engaging approach to rehabilitation, as they can provide interactive and motivating activities for stroke survivors (Norouzi-Gheidari et al. 2012). As the treatment is fundamentally incorrect, upper limb shoulder, elbow, and wrist may be important factors in restricting recovery. Robotic gadgets enable more rigorous practice and promote functional recovery after a stroke. To obtain the optimum advantages of robotic assistance, the patient must be actively involved throughout the training treatment. Hence, numerous robotic devices have been invented for this purpose because of the benefits of their support to upper limb rehabilitation treatment. Depending on the design, these devices are constructed of external mechanical linkages coupled to the patient at single or multiple joints (Krebs et al. 1998).

6.1.2 Cost of Stroke and Robotic Assistance for Rehabilitation

Stroke generally consumes a significant number of resources. This encompasses both direct and indirect expenses. The direct cost is connected to neuro-rehabilitation ted portions (Feigin et al. 2017). Rehabilitation using robotic devices has been demonstrated to have a significant influence on upper limb rehabilitation recovery. It aids therapists in providing high-intensity and repetition treatment. Along these lines, patients can get great benefits from neurorehabilitation progress while significantly lowering the therapist's labor (Kwakkel et al. 2008).

Robotic devices give patients recovery progress reports, which are correctly and consistently measured by the motor function of the patients to enhance their physiological capabilities. In this context, neurophysiological robotic aids were extensively researched to measure the intensity of therapy and to minimize cost compared to traditional treatment (Gupta et al. 2020, Frisoli et al. 2022). Hence, the motor function restoration system is extensively required and suggested for stroke patients. In recent times, there are lots of various robotic system equipment for upper limb rehabilitation assistance that have been shown, but only a few have been employed by stroke sufferers. They exhibited encouraging outcomes that warrant a significant development in the utilization of rehabilitative robotic devices during the previous decade (Das and Kumar 2023). Regaining the subject's functional capacity to execute the everyday duties needs the participation of the robot-assisted rehabilitation treatment.

Upper limb rehabilitation robots have garnered significant attention in recent years due to their potential to improve the recovery of stroke survivors. The studies demonstrate the use of upper limb rehabilitation robots for stroke rehabilitation indicates that these devices can be effective in improving upper limb function (Verma et al. 2020). One study conducted a systematic review and meta-analysis of randomized controlled trials examining the effects of robot-assisted therapy on upper limb function in stroke survivors. They found that robot-assisted therapy improved upper limb function more effectively than conventional therapy. The study analyzed data from 21 randomized controlled trials involving a total of 884 participants (Mehrholz et al. 2018). Another study conducted a systematic review of studies investigating the effectiveness of robotic devices for upper limb rehabilitation after stroke. They found that robotic devices improved upper limb motor function, range of motion, and spasticity compared to conventional therapy.

A more recent study investigated the use of a wearable exoskeleton for upper limb rehabilitation in stroke patients. Table 6.1 depicts the comparison of the Existing upper limb robots. The study found that the exoskeleton was effective in enhancing upper limb motor function, spasticity, and range of motion in stroke patients and was well-tolerated by patients.

TABLE 6.1
Comprehensive Analysis of Existing Rehabilitation Robots

Robot Name	Type of Robot	Degrees of Freedom	Range of Motion	End-Effector Type	Control Mode
ArmeoSpring (Adomavičienė et al. 2019)	Exoskeleton	7	Shoulder Flexion/Extension: 0°–180° Abduction/Adduction: 0°–45° Internal/External Rotation: 0°–90°	Hand-Grip device	Position and force
Bi-Manu-Track (Ivanova et al. 2017)	End-effector	4	Elbow Flexion/Extension: 0°–150° Wrist Flexion/ Extension: 0°–90° Wrist Abduction/ Adduction: 0°–30°	Pincer-Grasp Mechanism	Position and Force
InMotion ARM™ (Hsieh et al. 2017)	Exoskeleton	3	Shoulder Flexion/Extension: 0°–180° Abduction/Adduction: 0°–180° Internal/External Rotation: 0°–180°	Paddle-shaped Hand Grips	Impedance Control
Jintronix Rehabilitation System (Norouzi-Gheidari, Archambault, and Fung 2012)	End-effector	3	Shoulder Flexion/Extension: 0°–180° Abduction/Adduction: 0°–180° Internal/External Rotation: 0°–180°	Paddle-shaped Hand Grips	Motion-based Control
Kinova Jaco (Maheu et al. 2011)	End-effector	6	Elbow Flexion/Extension: 0°–135° Wrist Flexion/ Extension: 0°–130° Wrist Abduction/ Adduction: 0°–50°	Three-fingered Hand	Joystick or Motion-based Control
MIME Robotic System (Lum et al. 2005)	End-effector	3	Shoulder Flexion/Extension: 0°–180° Abduction/Adduction: 0°–180° Internal/External Rotation: 0°–180°	Grasp and Release Functionality	Motion-based Control
ReoGo (Hsieh et al. 2017),(CS et al. 2020)	Exoskeleton	3	Shoulder Flexion/Extension: 0°–180° Abduction/Adduction: 0°–180° Internal/External Rotation: 0°–180°	Hand-Grip Device	Impedance Control
RiceWrist (Pehlivan et al. 2014)	End-effector	1	Wrist Flexion/Extension: 0°–40°	Hand-Grip Device	Motion-based Control
T-WREX (Housman et al. 2007)	Exoskeleton	4	Elbow Flexion/Extension: 0°–140° Wrist Flexion/ Extension: 0°–90°	Grasp and Release Functionality	Motion-based Control

AI has the potential to revolutionize the field of rehabilitation by providing innovative solutions to help individuals recover from injuries or disabilities. AI-based rehabilitation systems have been developed (Kumar and Das 2024, Das et al. 2024) to enhance the efficacy of traditional rehabilitation approaches by incorporating real-time feedback and personalized training programs.

6.2 DESIGN AND DEVELOPMENT OF THE UPPER LIMB REHABILITATION ROBOT

To design a functional robot, it is crucial to ensure that the structure of its links and their assembly allow for the desired range of motion. The links of the robot were created individually and then assembled to verify that the desired range of motion was achievable. This approach allowed for

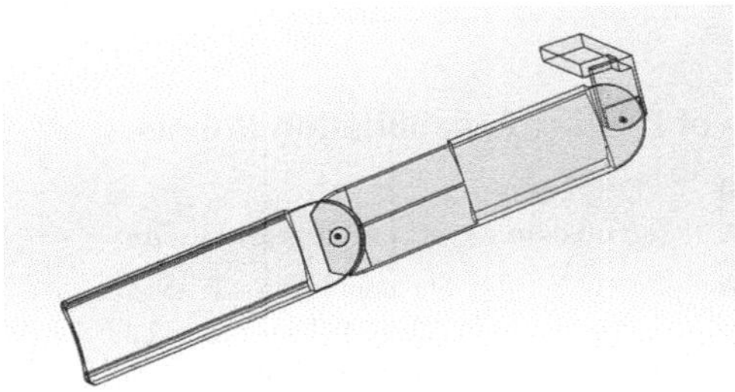

FIGURE 6.1 Assembled cad model.

the identification of any interferences or collisions between the links during the assembly process, which could be corrected before physical construction.

6.2.1 Design Process – Structure of Robot

The design of each link was based on the requirements for strength, rigidity, and weight. The material selection was also considered, and various options were evaluated to ensure that the connections could withstand the anticipated forces and stresses during operation. Finite Element Analysis (FEA) was used to validate the design and optimize the material usage. The assembly process was also analyzed using simulation tools to ensure that it was feasible and to identify any potential issues. The model was first constructed, which is shown in Figure 6.1.

6.2.2 Material Selection and Properties

The links are the primary components of the robot that connect the joints and determine the robot's range of motion. Rigid PVC (Polyvinyl Chloride) was selected as the material for links 1 and link 2. Because of its ease of machining and minimal cost. The material can be easily machined and shaped into the desired dimensions, which aided in the manufacturing process of the links. Moreover, the minimal cost of PVC made it an affordable option for the project budget. Thus, the combination of its mechanical properties, simplicity of machining, and low cost made rigid PVC an ideal material for the links (Verma et al. 2018). The support structure is the component that provides stability and support for the robot, aluminum was selected as the material for the support structure. Aluminum is a lightweight and strong metal that has outstanding mechanical properties. It is also highly corrosion-resistant, making it suitable for use in outdoor and harsh environments. Aluminum is also readily machinable, which allows for the creation of complex support structures with minimal effort.

Rigid PVC is a lightweight and low-cost material that is often used in structural applications. It has excellent rigidity, strength, and dimensional stability, making it an ideal choice for robot links. PVC is also easy to machine, meaning that the links can be manufactured with high precision and accuracy, which is essential for ensuring that the robot functions properly. Aluminum is a lightweight and durable metal that is often used in engineering applications. It has a high strength-to-weight ratio, meaning that it is powerful enough to support the robot but also light enough to avoid adding excessive weight to the overall structure. Aluminum is also corrosion-resistant, which is crucial for ensuring that the support structure remains stable over time.

6.2.3 Static Analysis

To assure the reliability and safety of the robot, it is essential to conduct stress and frequency simulations. The simulations serve to identify areas of the robot that are under high stress and could potentially collapse under load. During the simulation process, various loads and constraints are applied

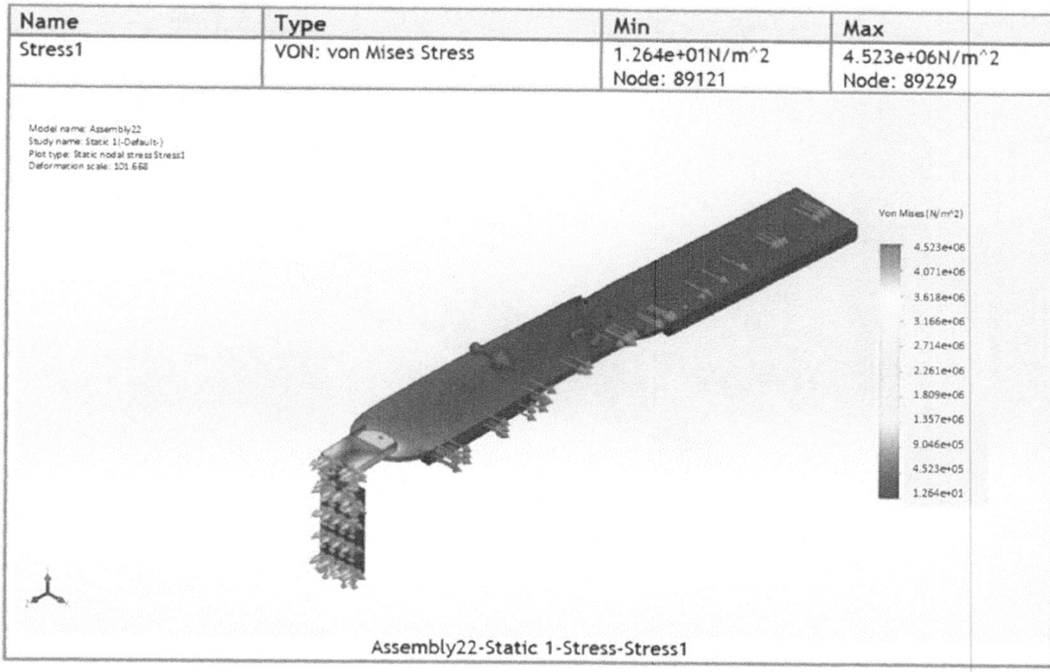

FIGURE 6.2 Image depicting stress application for FEA analysis.

to the model to simulate the expected real-world usage of the robot. This allowed us to see how the model would behave under various conditions and identify any areas of concern. Figure 6.2 shows a simulation for stress analysis. After analyzing the simulation results, areas of significant stress on the robot were identified, such as the joints and connection sites between the links. Figure 6.3 depicts the plot generated for strain analysis. Locations were also identified where the robot was more likely to experience malfunction or failure. This information was then used to make design modifications and enhancements to the robot's structure to increase its reliability and safety.

6.2.4 Frequency Analysis

Frequency analysis of a model involves analyzing the natural frequencies and mode shapes of the model to determine its structural behavior and identify potential design issues. The procedure begins by importing the three-dimensional (3D) model and generating a mesh of small elements that make up the model. Then, loads and boundary conditions are applied to simulate how the model will behave under varied conditions (Gupta et al. 2021). Once the simulation is run, a frequency response plot depicts the natural frequencies and mode shapes of the model. The natural frequencies are the frequencies at which the model will vibrate when excited, and the mode shapes are the patterns of vibration that the model will manifest at those frequencies.

After analyzing the frequency response, Figure 6.4 shows areas that were prone to high stresses and deformations, as well as the natural frequencies and mode structures of the model. Specifically, areas were identified where the model was likely to vibrate excessively, potentially leading to premature failure or damage.

6.2.5 Specifications of the Robot

Physical Dimensions – Table 6.2 displays the physical dimensions of the predominantly two-link model created, along with support to connect the chair and the links.

Name	Type	Min	Max
Strain1	ESTRN: Equivalent Strain	3.036e-10 Element: 51055	5.657e-04 Element: 29987

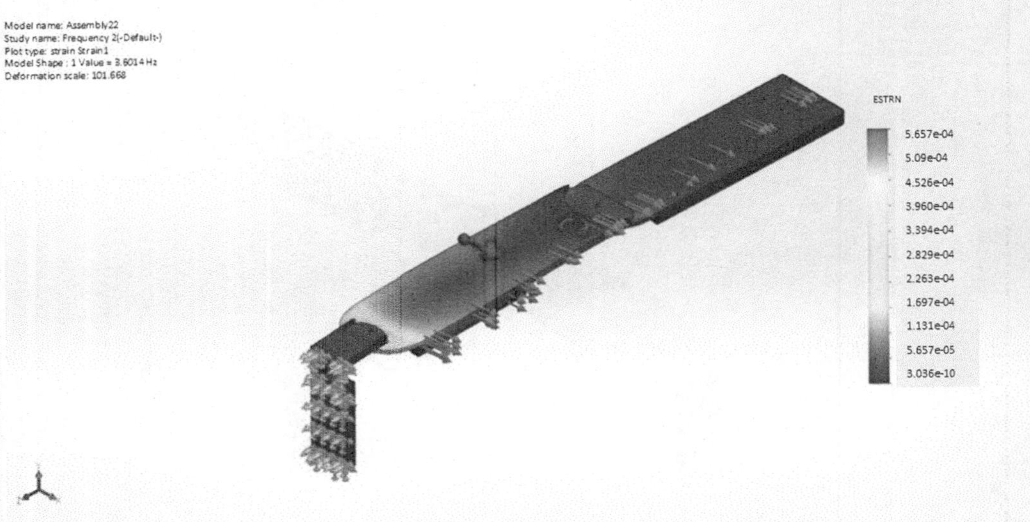

Assembly22-Static 1-Strain-Strain1

FIGURE 6.3 Image depicting strain application for FEA analysis.

Name	Type	Min	Max
Amplitude1	AMPRES: Resultant Amplitude Plot for Mode Shape: 1(Value = 3.6014 Hz)	0.000e+00 Node: 79461	2.012e+00 Node: 331

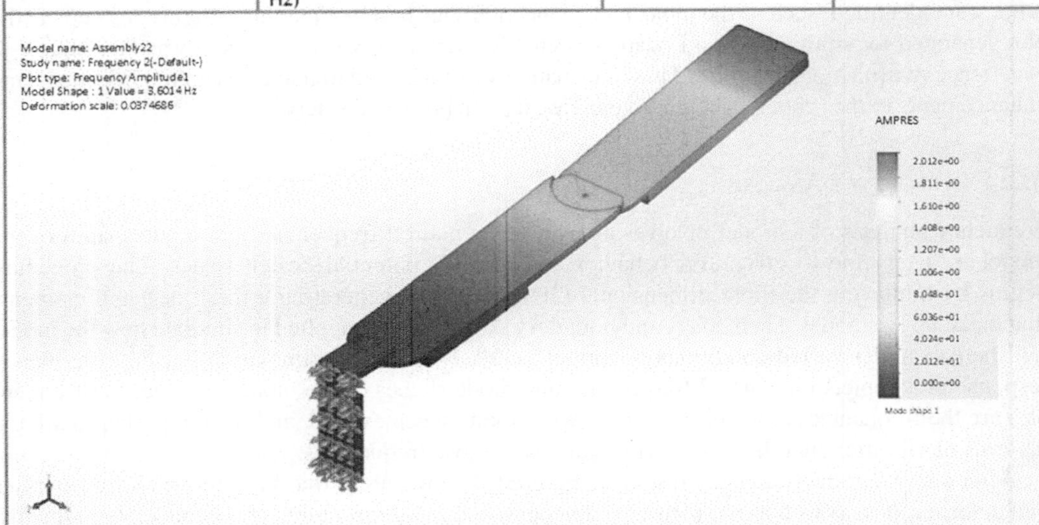

Assembly22-Frequency 2-Amplitude-Amplitude1

Name	Type	Min	Max
Amplitude2	AMPRES: Resultant Amplitude Plot for Mode Shape: 2(Value = 21.3477 Hz)	0.000e+00 Node: 79461	1.840e+00 Node: 1791

FIGURE 6.4 Analysis of the model's frequency characteristics.

TABLE 6.2
Dimensions of the model

Parameter	Dimension (mm) (L×B×T)	Remarks
Link 1	150×100×20	Connects to Joint 2
Link 2	220×100×20	Connects to Support
Support	110×75×10	90-degree bend
	180×75×10	To mount on chair

TABLE 6.3
Range of Motion of Model

Joint Number	Range of Motion (Degrees)
Joint 1	0–140
Joint 2	−60 to 180

TABLE 6.4
Exercises Executed in the Model

	Exercise Name	Movement Angle
Shoulder	FLEXION	0–180
Shoulder	EXTENSION	0 to −60
Elbow	FLEXION	0–140
Elbow	EXTENSION	140–0

6.2.6 Range of Motion

Table 6.3 provides the minimum and maximum angles of motion for a healthy human, as calculated and obtained from the range of motion data presented in the textbook "Orthopaedic Physical Assessment" by author David J. Magee.

6.2.7 List of Exercises

The inventory of exercises that can be done with the system is shown in Table 6.4 mainly.

6.2.8 Power Requirements

Table 6.5 shows the power requirements required for the model to function properly. As an added advantage, the system can operate in a dual mode. In case of any power failure, a 12v 10AH battery can be used for the correct working of the model.

6.3 DESIGN AND DEVELOPMENT

Figure 6.5 shows the complete circuit of the system. In the devised circuit, the input voltage of 220 V alternating current (AC) and 50 Hz is initially supplied to the main switch. Upon toggling on, the input voltage passes through the SMPS (Switched Mode Power Supply) to provide a stable output of 12 V direct current (DC). A DC-DC converter is then utilized to step down the voltage from 12 V to 5 V, which is used to power the controller (Das and Kumar 2024). An emergency valve is incorporated in the circuit to ensure immediate power cut-off in case of any emergencies. The 12 V output

TABLE 6.5
Power Requirements of the System

	Rating	Unit
Input supply	220	V_{AC}
	6	A
	50	Hz
Back up	12	V_{DC}
	10	AH

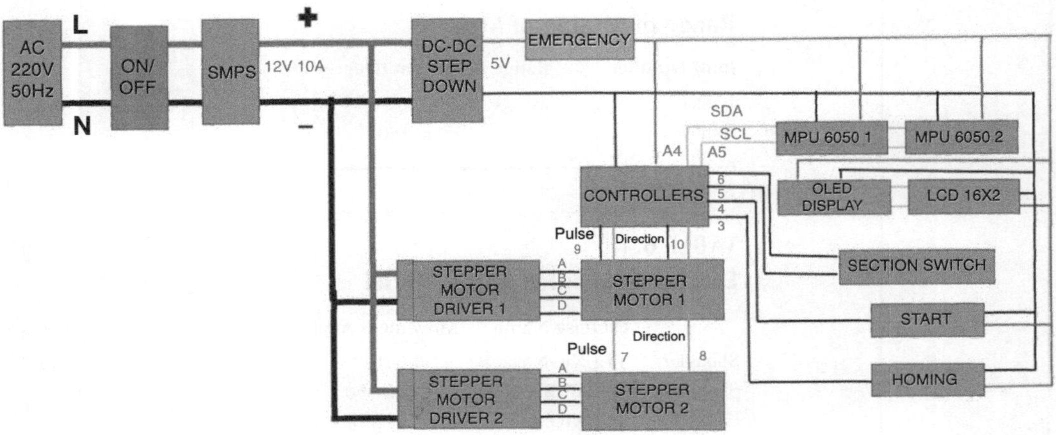

FIGURE 6.5 Circuit diagram of the system.

from the SMPS is directly supplied to the stepper motor driver, which is responsible for operating the stepper motor. All the sensors and switches in the circuit are energized by the 5 V DC output from the DC-DC converter. This ensures that all the sensors and controls in the circuit operate within their safe voltage limits.

6.4 SYSTEM FLOW

For the elbow exercise, the system checks if the angle is less than 140°, while for the shoulder exercise, it tests if the angle is less than 180°. If the angle is less than the specified value, the system then passes through the Proportional-Integral-Derivative (PID) control loop to calculate the number of pulses to be given to the motor. The computed step size is delivered to the motor, and the current angle value from the sensor is then passed to verify the condition again. The process sequence of the whole system is shown in Figure 6.6.

This process repeats until the joint angle is achieved, which signals the end of the flexion part of the exercise. After this, the system moves to the extension portion of the exercise, where it checks for 0° in the case of elbow exercise and −60° for shoulder exercise. If the angle is larger than 0° for elbow exercise or greater than −60° for shoulder exercise, the direction is reversed. The system then passes through the PID control loop to calculate the number of pulses to be given to the motor, and the current angle value from the sensor is verified again.

This procedure continues until the joint angle is obtained, which marks the end of the extension portion of the exercise. For shoulder exercise, the system needs to come to the origin, which is 0°, and thus the direction is reversed from the present direction, and the system tests for 0° when it reaches it. Once it reaches 0°, it completes one cycle of the exercise.

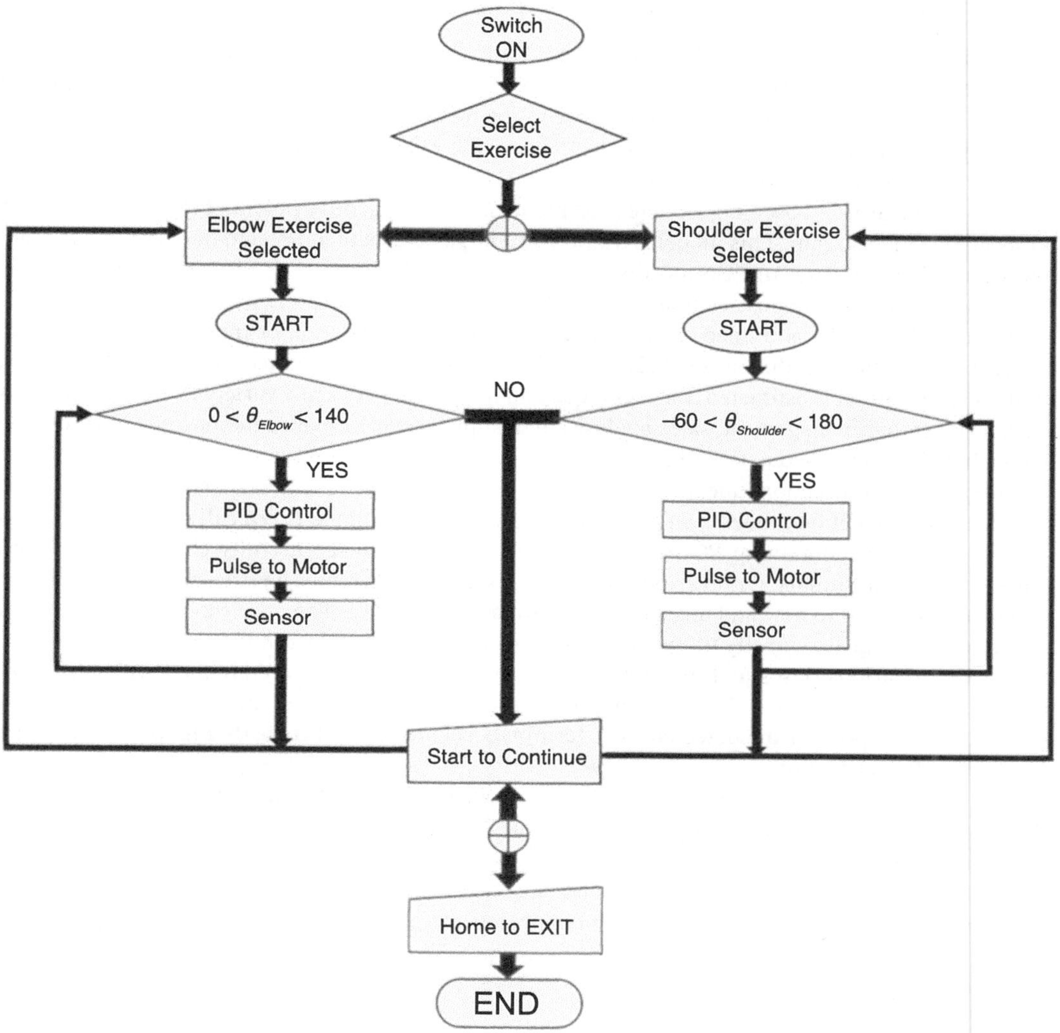

FIGURE 6.6 Process flow of the system.

6.5 REAL-TIME CONTROL AND EXERCISE TRACKING

MediaPipe is a powerful open-source cross-platform framework for creating real-time AI applications. It provides a wide range of perception, inference, and data processing capabilities that can be used to create applications such as augmented reality filters, gesture recognition, face detection, and more (Das and Kumar 2023). MediaPipe is designed to work with mobile, web, and desktop platforms, making it a versatile solution for developers seeking to build AI applications. One of the main features of MediaPipe is its support for machine learning models. The framework provides a set of pre-trained models for a variety of tasks such as object detection, face detection, landmark detection, and hand tracking. These models can be fine-tuned or retrained using custom datasets to obtain better performance for specific use cases.

MediaPipe also provides a rich set of tools and APIs that enable developers to easily integrate machine learning models into their applications. The framework supports a variety of popular machine learning libraries such as TensorFlow and TensorFlow Lite, making it simple to deploy and run models on mobile and edge devices.

6.5.1 Point of Sale (POS) Detection Using MediaPipe

Real-time POS (Point of Sale) detection using MediaPipe is an AI-based approach that seeks to improve the efficiency of retail operations by automating the process of detecting POS terminals in a store. The technique involves using computer vision models and machine learning algorithms provided by the MediaPipe framework to detect and locate POS terminals in real-time video streams (Kumar et al. 2022). The technique employs a two-stage process to detect POS terminals. In the first stage, a deep learning-based object detection model is used to identify potential POS terminal locations in the video stream. This model is trained on a large dataset of annotated images to understand the visual characteristics of POS terminals.

In the second stage, a pose estimation model is used to estimate the 3D pose of the detected POS terminals. This model is trained to predict the position and orientation of the POS terminal in 3D space, based on the two-dimensional (2D) bounding box detected in the first stage. Once the 3D pose of the POS terminal is estimated, the technique can be used to perform a variety of retail operations, such as inventory management, sales analysis, and employee performance monitoring. For example, the technique can be used to tally the number of transactions performed at each POS terminal, calculate the average transaction time, and analyze the sales data to identify trends and patterns.

The object detection model used in the first stage of the technique is typically trained on a large dataset of images containing POS terminals. The dataset must be carefully curated to include a variety of POS terminals, with various shapes, sizes, and orientations. This ensures that the model can generalize well to new and unseen POS terminals in the store. The pose estimation model used in the second stage is typically trained using synthetic data, derived by rendering 3D models of POS terminals in various poses and orientations. The synthetic data is then combined with real-world data to generate a large and diverse training dataset. This approach guarantees that the model can estimate the 3D pose of the detected POS terminals accurately and robustly Figure 6.7 shows the MediaPipe Pos Detection.

Once the object detection and pose estimation models have been trained, they are integrated into the MediaPipe framework to construct a real-time POS detection pipeline. The pipeline typically consists of several modules that analyze the video stream and detect POS terminals in real-time. These modules are designed to be modular and flexible, allowing developers to customize the pipeline to suit their specific needs. Figure 6.8 depicts the process flow of MediaPipe.

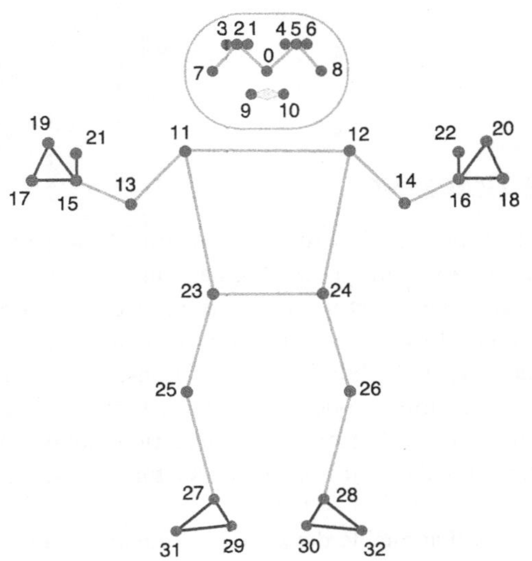

0. nose
1. right eye inner
2. right eye
3. right eye outer
4. left eye inner
5. left eye
6. left eye outer
7. right ear
8. left ear
9. mouth right
10. mouth left
11. right shoulder
12. left shoulder
13. right elbow
14. left elbow
15. right wrist
16. left wrist
17. right pinky knuckle #1
18. left pinky knuckle #1
19. right index knuclke #1
20. left index knuckle #1
21. right thumb knuckle #2
22. left thumb knuckle #2
23. right hip
24. left hip
25. right knee
26. left knee
27. right ankle
2g. left ankle
29. right heel
30. left heel
31. right foot index
32. left foot index

FIGURE 6.7 MediaPipe pos detection.

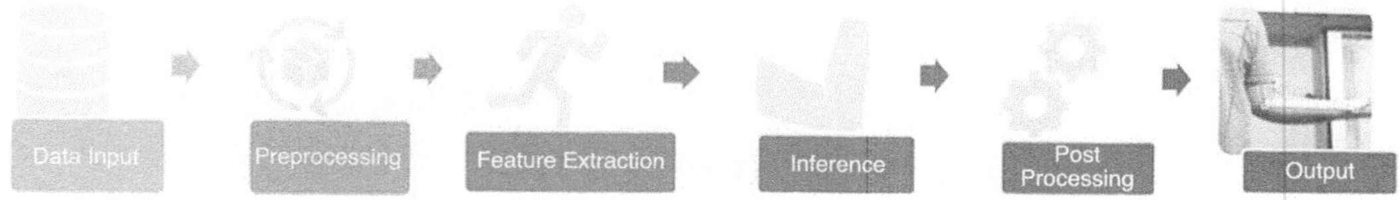

FIGURE 6.8 Flow of MediaPipe.

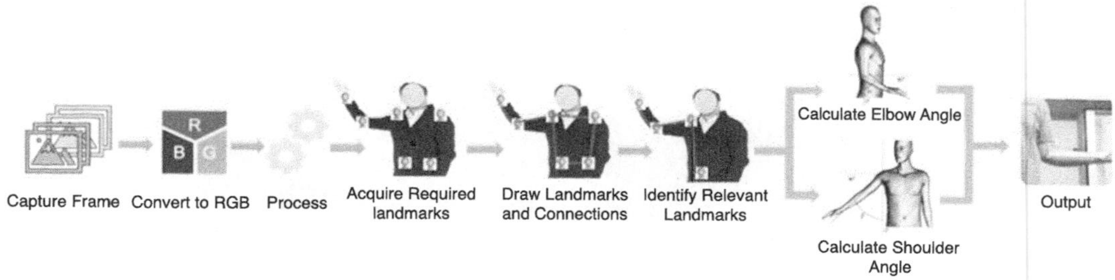

FIGURE 6.9 Angle calculation using MediaPipe framework.

6.5.2 Angle Measurement Using MediaPipe

Inputting an image or video stream, extracting body landmarks, identifying the relevant landmarks for the shoulders and elbows, calculating the elbow and shoulder angles using the atan2 function, and outputting the results. The Body Pose Estimation model is responsible for detecting and tracking the key points on the human body, and the extracted 2D landmark positions for the shoulders, elbows, and wrists are used to calculate the angles. Figure 6.9 illustrates the process of calculation of angle in elbow or shoulder.

The atan2 function is used to determine the angles between the forearm and upper arm for the elbow, and the upper arm and torso for the shoulder. The results can be displayed on the input image or video stream or written to a file or database, making them useful for physical therapy, sports performance analysis, and human-computer interaction applications. Figure 6.10 shows the output of elbow angle calculation.

6.5.3 Hardware Development

The integration of hardware components is a critical aspect of the 2-link upper limb rehabilitation robot. The system is designed with two microcontrollers, the Atmega328p and STMicroelectronics 32-bit microcontroller (STM32), which function as the brain of the system (Rawat and Kumar 2023). The Atmega328p is responsible for controlling the start and homing switches, while the STM32 is the principal controller of the system. The system's hardware components also include a normal DC switch for the start and homing switch, and a 220 V AC control switch for the main control of the system, a 16×2 display for showing messages and prompting patients to take appropriate actions, and an organic light-emitting diode (OLED) display for displaying the selected demo exercise. When the start button is pressed, the corresponding link begins moving, and the OLED display shows the demo exercise. The liquid crystal display (LCD) displays the current and final angle of movement during the exercise. This feedback helps patients monitor their progress and adjust their movements to achieve improved results.

Turn on the device and wait for the welcome message to appear on the display screen before utilizing the MOTION-MATE system. Before commencing the exercise, it is crucial to make sure

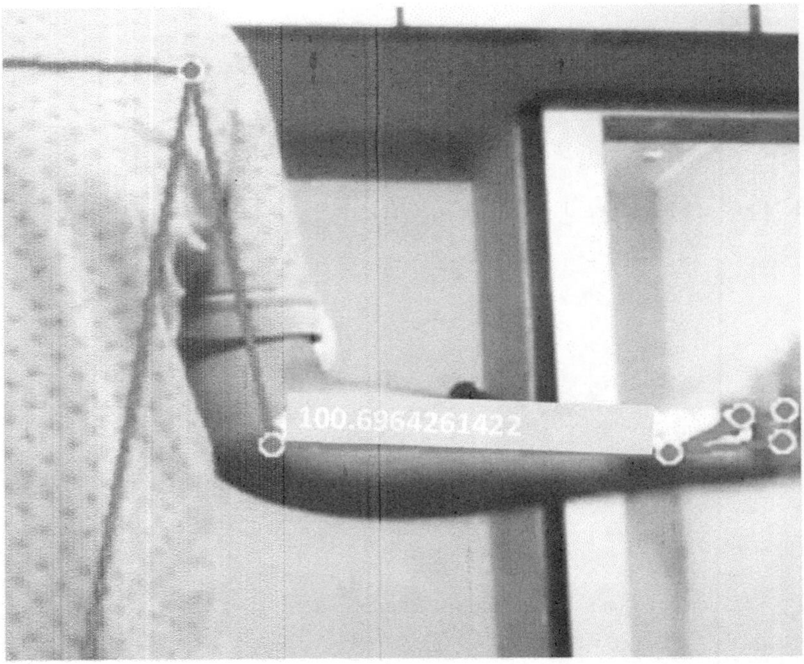

FIGURE 6.10 Elbow angle output of MediaPipe.

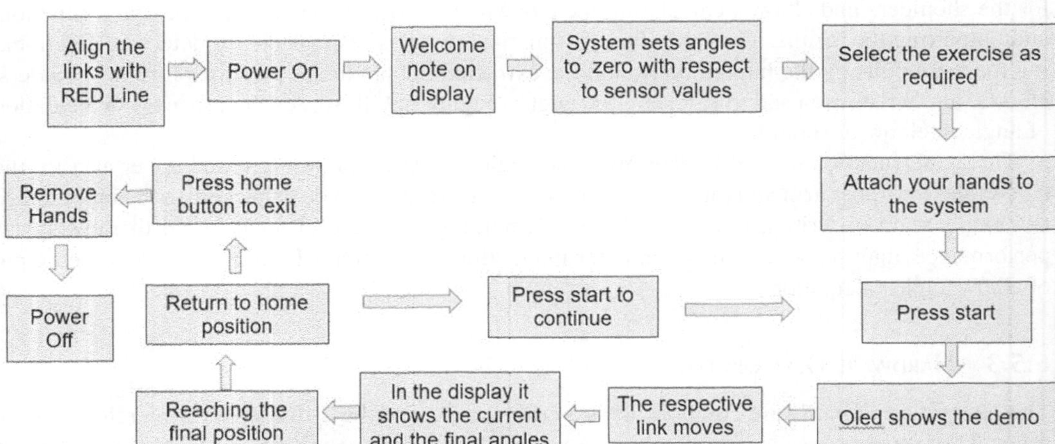

FIGURE 6.11 Flow of hardware model.

the REDLINE on the connection is aligned such that the sensor's value is reset to zero degrees. Choose the exercise that the patient needs after the system has been turned on and the sensors have been reset (Kumar et al. 2022). Once the activity has been confirmed on the display screen, secure the patient's hands to the links using the supplied velcro straps. Press the start button to initiate the exercise after that. Figure 6.11 depicts the flow of the hardware model.

The selected exercise will be demonstrated on the OLED display, and the corresponding connections will move in accordance with how well it is going. The patient can monitor their progress and modify their motions by seeing the present angle and the target angle on the display screen in real-time (Kumar et al. 2020). When the patient's hand reaches the last position of the exercise, it

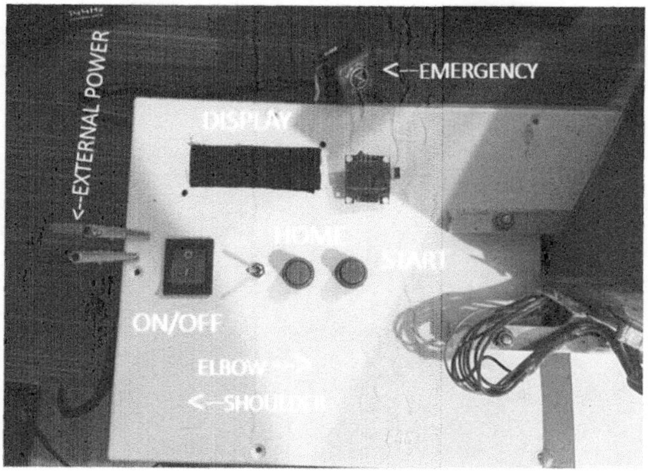

FIGURE 6.12 Control mechanisms and interfaces of the model.

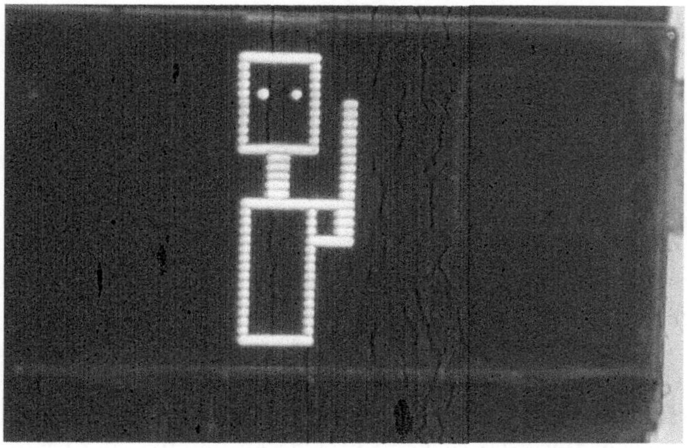

FIGURE 6.13 Demo exercise in OLED display.

will revert to its starting position, giving them the option of continuing the exercise or starting over from the beginning. Pressing the home button will terminate the exercise and turn off the power if the patient needs to cease. Figure 6.12 depicts the hardware model.

This display just shows the exercise demo for the exercise selected as this is a 2D plot there are limitations to show the exact, but it is still understandable that Figure 6.13 shows the OLED display output.

6.5.4 Software Integration

6.5.4.1 GUI for User

Graphical User Interface (GUI) for patients undergoing physical therapy. Figure 6.14 shows the overall GUI constructed. The GUI allows the patients to input their name and age in the respective tabs by pressing the "Start" button, which initiates the MediaPipe framework model for monitoring their exercise movements. The GUI also includes a "Selection" tab where patients can choose the specific exercise they want to perform and generate a report using the "Generate" icon.

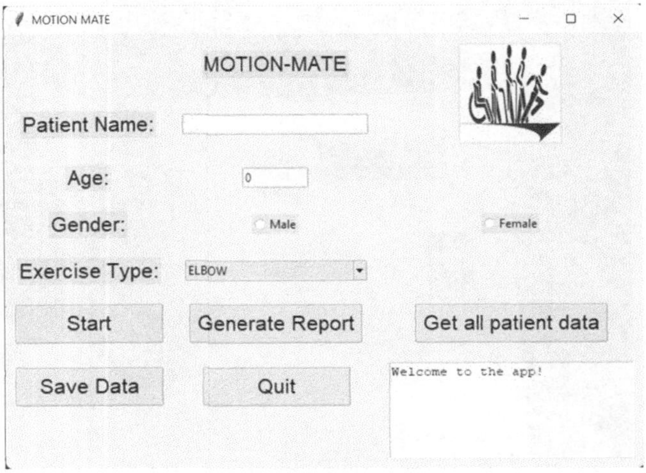

FIGURE 6.14 Overview Of GUI.

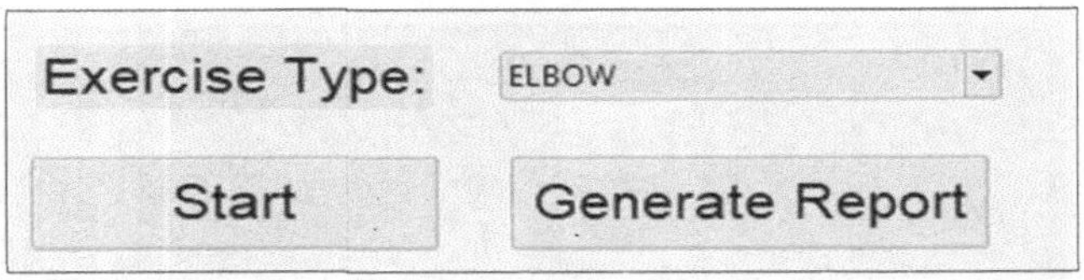

FIGURE 6.15 Exercise selection.

The report contains information such as the tally of exercises completed by the patient, which is obtained through the MediaPipe model's tracking capabilities. Additionally, the GUI includes a "Save Data" icon that allows the patients to save their data, such as their name and age and the exercise performed. The "Generate Report" button saves the report of the current patient in a file, and when the "Get all patient data" button is pressed, all the patient data is stored.

The implementation of this GUI seeks to provide an intuitive and user-friendly interface for patients to track their exercise progress easily. It also enables healthcare professionals to monitor and evaluate the patient's progress effectively. The GUI is designed to be simple to use and understand, making it accessible to patients of all ages and backgrounds. The GUI also includes a message window where messages related to the patients' exercise progress and system status are displayed. The message window is designed to provide patients with feedback on their exercise performance, such as the number of repetitions completed and the correctness of their movements.

The message window also displays status messages, such as errors encountered during system operation or issues with data input. For example, if any of the respective connections are not visible in the camera for the MediaPipe, it gives an error message. This enables patients to be aware of any issues with the system and helps them take the necessary corrective action to resolve the problem.

6.5.4.2 Exercise Selection Tab

The GUI provides patients with a selection menu where they can choose the type of exercise they want to perform. The available exercises are displayed as a drop-down list, making it simple for patients to select the desired exercise. Figure 6.15 displays the exercise selection.

When the patient selects the "Start" button in the GUI, a new window, as depicted in Figure 6.16, opens with the MediaPipe framework running in the background. This window is dedicated to measuring the angle of the selected exercise conducted by the patient. The MediaPipe framework

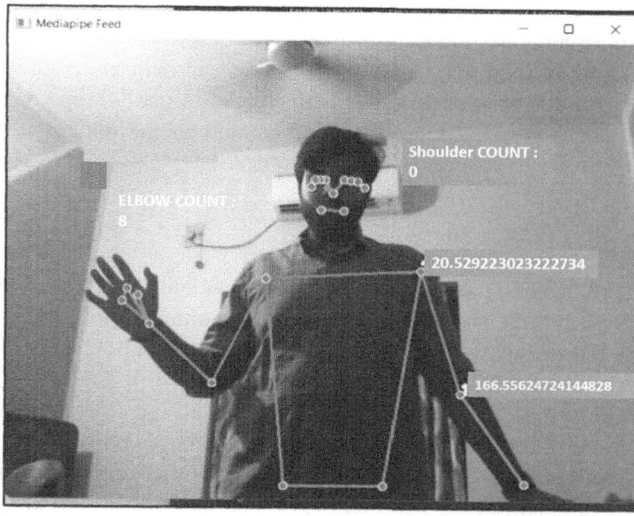

FIGURE 6.16 Window opens upon pressing the "Start" button.

NAME	AG	GENEDER	EXERCISE			
SOWRABH	23	Male	SHOULDER	AI model output	2023-04-05 23:24:25	
sowrabh	23	Male	Cardio			
siddhartha d	23	Male	Cardio			
AMAN BIJAL	23	Male	Strength Training			
sooryan	28	Male	ELBOW		25	2023-04.09 09:48:15
subramaniar	24	Male	ELBOW		5	2023-04-10 00:26:13

FIGURE 6.17 Model of getting all patient data.

utilizes a camera feed to monitor the patient's movements and calculate the angle of the joints involved in the exercise. As the patient performs the exercise, the angle measurements are continuously transmitted to the output window, where they are displayed to the patient. The output window provides real-time feedback to the patient on their exercise performance, enabling them to adjust their movements and enhance their technique. The output window also displays the count of exercises completed by the patient, which is calculated based on the angle measurements. Figure 6.16 shows the tab when the Start button is selected. To exit the pop-up window with the MediaPipe framework, the patient needs to select the "q" key. This key functions as an exit command for the MediaPipe framework, allowing the patient to exit the exercise session and return to the main GUI window.

6.6 GENERATE REPORT

When the patient selects the "Generate Report" button in the GUI, the system communicates with the database where all the patient data is stored. The relevant data, such as the patient's name, age, selected exercise, and exercise count, are retrieved from the database and consolidated into a Portable Document Format (PDF) file. The PDF file contains a summary of the patient's exercise performance, including the number of repetitions completed and the duration of the exercise session. A sample report generated from the GUI is shown in Figure 6.17. The PDF file is saved in the same file location as the GUI, making it simple for patients to access and share their exercise progress with their healthcare providers or family members. The filename is generated based on the patient's name and the exercise type, making it simple to identify the specific report for each patient and exercise. The report generation feature is an essential aspect of the GUI, as it provides patients with a tangible document of their exercise progress. This can help motivate them to continue their exercise routine and monitor their progress effectively. Additionally, the generated reports can be used by healthcare providers to evaluate the effectiveness of the patient's exercise regimen and make necessary adjustments to ensure optimal outcomes.

6.6.1 Get All Patient Data

The GUI also includes a "Get all patient data" button that patients can click to retrieve all their saved exercise data. When this button is selected, the GUI communicates with the database where all the patient data is stored and retrieves all the relevant exercise data. The data is then consolidated into a PDF report, which is saved in the same file location as the GUI. All patient data produced from the GUI is shown in Figure 6.17. This PDF report includes all the relevant exercise data, including the number of exercises completed, the duration of the exercise session, and the patient's exercise performance data, which includes angle measurements and other relevant metrics. The PDF report can be reviewed by the patient or their healthcare provider, providing vital insights into the patient's exercise routine and progress over time.

6.6.2 Data Base

The database component of the GUI functions as a central repository for storing all patient data. When a patient enters their information and starts an exercise session, the GUI communicates with the database to generate a new record for the patient, which includes their name, age, and any other relevant information.

During the exercise session, the GUI monitors the patient's progress and saves the data in the database, including the number of repetitions completed, the duration of the exercise session, and any errors or other issues encountered during the session. When a patient requests a report of their exercise history, the GUI communicates with the database to gather the relevant data and consolidates it into a PDF report, which is saved in the same location as the GUI. Additionally, patients can request to retrieve all their data, which is stored in Excel format, with each new addition added as a new row below the last saved row.

For the experiment, six male subjects were considered out of which 5 were in the age group 22–24 years and one subject was 28 years old. Four exercises were taken into consideration including Shoulder, Elbow, Cardio, and Strength Training Exercise.

6.7 CONCLUSION AND FUTURE SCOPE

The development of the two-link Upper Limb Rehabilitation Robot faced several challenges, including the need to ensure precise movement and range of motion while maintaining patient comfort and safety. Additionally, integrating real-time monitoring and feedback mechanisms presented technical and logistical hurdles. To address these challenges, a robust hardware design was implemented, featuring secure attachment mechanisms and flexible joints to accommodate a variety of patient needs. The incorporation of AI and machine learning algorithms facilitated real-time monitoring and personalized feedback, enhancing the effectiveness of rehabilitation sessions. Furthermore, the potential for telerehabilitation was explored, leveraging remote interaction capabilities to extend the reach of rehabilitation services. As a result of these decisions, the two-link Upper Limb Rehabilitation Robot demonstrated promising results in expediting upper limb rehabilitation for individuals with motor deficits. Its precise movements and adaptable design contributed to improved patient outcomes, including increased range of motion and enhanced motor function. The integration of AI-driven monitoring enhanced therapy effectiveness and patient engagement, leading to more efficient rehabilitation sessions. Moving forward, future development efforts will focus on optimizing the robot's hardware and software to further enhance its range of motion, versatility, and usability. This includes exploring the integration of VR technology to enhance patient engagement and motivation during rehabilitation sessions. Additionally, efforts will be made to expand the use of the robot for telerehabilitation, providing accessible rehabilitation services to patients in remote or underserved areas. By continually innovating and improving the two-link Upper Limb Rehabilitation Robot, we can advance the field of upper limb rehabilitation and improve outcomes for patients with motor impairments.

FUNDING

"The authors declare that no funds, grants, or other support were received during the preparation of this manuscript."

DECLARATIONS

Conflict of interest – The authors have no conflicts of interest to declare.

REFERENCES

Adomavičienė, Aušra, Kristina Daunoravičienė, Raimondas Kubilius, Lina Varžaitytė, and Juozas Raistenskis. 2019. "Influence of New Technologies on Post-Stroke Rehabilitation: A Comparison of Armeo Spring to the Kinect System." *Medicina* 55 (4): 98. https://doi.org/10.3390/medicina55040098

Bronzino, Joseph D. 2000. *Biomedical Engineering Handbook 2*. Vol. 2. Springer Science & Business Media. ISBN-13: 978-0849304620

Das, Kaushik, and Roushan Kumar. 2023. "Electric Vehicle Battery Capacity Degradation and Health Estimation Using Machine-Learning Techniques: A Review." *Clean Energy* 7 (6): 1268–81. https://doi.org/10.1093/ce/zkad054

Das, Kaushik, and Roushan Kumar. 2024. "A Comprehensive Review of Categorization and Perspectives on State-of-Charge Estimation Using Deep Learning Methods for Electric Transportation." *Wireless Personal Communications*, 1–20. https://doi.org/10.1007/s11277-023-10830-5

Das, Kaushik, Roushan Kumar, and Anurup Krishna. 2024. "Analyzing Electric Vehicle Battery Health Performance Using Supervised Machine Learning." *Renewable and Sustainable Energy Reviews* 189: 113967. https://doi.org/10.1016/j.rser.2023.113967

Feigin, Valery L, Bo Norrving, and George A Mensah. 2017. "Global Burden of Stroke." *Circulation Research* 120 (3): 439–48. https://doi.org/10.1161/CIRCRESAHA.116.308413

Feigin, Valery L, Rita V Krishnamurthi, Priya Parmar, Bo Norrving, George A Mensah, Derrick A Bennett, Suzanne Barker-Collo, et al. 2015. "Update on the Global Burden of Ischemic and Hemorrhagic Stroke in 1990–2013: The GBD 2013 Study." *Neuroepidemiology* 45 (3): 161–76. https://doi.org/10.1159/000441085

Frisoli, Antonio, Michele Barsotti, Edoardo Sotgiu, Giuseppe Lamola, Caterina Procopio, and Carmelo Chisari. 2022. "A Randomized Clinical Control Study on the Efficacy of Three-Dimensional Upper Limb Robotic Exoskeleton Training in Chronic Stroke." *Journal of Neuroengineering and Rehabilitation* 19 (1): 14.

Gupta, Akash, Amit Kumar Mondal, and Mukul Kumar Gupta. 2019. "Kinematic, Dynamic Analysis and Control of 3 DOF Upper-Limb Robotic Exoskeleton." *Journal Européen Des Systèmes Automatisés* 52 (3): 297–304. https://doi.org/10.18280/jesa.520311

Gupta, Akash, Anshuman Singh, Varnita Verma, Amit Kumar Mondal, and Mukul Kumar Gupta. 2020. "Developments and Clinical Evaluations of Robotic Exoskeleton Technology for Human Upper-Limb Rehabilitation." *Advanced Robotics* 34 (15): 1023–40. https://doi.org/10.1080/01691864.2020.1749926

Gupta, Mukul Kumar, Roushan Kumar, Varnita Verma, and Abhinav Sharma. 2021. "Robust Control Based Stability Analysis and Trajectory Tracking of Triple Link Robot Manipulator." *Journal Européen des Systèmes Automatisés* 54: 641–47. https://doi.org/10.18280/jesa.540414

Housman, Sarah J, Vu Le, Tariq Rahman, Robert J Sanchez, and David J Reinkensmeyer. 2007. "Arm-Training with T-WREX after Chronic Stroke: Preliminary Results of a Randomized Controlled Trial." In *2007 IEEE 10th International Conference on Rehabilitation Robotics*, 562–68. https://doi.org/10.1109/icorr.2007.4428481

Hsieh, Yu-Wei, Tsai-Yu Shih, Keh-Chung Lin, and CY Wu. 2017. "Upper-Extremity Robot-Aided Rehabilitation after Stroke: A Comparison of the Arm and Wrist Robots." *Journal of the Neurological Sciences* 381: 599. https://doi.org/10.1016/j.jns.2017.08.1688

Ivanova, Ekaterina, Axel Krause, Marie Schälicke, Franziska Schellhardt, Natalie Jankowski, Josy Achner, Henning Schmidt, Michael Joebges, and Jörg Krüger. 2017. "Let's Do This Together: Bi-Manu-Interact, a Novel Device for Studying Human Haptic Interactive Behavior." In *2017 International Conference on Rehabilitation Robotics (ICORR)*, 708–13, London, UK.

Krebs, H Igo, Neville Hogan, Mindy L Aisen, and Bruce T Volpe. 1998. "Robot-Aided Neurorehabilitation." *IEEE Transactions on Rehabilitation Engineering* 6 (1): 75–87. https://doi.org/10.1109/86.662623

Kumar, Roushan, Adesh Kumar, Mukul Kumar Gupta, Jitendra Yadav, and Arpit Jain. 2022. "Solar Tree-Based Water Pumping for Assured Irrigation in Sustainable Indian Agriculture Environment." *Sustainable Production and Consumption* 33: 15–27. https://doi.org/10.1016/j.spc.2022.06.013

Kumar, Roushan, and Kaushik Das. 2024. "Lithium Battery Prognostics and Health Management for Electric Vehicle Application--A Perspective Review." *Sustainable Energy Technologies and Assessments* 65: 103766. https://doi.org/10.1016/j.seta.2024.103766

Kumar, Roushan, Neelu J Ahuja, and Mukesh Saxena. 2018. "Improvement and Approval of Impediment Recognition and Activity for Power Window." In *Intelligent Communication, Control and Devices*, 855–64. Springer. https://doi.org/10.1007/978-981-10-5903-2_89

Kumar, Roushan, Neelu Jyoti Ahuja, Mukesh Saxena, and Adesh Kumar. 2020. "Automotive Power Window Communication with DTC Algorithm and Hardware-in-the Loop Testing." *Wireless Personal Communications* 114 (4): 3351–66. https://doi.org/10.1007/s11277-020-07535-4

Kumar, Roushan, Rupendra Kumar Pachauri, Pankaj Badoni, Deepak Bharadwaj, Udayveer Mittal, and Abhishek Bisht. 2022. "Investigation on Parallel Hybrid Electric Bicycle along with Issuer Management System for Mountainous Region." *Journal of Cleaner Production* 362 (June): 132430. https://doi.org/10.1016/j.jclepro.2022.132430

Kwakkel, Gert, Boudewijn J Kollen, and Hermano I Krebs. 2008. "Effects of Robot-Assisted Therapy on Upper Limb Recovery after Stroke: A Systematic Review." *Neurorehabilitation and Neural Repair* 22 (2): 111–21. https://doi.org/10.1177/1545968307305457

Lum, Peter S, Charles G Burgar, Machiel der Loos, Peggy C Shor, Matra Majmundar, and Ruth Yap. 2005. "The MIME Robotic System for Upper-Limb Neuro-Rehabilitation: Results from a Clinical Trial in Subacute Stroke." In *9th International Conference on Rehabilitation Robotics, 2005. ICORR 2005*, 511–14. https://doi.org/10.1109/icorr.2005.1501153

Maheu, Veronique, Philippe S Archambault, Julie Frappier, and François Routhier. 2011. "Evaluation of the JACO Robotic Arm: Clinico-Economic Study for Powered Wheelchair Users with Upper-Extremity Disabilities." In *2011 IEEE International Conference on Rehabilitation Robotics*, 1–5. https://doi.org/10.1109/icorr.2011.5975397

Mehrholz, Jan, Marcus Pohl, Thomas Platz, Joachim Kugler, and Bernhard Elsner. 2018. "Electromechanical and Robot-Assisted Arm Training for Improving Activities of Daily Living, Arm Function, and Arm Muscle Strength after Stroke." *Cochrane Database of Systematic Reviews* 9. https://doi.org/10.1002/14651858.cd006876.pub4

Norouzi-Gheidari, Nahid, Philippe S Archambault, and Joyce Fung. 2012. "Effects of Robot-Assisted Therapy on Stroke Rehabilitation in Upper Limbs: Systematic Review and Meta-Analysis of the Literature." https://doi.org/10.1682/jrrd.2010.10.0210

Park, Si-Woon, Jae-Hyung Kim, and Yun-Jung Yang. 2018. "Mental Practice for Upper Limb Rehabilitation after Stroke: A Systematic Review and Meta-Analysis." *International Journal of Rehabilitation Research* 41 (3): 197–203. doi: 10.1097/MRR.0000000000000298

Pehlivan, Ali Utku, Fabrizio Sergi, Andrew Erwin, Nuray Yozbatiran, Gerard E Francisco, and Marcia K O'Malley. 2014. "Design and Validation of the RiceWrist-S Exoskeleton for Robotic Rehabilitation after Incomplete Spinal Cord Injury." *Robotica* 32 (8): 1415–31. https://doi.org/10.1017/s0263574714001490

Pollock, Alex, Sybil E Farmer, Marian C Brady, Peter Langhorne, Gillian E Mead, Jan Mehrholz, and Frederike van Wijck. 2014. "Interventions for Improving Upper Limb Function after Stroke." *Cochrane Database of Systematic Reviews* 11. https://doi.org/10.1002/14651858.CD010820.pub2

Rawat, Kulbeer Singh, and Roushan Kumar. 2023. "Insight into the Novel Low Cost Green Air Pollution Monitoring and Control Systems: A Technological Solution from Concept to Market." *Journal of Cleaner Production* 427 (August): 139218. https://doi.org/10.1016/j.jclepro.2023.139218

Solomon, Patricia, and Sue Baptiste. 2005. *Innocations in Rehabilitation Science Education: Preparing Leaders for the Future.* Springer, Berlin, Heidelberg.

Verma, Varnita, A Gupta, M K Gupta, and P Chauhan. 2020. "Performance Estimation of Computed Torque Control for Surgical Robot Application." *Journal of Mechanical Engineering and Sciences* 14 (3): 7017–28. https://doi.org/10.15282/jmes.14.3.2020.04.0549

Verma, Varnita, Vinay Chowdary, Mukul Kumar Gupta, and Amit Kumar Mondal. 2018. "IoT and Robotics in Healthcare." In *Medical Big Data and Internet of Medical Things*, 245–69. CRC Press. https://doi.org/10.1201/9781351030380

7 Mortality Prediction in Non-Alcoholic Fatty Liver Disease Using Machine Learning

Bikash Sadhukhan, Anandarupa Neogi, Jyoti Anand, Anubhav Jaiswal, and Ankush Kumar

7.1 INTRODUCTION

The liver plays a pivotal role in human physiology, serving as a central organ responsible for a diverse array of functions essential for metabolic processes, digestion, immunity, and detoxification (Kalra et al. 2024). It constitutes approximately 2% of an adult's total body weight. The etiology of liver diseases is intricate and influenced by a myriad of factors, such as sex, ethnicity, genetic predisposition, exposure to toxins, body mass index, and the presence of diabetes. NAFLD has emerged as a leading cause of liver-related disorders worldwide. NAFLD significantly increases the risk of various health complications, including cardiovascular diseases, liver failure, fibrosis, cirrhosis, and type 2 diabetes (Maurice and Manousou 2018). This disease includes a variety of liver abnormalities, ranging from excess fat deposition (steatosis) to increasingly severe conditions such as nonalcoholic steatohepatitis (NASH), characterized by hepatocellular damage and inflammation, and its impact is substantial. The prevalence of NAFLD was notably high in 2019, affecting approximately 1.6 billion individuals globally, representing nearly 22%–30% of the adult population across developed and developing nations. This condition is particularly common in individuals aged 40–60 years (Teng et al. 2023).

Several factors cause NAFLD, a disorder in which liver cells accumulate extra fat, among people who drink little or no alcohol. The contributing factors include insulin resistance and rapid weight gain leading to fat deposition, among others. The potential complications of NAFLD are severe and may lead to mortality, notably liver failure or liver cancer. Mortality-related symptoms typically manifest in advanced stages and complications, including ascites, sepsis, hepatorenal syndrome, and hepatocellular carcinoma (HCC) (Benedict and Zhang 2017). While individuals can live for many years with NAFLD, approximately 30% progress to nonalcoholic steatohepatitis (NASH) and subsequent scarring. Among these patients, approximately 20% develop end-stage cirrhosis, which increases the chance of cancer and liver failure (Fernando et al. 2019).

Over the past few decades, the occurrence of NAFLD has notably increased, making it an important area of study in hepatology. Among NAFLD patients, a substantial proportion progress to nonalcoholic steatohepatitis (NASH), a more severe inflammatory phase associated with fibrosis and eventual end-stage liver disease (Fernando et al. 2019). Currently, the diagnosis of NASH relies on invasive procedures such as liver biopsy, which poses challenges in clinical management. The increasing prevalence of NAFLD and its potential progression to NASH and advanced liver disease underscore the urgent need for enhanced diagnostic and prognostic approaches. Accurate identification of individuals at risk of disease progression and adverse outcomes is crucial for timely intervention. Furthermore, the availability of noninvasive diagnostic methods for NASH diagnosis remains an area of active research interest.

DOI: 10.1201/9781003486640-7

7.1.1 Wearable Technologies in Healthcare

There has been a significant increase in wearable technology in recent years. These technologies include a wide variety of gadgets carried by users, such as glasses, wristwatches, rings, chest straps, and prosthetic sockets. The internet of Medical Things (IoMT) comprises implantable, ambient, and fixed technologies utilized in healthcare settings. Wearable devices are an essential part of this ecosystem. Wearable gadgets are outfitted with a variety of sensors, including accelerometers, temperature sensors, biometric sensors, and optical sensors. These sensors allow devices to constantly monitor a wide range of human signals. Although the accuracy of sensor readings from wearable devices may not always match that of stationary hospital devices, they are often deemed acceptable depending on the specific application (Delmastro et al. 2020). The interaction between sensors included in IoMT devices and individual users generates a substantial flow of data, from which pertinent attributes can be extracted using machine learning algorithms to detect and comprehend significant patterns. This dataset has considerable promise in several healthcare and senior care domains, such as detecting activities to assess health status, identifying falls, detecting stress, tracking fitness, monitoring vital signs, and diagnosing diseases (Sabry et al. 2022). The utilization of machine learning methodologies to assess and extract information from physiological signals obtained by wearable devices has been a thriving area of research in the last 10 years, with a multitude of published works making significant contributions to this subject. Although there has been significant research and a rapid increase in the use of wearable devices, namely, smartwatches, in daily life, only a few machine learning applications for these devices have successfully made them available on the market.

Recent research has highlighted the ability of wearable devices to serve as effective electronic diagnostic tools for detecting different illnesses. Wearables have become an excellent tool for diagnosing physiological disorders due to their ability to remotely access, monitor, and continuously collect individualized data in real time. The physiological parameters obtained from these biosensors have been shown to be effective in detecting a range of medical conditions, including Lyme disease (Li et al. 2017), respiratory infections, cardiovascular disorders (Wang et al. 2022; Torres-Soto and Ashley 2020), neurological disorders (Tang et al. 2021), coronavirus diseases (Mishra et al. 2020), Parkinson's disease (Ancona et al. 2022), diabetes, and liver diseases. Wearables not only have the ability to identify physical illnesses but can also be used to diagnose mental states. The utilization of wearable biosensors to provide real-time and precise physiological data is currently and will continue to have a significant influence on our everyday lives in the future. Utilizing wearables as diagnostic instruments has various challenges, such as attaining and sustaining accuracy, managing power consumption, and ensuring connectivity. The manufacture of these devices presents challenges due to the need for downsizing and the integration of many sensors (Vijayan et al. 2021). Compared to traditional diagnostic methods conducted in a laboratory, these tailored diagnostic approaches, which can be monitored remotely, create concerns about the security, sharing, and storage of data (Brönneke et al. 2021).

7.1.2 Advances in the Detection of Liver Disease Using Machine Learning

Recent developments in machine learning have demonstrated optimistic outcomes in the prediction of NAFLD and its progression through a variety of parameters. Machine learning serves as a supportive tool for developing predictive models for assessing mortality risk in individuals diagnosed with NAFLD. These models aid in determining the remaining duration for further treatment and decision-making. Additionally, healthcare professionals can utilize the generated data to monitor patients' conditions, recommend lifestyle modifications, and administer appropriate treatments as necessary.

Machine learning models for liver disease detection represent a promising frontier in healthcare innovation. Wearable devices have revolutionized healthcare by enabling continuous monitoring of critical symptoms and relevant physiological parameters in real time. With their built-in sensors, these devices are capable of capturing data such as heart rate, blood pressure, and glucose levels and providing valuable information about patients' health status. In the context of liver disease detection, wearable devices play a crucial role in collecting relevant data points that allow for the application of machine learning models to predict and diagnose various liver conditions. The integration of machine learning models can lead to significant improvements in the early detection of liver diseases. For instance, a study conducted at a leading healthcare institution demonstrated how real-time monitoring of liver enzyme levels using wearable biosensors enabled early detection of liver diseases in high-risk patients (AL Abed and Alameri 2019; Chuang et al. 2011). By continuously tracking changes in enzyme levels and correlating them with other clinical parameters, the machine learning model achieved remarkable accuracy in predicting liver disease progression and identifying patients in need of immediate intervention (Schattenberg et al. 2023). Cirrhosis and other chronic liver diseases can be monitored using wearable devices (Buckholz and Rosenblatt 2023). By collecting data on factors such as fluid intake, physical activity, and medication adherence, researchers successfully formulated individualized care strategies customized to the specific requirements of each patient. This proactive strategy not only enhanced patient outcomes but also decreased healthcare expenses by preventing hospitalizations.

This research aimed to bridge critical knowledge gaps by investigating the relationship between NAFLD and various body metrics within a retrospective cohort spanning nearly two decades. Our primary aim was to construct predictive models that estimate the risk of mortality among patients with NAFLD by utilizing the integration of machine learning algorithms. Our objective was to optimize treatment outcomes for individuals with NAFLD by integrating sensor-derived data analysis with clinical parameter assessment in the field of hepatology. This study has two primary objectives:

1. The relationships between NAFLD and several body parameters in persons who were diagnosed with NAFLD were examined. The objective of this research was to investigate the relationships between NAFLD and factors such as age, weight, height, BMI, lipid profiles, and other pertinent physical and metabolic features using machine learning approaches.
2. Various machine learning models capable of accurately predicting the risk of mortality in patients diagnosed with NAFLD have been developed and validated. By integrating machine learning algorithms, this study aimed to leverage extensive datasets to construct predictive models that incorporate clinical and demographic factors, facilitating the identification of patients at greater risk of mortality due to NAFLD-related complications.

This research builds on the authors' earlier work (Neogi et al. 2024), aiming to provide significant insights into the clinical implications of NAFLD. It seeks to enhance risk stratification strategies and facilitate personalized patient management approaches for individuals affected by this prevalent liver condition.

The rest of the manuscript is organized as follows: Section 7.2 introduces a comprehensive summary of existing methods for predicting mortality and highlights the growing role of ML in healthcare. Section 7.3 describes the specifics of the dataset, including patient characteristics, the machine learning algorithms chosen, and the preprocessing steps taken to ensure data quality. Section 7.4 presents the findings of mortality risk prediction using different machine learning models, accompanied by an in-depth discussion of the performance metrics. Finally, Section 7.5 briefly summarizes the key findings of the study, emphasizing their significance in clinical practice and outlining avenues for future research and improvement.

7.2 LITERATURE SURVEY

NAFLD is a major global public health issue, and its incidence has consistently risen in recent decades. Early detection and accurate prediction of NAFLD severity are crucial for effective management and prevention of disease progression. Physical inactivity is the primary factor contributing to all liver disorders. Individuals can monitor their physical activity with a high degree of precision using wearable devices. Individuals with non-NAFLD liver disease and hepatocellular carcinoma (HCC) can benefit from the dual role of these wearable devices in diagnosing liver disorders and tracking beneficial physical activity. Therefore, data collected from wearable devices serve as a reliable measure of wellbeing for patients afflicted with liver disorders. Enhancing physical activity results in enhanced cardiorespiratory fitness, which can be assessed using the cardiopulmonary exercise test (CPET). In the field of transplant hepatology, CPET has proven to be useful for risk assessment (Dunn et al. 2021). Kim et al. (2020) tracked patients using Neofit, a device that records metrics such as calories burned, heart rate, step count, and activity duration. After 12 weeks of adhering to the workout plan, the HCC patients who finished their treatments exhibited noticeable improvements in body composition and fitness. In a study conducted by Schneider et al. (2021), participants' physical activity was measured using a wrist accelerometer. The study showed that liver disease decreased as people became more active, and the decrease was directly related to the amount of exercise. This reduction in liver disease was unrelated to body fat levels.

Machine learning (ML) algorithms have recently gained prominence as valuable tools for predicting NAFLD and other liver-related diseases. Machine learning (ML) is being used extensively to construct NAFLD diagnostic models utilizing imaging, biomarker, or clinical data (Haas et al. 2021). ML approaches involve a variety of algorithms that vary in complexity, accuracy, processing demands, and application-specific details; these methods can be applied alone or in combination with statistical methods. Clinical testing and noninvasive imaging approaches have significantly lower accuracies owing to technological limitations; however, ML algorithms have the potential to overcome these issues and outperform traditional manual diagnosis methods for NAFLD. Voss et al. (Voss et al. 2022) investigated how a wearable electronic nose built on gas sensors could be used to detect and measure liver dysfunction. An electronic nose equipped with three sensor modules containing nine different MOx layers was used to detect gases indicative of liver dysfunction. Complex data analysis techniques, focusing on time and nonlinear dynamics domains, were applied to identify patterns in the recorded time series of respiration gas levels. This study demonstrated exceptional sensitivity, specificity, and accuracy in identifying patients with hepatic cirrhosis. The most promising results were obtained with the AdaBoost machine learning model, demonstrating near-perfect accuracy and F1 scores. Aslam et al. (2022) demonstrated that ML algorithms such as logistic regression, random forest (RF), support vector machine (SVM), naïve Bayes, and multilayer perceptron are effective in predicting NAFLD severity. Notably, SVM and RF achieved the highest accuracy of 99%, indicating excellent potential for the early detection and risk assessment of NAFLD. Additionally, the study highlighted the significance of feature selection and dataset balancing methods for enhancing prediction accuracy. Razmpour et al. (2023) utilized ML techniques, such as neural networks, RF, and SVM, to predict NAFLD using physical measurements and body composition indices. This study demonstrated an accuracy of 82% with the RF model in identifying NAFLD. Furthermore, this research emphasizes the potential of ML-based systems in assisting NAFLD diagnosis, especially in areas with limited access to qualified physicians.

Ben-Assuli et al. (2022) employed time series modeling methods to stratify NAFLD patients into risk groups for fibrosis progression. By analyzing data from more than 5,500 individuals over a 10-year period, this study utilized a hidden Markov model and group-based trajectory modeling to classify individuals based on fibrosis risk stage trajectory. This research underscores the importance of long-term follow-up and suggests that these models be integrated into clinical decision support systems for personalized NAFLD management. Using NHANES data, (Atsawarungruangkit et al. 2021) focused on developing ML algorithms to predict NAFLD predisposition in the US population. This study applied various ML algorithms and features related to NAFLD, identifying factors such as waist circumference and fasting C-peptide levels as predictors of NAFLD. Despite limitations such as missing data and a reliance on ultrasonography for diagnosis, this research provided valuable insights for updating NAFLD risk prediction models. Ji et al. (2022) developed and validated machine learning models utilizing data from 304,145 adults to accurately screen for NAFLD, with XGBoost exhibiting the highest accuracy of 88%, precision of 80%, recall of 89%, F1 score of 88%, and AUC of 95%. The significance rankings of the detected covariates, such as age, BMI, waist circumference, and numerous health indicators, offer useful perceptions for the prevention and treatment of NAFLD. Weng et al. (2023) developed ML models for the initial identification of fatty liver disease (FLD) in China utilizing data from 30,574 individuals. Among the eight models, the XGBoost model demonstrated the greatest accuracy, attaining a score of 89.77%, emphasizing the significance of body mass index, triglycerides, and alanine aminotransferase as key predictors of FLD. Sorino et al. (2021) developed and validated a simple neural network-based web app for predicting NAFLD, particularly its absence, achieving an accuracy of 77% and an AUC of 82%. The web app demonstrated good performance with a specificity of 1.00 and sensitivity of 0.73, offering a cost-effective solution for NAFLD diagnosis and reducing healthcare burdens. Naderi Yaghouti et al. (2024) developed a machine learning application that predicts NASH using clinical data, including blood parameters and the NAFLD activity score, achieving an accuracy of 81.32%±6.43% with random forest and sequential forward selection feature selection. The results show that ML could be useful for detecting NASH noninvasively, as it offers a promising alternative to conventional diagnostic methods and paves the way for scalable approaches to enhance the screening and monitoring of the progression of NASH. An NAFLD risk prediction model was devised and validated in Chinese adults over the age of 60 years in another study (Pan et al. 2023) utilizing multivariate logistic regression and random forest analysis. The optimal model, which included BMI, triglyceride level, alanine aminotransferase level, and lymphocyte count, demonstrated superior performance compared to existing models, providing a basis for personalized health interventions to reduce NAFLD incidence in this population segment. This systematic review (Zhao et al. 2023) analyzed 15 studies assessing image-based artificial intelligence (AI) for diagnosing fatty liver, yielding a pooled sensitivity of 92% and specificity of 94%.

Finally, the literature review revealed that, utilizing wearable devices and machine learning algorithms, NAFLD can be accurately predicted and detected at an early stage. Research has demonstrated that wearable devices can be used to effectively track physical activity, which is linked to liver health. These devices have also shown promise in improving patient outcomes. The use of ML algorithms to predict the severity of NAFLD and the risk of mortality has also shown encouraging results, providing important information for individualized treatment plans. Improving NAFLD diagnosis, risk assessment, and treatment through the integration of machine learning has enormous potential to lead to better patient care and outcomes. Translating these findings into clinical practice and addressing the growing global burden of NAFLD will require collaborative efforts between clinicians, data scientists, and technology developers as this field of study continues to advance.

7.3 METHODOLOGY

The methodology employed in this research aimed to comprehensively analyze the influence of NAFLD on long-term health outcomes among adult individuals diagnosed with NAFLD. This study focused on elucidating associations between NAFLD and various demographic and physical measurements and metabolic factors, with a particular emphasis on predicting mortality risk using ML algorithms.

7.3.1 Dataset

This research employs a dataset that includes data from a community cohort of 17,549 adult individuals suffering from NAFLD in Olmsted County, Minnesota, from 1997 to 2014. Data from the Rochester Epidemiology Project database were used to establish this cohort. Guided by the

TABLE 7.1
Physiological Metrics

Column	Description
ID	Identifier
Age	Age when they joined the study
Male	0 means female, 1 means male
Weight	Weight in kilograms
Height	Height in centimeter
BMI	Body mass index
Futime	Survival time till death or the most recent follow-up.
Status	0 indicates that the individual was alive at the previous follow-up, whereas 1 indicates that the individual has passed away.

TABLE 7.2
Metabolic Metrics

Column	Description
ID	Identifier
Days	No. of days passed since the index date.
Test	Recorded value's type (hdl, sbp, dbp, fib4, smoke)
Value	The numeric value

principles outlined in (Allen et al. 2018), the dataset focuses on assessing the impact of NAFLD on long-term health outcomes. NAFLD, characterized by hepatic steatosis without alcohol consumption, impacts a substantial part of the global population and is associated with conditions such as nonalcoholic steatohepatitis (NASH) and liver fibrosis.

The dataset included demographic factors such as age and sex, as well as physiological measurements such as weight, height, and BMI, as described in Table 7.1. Additionally, metabolic data, as described in Table 7.2, including cholesterol levels, high density lipoprotein (HDL) levels, low density lipoprotein (LDL) levels, systolic and diastolic blood pressure (SBP, DBP), smoking status, and fibrosis-4 (FIB-4) scores, were collected. Each participant's data were recorded multiple times over the study period, resulting in a total of 400,123 observations. Missing values for height, weight, and BMI were imputed using median values. To assess the efficacy of the machine learning model, the dataset was partitioned into training and testing subsets at a 70:30 ratio. To ensure model impartiality and accuracy, the dataset underwent meticulous preprocessing steps. This included balancing the dataset to address class imbalances and removing inconsistencies and null values. Additionally, the dataset covered a wide age spectrum, ensuring that the models could accurately predict outcomes across different age groups. Height, weight, and BMI values that were not available were replaced with median values. The distributions after this replacement were checked for normality to assure reliable statistical analysis.

This research attempts to establish associations between NAFLD and various health metrics, predict mortality risk using machine learning algorithms, and explore the effectiveness of different predictive models in identifying long-term health outcomes associated with NAFLD. Python was used for data preprocessing and statistical analysis. Figure 7.1 shows a pair plot, offering a comprehensive visual representation of the relationships between different variables in the dataset. This visual representation offers insight into the correlations and patterns among the different variables, providing a comprehensive overview of their interactions.

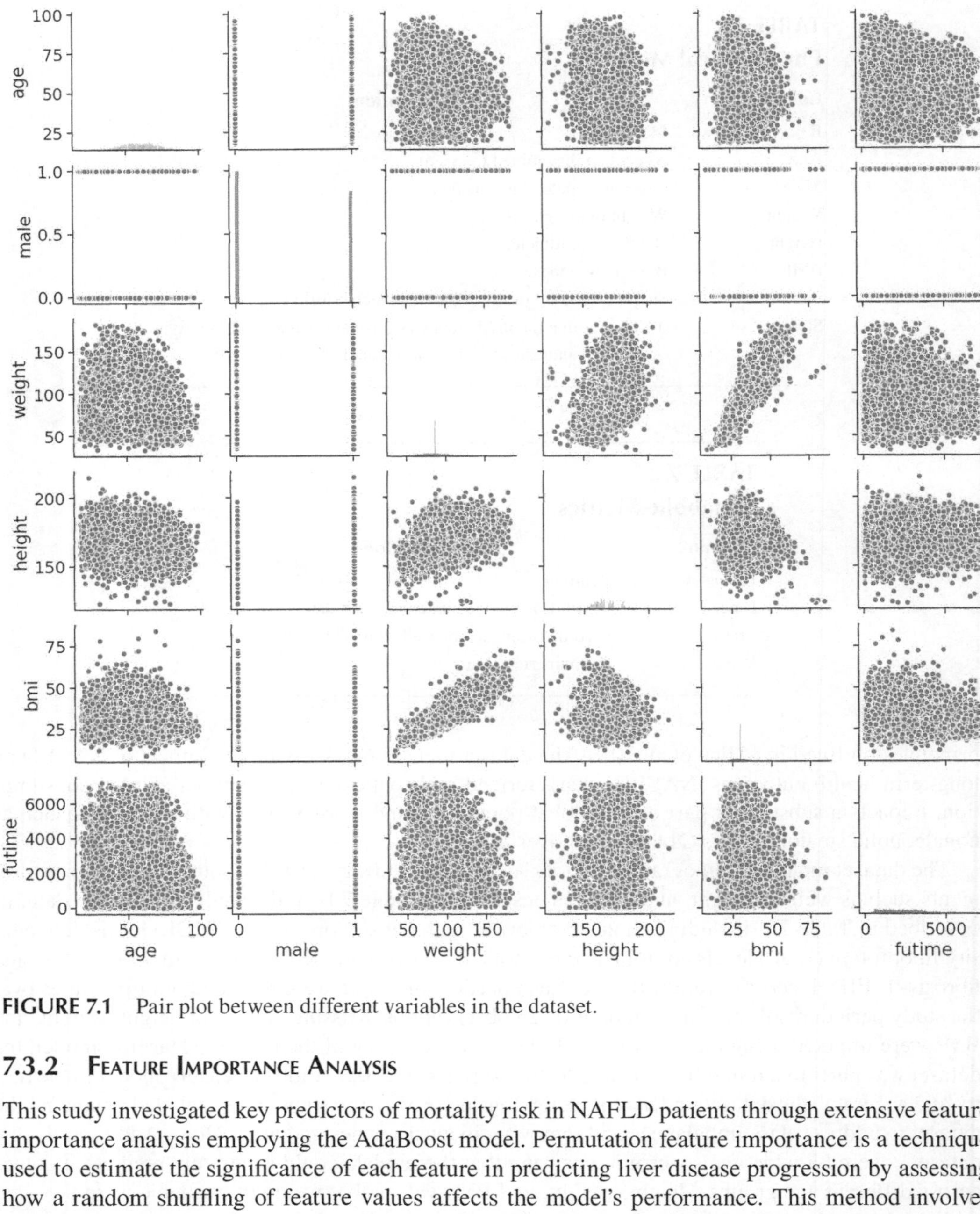

FIGURE 7.1 Pair plot between different variables in the dataset.

7.3.2 Feature Importance Analysis

This study investigated key predictors of mortality risk in NAFLD patients through extensive feature importance analysis employing the AdaBoost model. Permutation feature importance is a technique used to estimate the significance of each feature in predicting liver disease progression by assessing how a random shuffling of feature values affects the model's performance. This method involves training the model on the original dataset and evaluating its performance on a validation set to establish a baseline metric. For each feature, the values are shuffled in a copy of the validation set, and the model's performance is re-evaluated. The change in performance is measured and averaged over multiple iterations to provide a stable estimate of the feature's importance. The analysis revealed several notable factors that have a major impact on the risk of mortality in this group of patients:

Fibrosis Stage: The FIB-4 score has been recognized as a crucial predictor for assessing the severity of liver fibrosis. Advanced liver fibrosis is widely acknowledged as a crucial factor in determining the risk of death among patients with NAFLD. The FIB-4 score is a

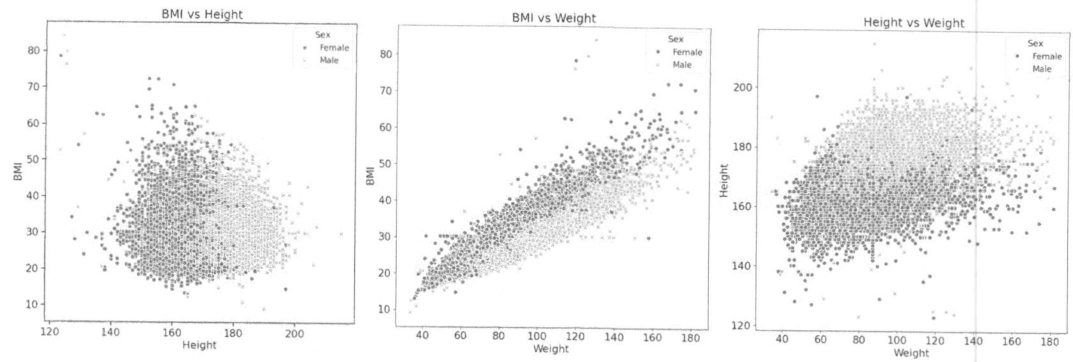

FIGURE 7.2 Relationships among height, weight and BMI.

reliable measure of the severity of liver fibrosis. It allows clinicians to accurately evaluate the prognosis and risk of death associated with NAFLD.

Metabolic Profile: Abnormal cholesterol levels, along with high blood pressure (both systolic and diastolic), have been identified as important factors contributing to the risk of death in NAFLD patients. Metabolic abnormalities are intricately connected to cardiovascular risk factors, which greatly increase the chances of negative cardiovascular events and death in individuals with NAFLD. Hence, it is crucial to implement thorough control of dyslipidemia and hypertension to effectively reduce the risk of mortality among individuals with NAFLD.

Body Mass Index (BMI): Obesity, indicated by a high BMI, has become a notable risk factor for both the onset of NAFLD and its related consequences. An elevated BMI is intricately linked to the pathogenesis of NAFLD, predisposing individuals to hepatic steatosis and subsequent progression to more severe stages of the disease. Moreover, obesity exacerbates metabolic dysfunction and systemic inflammation, further augmenting the risk of adverse outcomes and mortality in NAFLD patients. Figure 7.2 illustrates the relationships among height, weight, and BMI, showing how these physiological measures correlate with each other. This visual representation provides insight into how changes in height and weight influence BMI, a key indicator of body composition and overall health.

Analyzing the significance of these characteristics provides valuable understanding of the clinical factors that are most relevant to mortality associated with NAFLD. Clinicians can optimize interventions and therapeutic strategies for NAFLD patients by identifying and comprehending these crucial predictors. This will effectively reduce mortality risk and improve overall prognosis and outcomes.

7.3.3 Machine Learning Models

Decision Tree (DT): Decision tree algorithms are pivotal in partitioning the data space iteratively, thereby creating subsets based on input features and values to establish homogeneous groups associated with the target variable (Zhang et al. 2021). These algorithms meticulously select features that offer the optimal segregation of data, either by maximizing information gain or minimizing impurity. The iterative process persists until specific termination conditions, such as attaining the maximum depth or reaching a predetermined level of purity, are satisfied. Consequently, decision trees form a hierarchical tree-like structure, where nodes are decision points and leaf nodes provide the final predicted outputs (Bhakta et al. 2023). Decision trees are crucial for accurately categorizing individuals with liver disease by considering many demographic, physiological, and metabolic aspects. This aids in precise diagnosis and treatment.

Algorithm: Decision Tree

1. Begin with the complete dataset as the root node.
2. For each feature, calculate the information gain or Gini index for all possible splits.
3. Choose the feature and the split point that provides the maximum information gain or minimum Gini index.

   The Gini impurity for a node t is calculated as

$$G(t) = 1 - \sum_{i=1}^{c} p(i|t)^2$$

   Where $p(i|t)$ is the probability of class i at node t, and c is the number of classes.

   The information gain for a split A at node t is

$$\text{Gain}(A,t) = G(t) - \sum_{v \in \text{values}(A)} \frac{|t_v|}{|t|} G(t_v)$$

   Where t_v is the subset of t for which feature A has value v.
4. Divide the dataset into two subsets using the selected feature and split point.
5. Iteratively perform steps 2–4 for each subset until a specified stopping condition is reached.
6. Determine the class label for each leaf node by selecting the class that is most frequently represented among the samples in that node.

   The outcome is a hierarchical arrangement in which every internal node signifies a decision made according to a specific characteristic, each branch signifies the consequence of that decision, and each leaf node signifies a classification label.

   Random Forest (RF): RF is a well-known approach in which numerous decision trees are constructed during the training phase, each utilizing a random subset of features and data points (Ho 1995). This diversity ensures that each individual tree captures unique aspects of the dataset, thereby mitigating biases and reducing variance. During the prediction phase, the RF aggregates predictions from each individual tree, typically through averaging or voting mechanisms. This ensemble approach not only minimizes the risk of overfitting but also improves the model's capacity to extrapolate to unfamiliar data (Laha et al. 2023). Random forests are highly proficient at analyzing a wide range of characteristics and accurately predicting the severity of liver illness or the likelihood of developing complications, particularly in the field of liver disease detection.

Algorithm: Random Forest

1. Randomly select B bootstrap samples from the original training data. Each sample is drawn with replacement and is of the same size as the original dataset.
2. For each bootstrap sample b (where $b = 1, 2, \ldots, B$):

   Create a decision tree T_b using the following process:

   At each node, randomly select a subset of m features from the total p features. The value of m is a hyperparameter and is usually $\sqrt{p}$ or $\log_2(p)$

   Among the m selected features, choose the best feature and split point based on a splitting criterion to split the node.

   Grow the tree to the largest extent possible (i.e., until a stopping criterion is met, such as maximum depth or minimum samples per leaf).
3. The final predicted class label for the input instance x is determined by majority voting among the B predicted class labels.

   The final predicted class $\hat{y}$ for an instance x is:

$$\hat{y} = \text{mode}\{T_b(x) : b = 1, 2, \ldots., B\}$$

here $T_b(x)$ is the predicted class by the bth decision tree for input x.

***K*-Nearest Neighbors (KNNs):** KNN algorithms are renowned for their simplicity and effectiveness, particularly in classification tasks. They are widely recognized for addressing regression and classification problems involving datasets of varying sizes, numbers of labels, noise levels, ranges, and contexts. The essence of KNN lies in its ability to identify the '*k*' nearest training data points to a given query instance, typically based on a specified distance measure such as Euclidean distance (Guo et al. 2003). Consequently, the prediction for the query instance is determined by considering the most common class or the average value of the '*k*' closest neighbors. The KNN algorithm excels in liver disease detection by effectively categorizing patients according to their similarity to others with identifiable traits of liver disease. This capability facilitates precise diagnosis and risk assessment.

Algorithm: *K*-Nearest Neighbors

1. Select the desired number of neighbors k.
2. For each input sample:
   Compute the Euclidean distance metric between the input sample and all training samples to get the distance.
   Euclidean distance between two instances x_i andx_j

$$d\left(x_i, x_j\right) = \sqrt{\sum_{l=1}^{n}\left(x_i, l - x_{j,l}\right)^2}$$

   where n is the total number of features, and $x_i, l\ x_{j,l}$ are the feature values of instances x_i and x_j, respectively.
3. For a new instance x, compute the distance between x and all instances in the training set.
   Arrange the distances in order of ascending.
   Select the k instances that have the smallest distances to x. These k instances are the nearest neighbors.
4. Assign the class label to the new instance x based on the majority class among its k-nearest neighbors.
   Let $N_k(x)$ be the set of the k -nearest neighbors of instance$x$
   The predicted class $\hat{y}$ for instance x is

$$\hat{y} = \arg\max_{c} \sum_{x_i \in N_k(x)} 1\left(y_i = c\right)$$

   where y_i is the class label of neighbor x_i, and 1 is the indicator function which equals 1 if $y_i = c$ and 0 otherwise.

Support Vector Machine (SVM): For classification tasks, SVM is an effective machine learning model that establishes a clear boundary between two categories to predict labels using one or more sets of feature vectors (Noble 2006). This decision boundary—known as the hyperplane—is positioned to maximize the separation between the closest data points of each class. These critical data points are called support vectors. SVMs can efficiently handle both linear and nonlinear classification problems by employing various kernel functions to map input features into higher-dimensional spaces (Shmilovici 2005). SVM algorithms are highly effective in categorizing patients with liver diseases into specific disease groups by analyzing complex patterns in their demographic, physiological, and metabolic profiles. This capability supports accurate diagnosis and prediction.

Algorithm: Support Vector Machine

1. Initialize the parameters of the SVM such as regularization parameter C, kernel type).
2. For the linear case:
   Find the hyperplane that optimizes the distance between the two classes. The margin is the precise measurement of the distance that exists between the hyperplane and the closest samples (support vectors) from every class.
3. For the nonlinear case:
   Apply a kernel function (such as polynomial or RBF) on the input data in order to convert it into a space with a higher number of dimensions.
   Determine the hyperplane that optimizes the margin in the transformed space.
4. Use the hyperplane to classify new samples.

Logistic Regression (LR): Logistic regression serves as a cornerstone in binary classification tasks, specifically in the prediction of the likelihood that an instance will belong to a particular class (Nusinovici et al. 2020). Unlike linear regression, logistic regression models the probability using the logistic function, thereby transforming the linear combination of features into a probability score ranging between 0 and 1. The coefficients acquired during the training phase are optimized to minimize the difference between the predicted probability and the actual class labels (Pathak et al. 2023). In liver disease detection, logistic regression models are adept at predicting the likelihood of individuals having certain liver disease conditions based on their comprehensive demographic, physiological, and metabolic profiles.

Algorithm: Logistic Regression

1. Initialize the weights w and bias$b$.
2. For each iteration until convergence:
   Calculate the linear combination of input features and weights:

$$z = w.x + b$$

   Apply the sigmoid function to z, to get the predicted probability:

$$\hat{y} = \sigma(z), \text{ where}$$

$$\sigma(z) = \frac{1}{1+e^{-z}}$$

   Compute the loss using the binary cross-entropy loss function:

$$\text{Loss} = -\frac{1}{N}\sum_{i=1}^{N}\left[y_i \log(\hat{y}) + (1-y_i)\log(1-\widehat{y_i})\right]$$

   Update the weights and bias using gradient descent:

$$w := w - \eta\frac{\partial \text{Loss}}{\partial w}$$

$$b := b - \eta\frac{\partial \text{Loss}}{\partial w}$$

   where η is the learning rate.
3. Use the learned weights and bias to make predictions on new samples.

AdaBoost Model: AdaBoost, also known as adaptive boosting, is a robust ensemble learning strategy that merges several weak learners to form a strong learner. The model iteratively performs training on weak models to correct errors made by preceding models, assigning higher weights to misclassified instances (Chengsheng et al. 2017). The final prediction is obtained by aggregating the predictions derived from these weak models. In liver disease detection, AdaBoost models leverage the diversity among weak learners to predict disease severity or the risk of developing complications based on multifaceted sets of patient features (Bhakta et al. 2023). This amalgamation of diverse models enhances the overall predictive performance and resilience of liver disease detection models.

Algorithm: AdaBoost

1. Initialize the weights of the training samples uniformly.
2. For each iteration t

   Train a weak classifier $h_t(x)$ on the weighted training samples.

   Calculate the error rate ϵ_t of $h_t(x)$

   Compute the classifier weight $\alpha_t = \frac{1}{2}\log\left(\frac{1-\epsilon_t}{\epsilon_t}\right)$

   Update the weights of the training samples

$$w_i := w_i \exp\left(-\alpha_t y_i h_t(x_i)\right)$$

   Normalize the weights.
3. Combine the weak classifiers to form the final strong classifier:

$$H(x) = \text{sign}\left(\sum_{t=1}^{T}\alpha_t\ h_t(x)\right)$$

4. Use the final strong classifier to make predictions on new samples.

7.4 PERFORMANCE METRICS

To evaluate the effectiveness of ML models, various metrics have been employed. The primary measures used to assess the performance of the model include accuracy, precision, recall, and F1-score. Each of these indicators offers distinct perspectives on the model's performance.

a. **Accuracy:** This metric measures the general reliability of a model by counting the number of instances for which the model produced correct outcomes relative to the total number of cases.

$$\text{Accuracy} = \frac{\text{TP}+\text{TN}}{\text{TP}+\text{TN}+\text{FP}+\text{FN}} \tag{7.1}$$

   where:

   TP: Count of positive cases accurately forecasted.

   TN: Count of negative cases correctly forecasted.

   FP: count of negative cases incorrectly forecasted.

   FN: Count of positive cases incorrectly forecasted.

b. **Precision:** Precision quantifies the degree of correctness of optimistic forecasts. This measure calculates how many positive cases were correctly predicted compared to the aggregate count of positive occurrences.

$$\text{Precision} = \frac{\text{TP}}{\text{TP}+\text{FP}} \tag{7.2}$$

c. **Recall:** The model's capacity to identify all positive cases is evaluated by this metric. It is determined by the ratio of TP to the total number of positives.

$$\text{Recall} = \frac{\text{TP}}{\text{TP} + \text{FN}} \tag{7.3}$$

c. **F1-Score:** This metric provides a fair evaluation of the relative importance of recall and precision by calculating their harmonic mean. This approach is especially beneficial when there is an uneven distribution of classes.

$$\text{F1-Score} = 2 \times \frac{\text{Precision} \times \text{Recall}}{\text{Recision} + \text{Recall}} \tag{7.4}$$

7.5 RESULTS AND ANALYSIS

The objective of this analysis was to investigate the intricate correlation between clinical factors and mortality risk in NAFLD patients. By conducting thorough data analysis and utilizing sophisticated ML algorithms, valuable insights were gained into the factors that can predict mortality in this specific set of patients. Six distinct ML models—DT, K-NN, RF, LR, SVM, and AdaBoost—were assessed for their effectiveness in predicting mortality likelihood among NAFLD patients diagnosed from 1997 to 2014. Various physical and biochemical metrics (e.g., HDL, LDL, SBP, DBP, FIB-4 index) and demographic factors (e.g., age, sex, weight, height, BMI) were included in the analysis. Figure 7.3 illustrates the correlation matrix that represents the correlations (ranging from −1 to 1) between different variables in the dataset. In addition, a train-test split of 70/30 was used to ensure that the model could be applied to new data. The confusion matrices for the different models are presented in Figure 7.4. Each subfigure corresponds to a specific model: (a) DT, (b) K-NN, (c) RF, (d) LR, (e) SVM, or (f) AdaBoost. Confusion matrices provide a graphical depiction

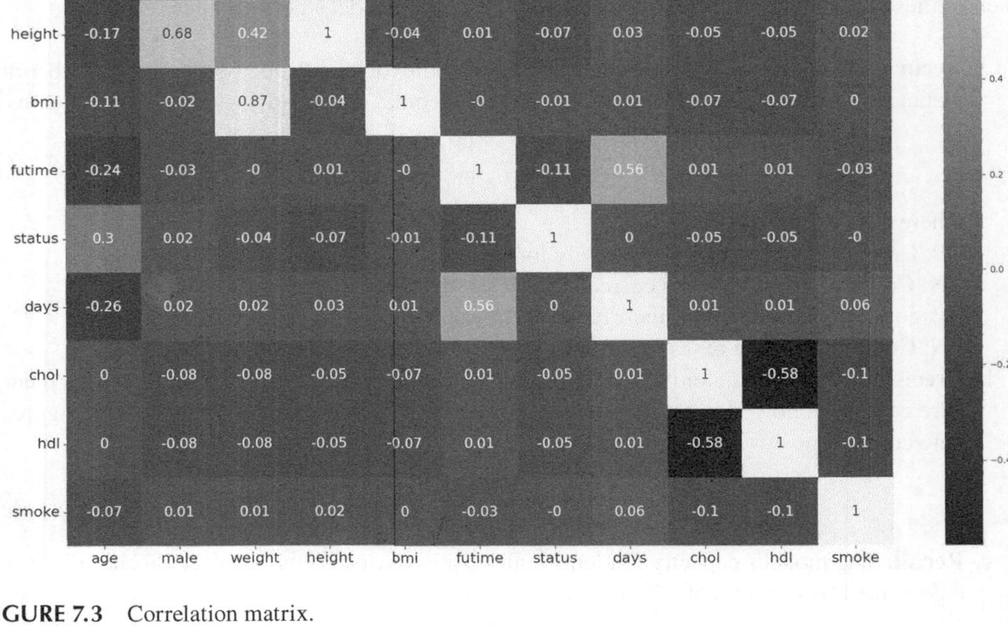

FIGURE 7.3 Correlation matrix.

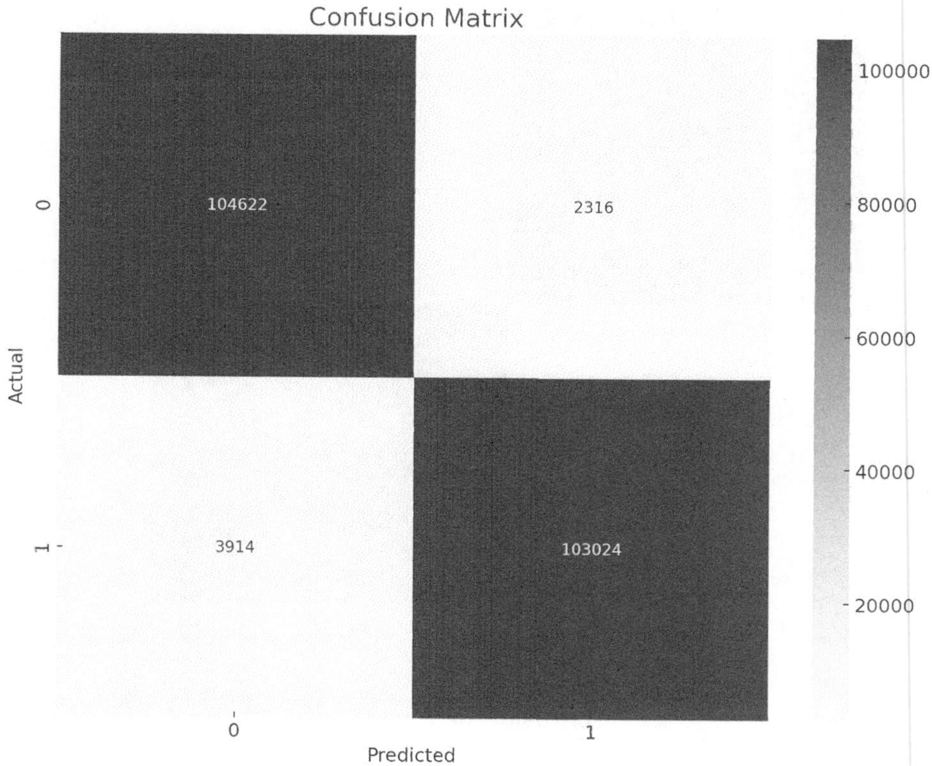

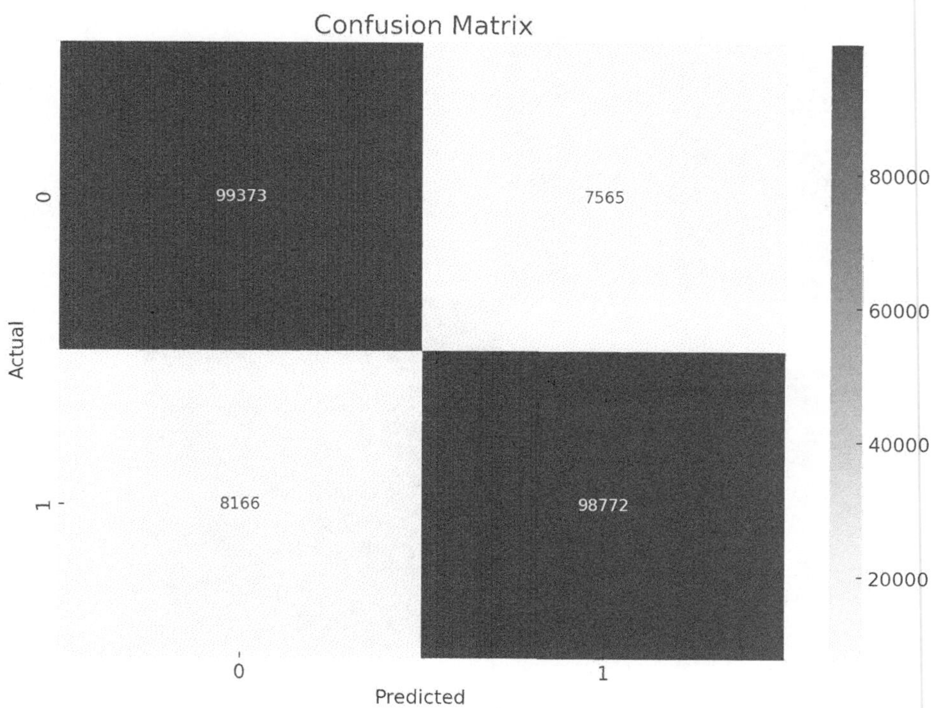

FIGURE 7.4 (a) Confusion matrix for the Decision Tree Model. (b) Confusion matrix for the K-NN Model. (c) Confusion matrix for the RF model. (d) Confusion matrix for the LR model. (e) Confusion matrix for the SVM model. (f) Confusion matrix for the AdaBoost model.

(Continued)

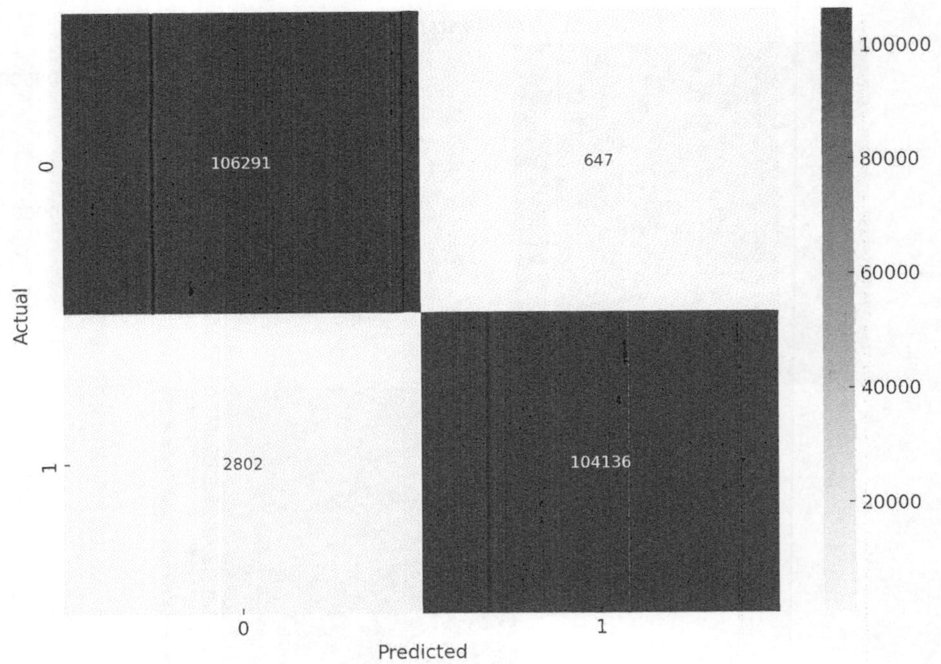

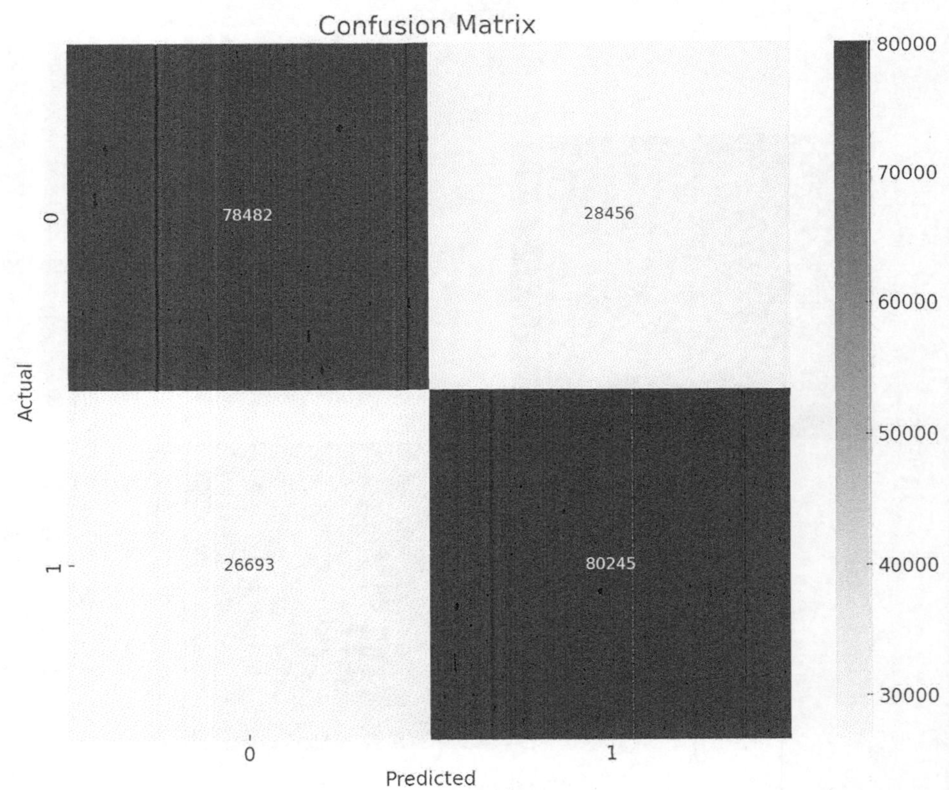

FIGURE 7.4 (*Continued*) (a) Confusion matrix for the Decision Tree Model. (b) Confusion matrix for the K-NN Model. (c) Confusion matrix for the RF model. (d) Confusion matrix for the LR model. (e) Confusion matrix for the SVM model. (f) Confusion matrix for the AdaBoost model.

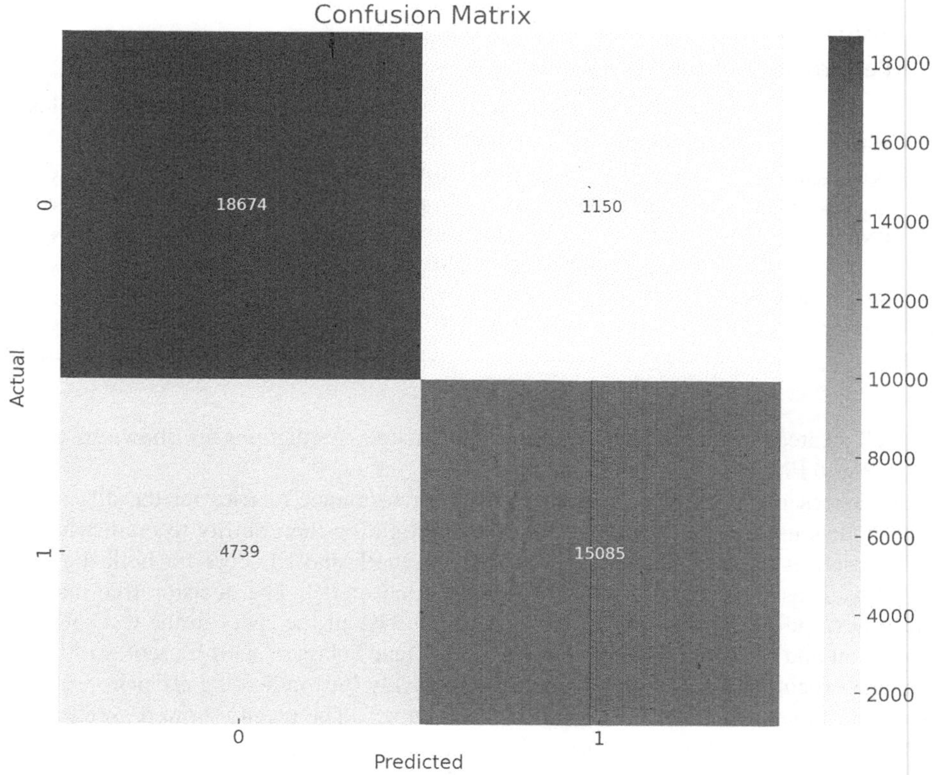

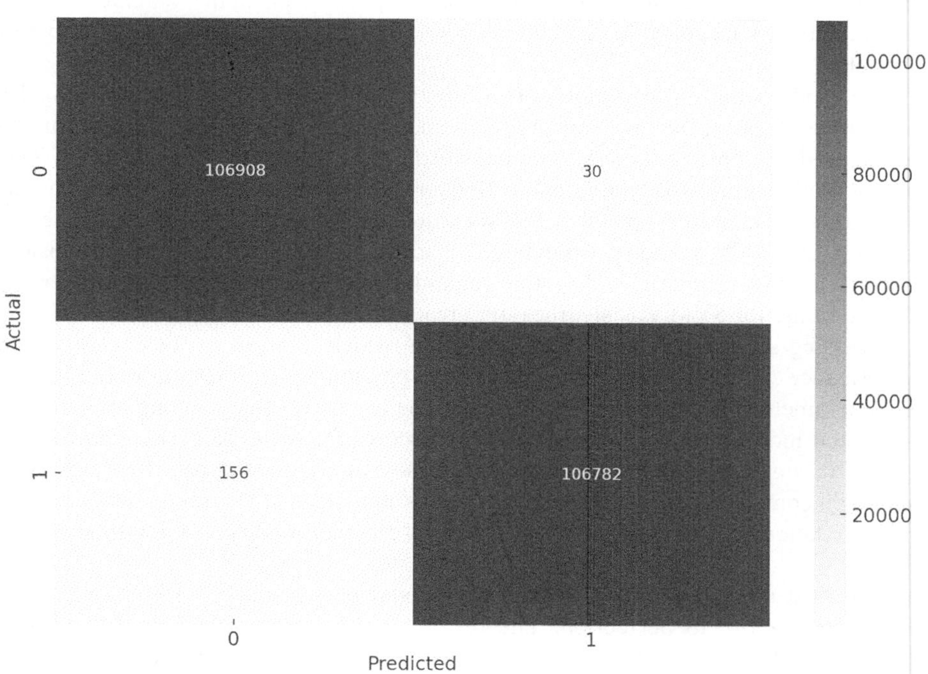

FIGURE 7.4 (*Continued*) (a) Confusion matrix for the Decision Tree Model. (b) Confusion matrix for the K-NN Model. (c) Confusion matrix for the RF model. (d) Confusion matrix for the LR model. (e) Confusion matrix for the SVM model. (f) Confusion matrix for the AdaBoost model.

TABLE 7.3
Performance of the ML Models

		Precision		Recall		F1-score		Execution Time
Model	**Accuracy**	*Alive*	*Dead*	*Alive*	*Dead*	*Alive*	*Dead*	
Decision tree	0.97	0.96	0.98	0.98	0.96	0.97	0.97	5.128 s
Random forest	0.98	0.97	0.99	0.99	0.97	0.98	0.98	115.542 s
KNN	0.93	0.92	0.93	0.93	0.92	0.93	0.93	82.704 s
SVM	0.85	0.80	0.93	0.94	0.76	0.86	0.84	402.345 s
Logistic regression	0.74	0.75	0.74	0.73	0.75	0.74	0.74	0.999 s
AdaBoost	99.91	0.99	0.99	0.99	0.99	0.99	0.99	648.994 s

of how well a categorization model performs. The models' predictions are shown by the counts of TP, TN, FP, and FN.

Table 7.3 presents a thorough summary of the performance metrics for the different machine learning models used in our study, specifically highlighting their ability to predict NAFLD mortality. The metrics include the accuracy, precision, recall, and F1-score for both the "Alive" and "Dead" classes, as well as the execution time for each model. The decision tree model attained 97% accuracy, indicating that it accurately classified 97% of the cases in the test set. It exhibited high precision and recall for both the "Alive" and "Dead" classes, with F1-scores of 0.97 for both classes. The execution time for this model was relatively low, indicating efficient processing. The RF model surpassed the DT model, with a 98% accuracy. The results showed excellent precision, recall, and F1-scores for both categories, demonstrating strong performance in predicting the risk of mortality. The execution time for the random forest was greater than that for the decision tree, which is expected due to the use of the ensemble learning technique in the random forest. However, the trade-off between accuracy and execution time seems justified given the superior performance of the model.

The KNN model achieved an accuracy of 93%, with slightly lower precision, recall, and F1-scores than those of the decision tree and random forest models. However, KNN still performed reasonably well in predicting mortality risk, with balanced performance for both categories. The execution time for KNN was relatively high, indicating a longer processing time compared to that of the decision tree and random forest methods. SVM exhibited lower accuracy than did the decision tree, random forest, and KNN methods, achieving 85% accuracy. It also showed lower precision, recall, and F1-scores for both categories, suggesting suboptimal performance in predicting mortality risk. The execution time for SVM was significantly greater than that of the other models, suggesting a slower processing speed. Although SVMs have been widely used in various classification tasks, their performance in this study was relatively weak, possibly due to the complexity of the dataset and model parameters. Logistic regression yielded the lowest accuracy among all models, at 74%. It demonstrated moderate precision, recall, and F1-scores for both categories, showing mediocre performance in mortality risk prediction. However, logistic regression had the shortest execution time, making it computationally efficient. Despite its simplicity, logistic regression may not capture the complex relationships in the dataset as effectively as other models, leading to lower predictive performance.

The AdaBoost algorithm demonstrated exceptional performance, with an accuracy rate of 99.91%, which is close to perfection. The results showed outstanding precision, recall, and F1-scores for both classes, suggesting excellent performance in predicting mortality risk. Although AdaBoost had the highest execution time among all models, the trade-off between accuracy and processing time is justified given its outstanding performance. The AdaBoost ensemble learning technique efficiently combines weak learners to generate powerful learners,

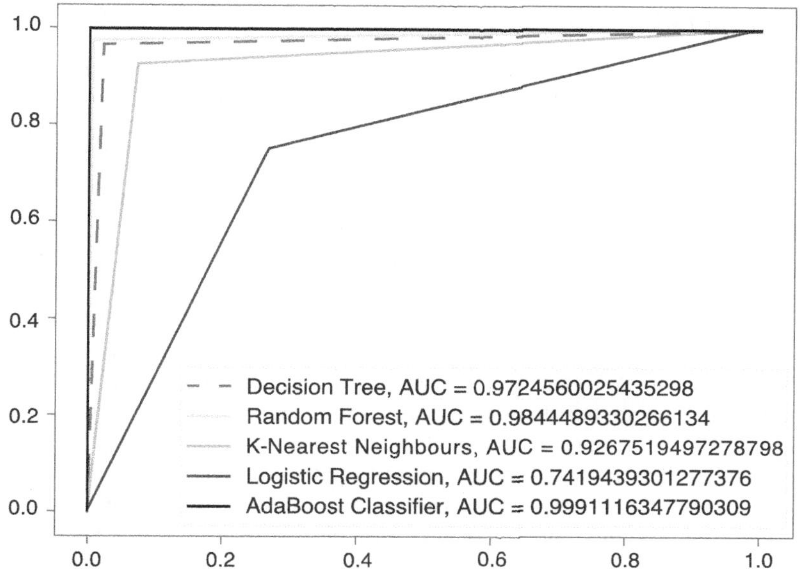

FIGURE 7.5 ROC curves for different ML models.

resulting in highly accurate predictions. The importance of our study lies in the nearly flawless accuracy and F1-score, highlighting the capacity of machine learning models to accurately predict NAFLD mortality. However, a constraint arises from the dataset's insufficient inclusion of various ethnic groups, potentially affecting the applicability of our results. Therefore, it is important for future research efforts to prioritize incorporating diverse datasets to strengthen the reliability of models and improve their ability to make accurate predictions, especially in regard to various ethnic populations. The Receiver Operating Characteristic (ROC) curves of several machine learning models are shown in Figure 7.5. Through plotting of the true positive rate against the false positive rate at various threshold values, the ROC curve illustrates the diagnostic performance of each model. A larger area under the curve (AUC) implies superior performance, with the curve positioned closer to the top-left corner reflecting greater sensitivity and specificity. This comparison demonstrates the efficacy of each model in forecasting outcomes in individuals with NAFLD.

The implications of the results are important for the evaluation of risk in clinical settings and the creation of tailored approaches to managing patients with NAFLD. By employing ML algorithms and understanding key mortality indicators, healthcare practitioners can quickly identify individuals with a high risk of death in the early stages of a disease and provide targeted interventions to minimize adverse outcomes. Strategies focused on managing liver fibrosis, optimizing metabolic parameters, and addressing obesity are crucial for decreasing the risk of mortality and improving the long-term prognosis of patients with NAFLD.

Although our study offers valuable insights into predicting mortality in NAFLD patients, it has limitations. The findings of our study may have limited generalizability due to the retrospective nature of the dataset and the inherent biases associated with observational studies. Moreover, additional investigations are necessary to validate the predictive models for various patient demographics and evaluate their practical value in real-life scenarios. Further research should investigate the incorporation of innovative biomarkers and imaging techniques to increase the precision of mortality prediction models for NAFLD patients.

7.6 CONCLUSIONS

This research has underscored the remarkable efficacy of machine learning models in accurately predicting mortality risk among NAFLD patients. Initial challenges included selecting the most suitable ML model among several options and ensuring the integration of diverse patient data. Through meticulous analysis and comparison, AdaBoost emerged as the optimal model, achieving outstanding performance with an accuracy, precision, recall, and F1 score of 99%. Decisions regarding model selection and feature incorporation are pivotal in achieving these outcomes. The successful integration of a wide array of physical, biochemical, and demographic measurements enabled precise mortality forecasts. The outcomes highlight the potential of AdaBoost in clinical settings for risk categorization and early intervention strategies among NAFLD patients.

Future research should focus on integrating multimodal data, such as genetic, proteomic, metabolomic, imaging, and clinical data, to enhance diagnostic accuracy and provide deeper insights into the disease. Advancements in imaging techniques and longitudinal studies could improve early detection and monitoring of disease progression. The development of personalized treatment plans facilitated by predictive models could optimize patient outcomes. Additionally, exploring the integration of wearable technology, enhancing screening programs, implementing real-time data analysis and feedback systems, and using telemedicine for remote monitoring and management could significantly advance the field. The development of predictive models for complications and the creation of robust algorithms for remote consultations could further improve access to care and patient engagement.

REFERENCES

AL Abed, Hadeel S., and Layla M. Alameri. 2019. "Detection of the Level of Human ALT Liver Enzyme Concentration by Using Laser Biosensor Multimode Fibres (MMF)." *Biochemical & Cellular Archives.*

Allen, Alina M., Terry M. Therneau, Joseph J. Larson, Alexandra Coward, Virend K. Somers, and Patrick S. Kamath. 2018. "Nonalcoholic Fatty Liver Disease Incidence and Impact on Metabolic Burden and Death: A 20 Year-Community Study." *Hepatology* 67 (5): 1726–36. https://doi.org/10.1002/hep.29546

Ancona, Stefania, Francesca D. Faraci, Elina Khatab, Luigi Fiorillo, Oriella Gnarra, Tobias Nef, Claudio L. A. Bassetti, and Panagiotis Bargiotas. 2022. "Wearables in the Home-Based Assessment of Abnormal Movements in Parkinson's Disease: A Systematic Review of the Literature." *Journal of Neurology* 269 (1): 100–110. https://doi.org/10.1007/s00415-020-10350-3

Aslam, Muhamamd Haseeb, Syed Fawad Hussain, and Raja Hashim Ali. 2022. "Predictive Analysis on Severity of Non-Alcoholic Fatty Liver Disease (NAFLD) Using Machine Learning Algorithms." In *2022 17th International Conference on Emerging Technologies (ICET)*, 95–100. https://doi.org/10.1109/ICET56601.2022.10004660

Atsawarungruangkit, Amporn, Passisd Laoveeravat, and Kittichai Promrat. 2021. "Machine Learning Models for Predicting Non-Alcoholic Fatty Liver Disease in the General United States Population: NHANES Database." *World Journal of Hepatology* 13 (10): 1417–27. https://doi.org/10.4254/wjh.v13.i10.1417

Ben-Assuli, Ofir, Arie Jacobi, Orit Goldman, Shani Shenhar-Tsarfaty, Ori Rogowski, David Zeltser, Itzhak Shapira, Shlomo Berliner, and Shira Zelber-Sagi. 2022. "Stratifying Individuals into Non-Alcoholic Fatty Liver Disease Risk Levels Using Time Series Machine Learning Models." *Journal of Biomedical Informatics* 126 (February):103986. https://doi.org/10.1016/j.jbi.2022.103986

Benedict, Mark, and Xuchen Zhang. 2017. "Non-Alcoholic Fatty Liver Disease: An Expanded Review." *World Journal of Hepatology* 9 (16): 715–32. https://doi.org/10.4254/wjh.v9.i16.715

Bhakta, Susmit Sekhar, Bikash Sadhukhan, and Nabanita Das. 2023. "Enhancing Early Detection of Cardiovascular Diseases Using Machine Learning Techniques: A Comparative Study." In *2023 3rd International Conference on Innovative Mechanisms for Industry Applications (ICIMIA)*, 875–80. https://doi.org/10.1109/ICIMIA60377.2023.10426035

Bhakta, Susmit Sekhar, Sangita Ghosh, and Bikash Sadhukhan. 2023. "Credit Card Fraud Detection Using Machine Learning: A Comparative Study of Ensemble Learning Algorithms." In *2023 9th International Conference on Smart Computing and Communications (ICSCC)*, 296–301. https://doi.org/10.1109/ICSCC59169.2023.10335075

Brönneke, Jan Benedikt, Jennifer Müller, Konstantinos Mouratis, Julia Hagen, and Ariel Dora Stern. 2021. "Regulatory, Legal, and Market Aspects of Smart Wearables for Cardiac Monitoring." *Sensors* 21 (14): 4937. https://doi.org/10.3390/s21144937

Buckholz, Adam P., and Russell Rosenblatt. 2023. "Remote Monitoring of Cognition in Cirrhosis and Encephalopathy: Future Opportunity and Challenge." *Metabolic Brain Disease* 38 (5): 1737–47. https://doi.org/10.1007/s11011-022-01134-x

Chengsheng, Tu, Liu Huacheng, and Xu Bing. 2017. "AdaBoost Typical Algorithm and Its Application Research." *MATEC Web of Conferences* 139: 00222. https://doi.org/10.1051/matecconf/201713900222

Chuang, Ya-Hsuan, Yun-Tzu Chang, Kuo-Liang Liu, Hwan-You Chang, and Tri-Rung Yew. 2011. "Electrical Impedimetric Biosensors for Liver Function Detection." *Biosensors and Bioelectronics* 28 (1): 368–72. https://doi.org/10.1016/j.bios.2011.07.049

Delmastro, Franca, Flavio Di Martino, and Cristina Dolciotti. 2020. "Cognitive Training and Stress Detection in MCI Frail Older People through Wearable Sensors and Machine Learning." *IEEE Access* 8: 65573–90. https://doi.org/10.1109/ACCESS.2020.2985301

Dunn, Michael A., Matthew R. Kappus, Pamela M. Bloomer, Andres Duarte-Rojo, Deborah A. Josbeno, and John M. Jakicic. 2021. "Wearables, Physical Activity, and Exercise Testing in Liver Disease." *Seminars in Liver Disease* 41 (2): 128–35. https://doi.org/10.1055/s-0040-1716564

Fernando, Dinali H., Josephine M. Forbes, Peter W. Angus, and Chandana B. Herath. 2019. "Development and Progression of Non-Alcoholic Fatty Liver Disease: The Role of Advanced Glycation End Products." *International Journal of Molecular Sciences* 20 (20): 5037. https://doi.org/10.3390/ijms20205037

Guo, Gongde, Hui Wang, David Bell, Yaxin Bi, and Kieran Greer. 2003. "KNN Model-Based Approach in Classification." In *On the Move to Meaningful Internet Systems 2003: CoopIS, DOA, and ODBASE*, edited by Robert Meersman, Zahir Tari, and Douglas C. Schmidt, 986–96. Lecture Notes in Computer Science. Berlin, Heidelberg: Springer. https://doi.org/10.1007/978-3-540-39964-3_62

Haas, Mary E., James P. Pirruccello, Samuel N. Friedman, Minxian Wang, Connor A. Emdin, Veeral H. Ajmera, Tracey G. Simon, et al. 2021. "Machine Learning Enables New Insights into Genetic Contributions to Liver Fat Accumulation." *Cell Genomics* 1 (3): 100066. https://doi.org/10.1016/j.xgen.2021.100066

Ho, Tin Kam. 1995. "Random Decision Forests." In *Proceedings of 3rd International Conference on Document Analysis and Recognition*, vol. 1, 278–82. Montreal, Que., Canada: IEEE Comput. Soc. Press. https://doi.org/10.1109/ICDAR.1995.598994

Ji, Weidong, Mingyue Xue, Yushan Zhang, Hua Yao, and Yushan Wang. 2022. "A Machine Learning Based Framework to Identify and Classify Non-Alcoholic Fatty Liver Disease in a Large-Scale Population." *Frontiers in Public Health* 10:846118. https://doi.org/10.3389/fpubh.2022.846118

Kalra, Arjun, Ekrem Yetiskul, Chase J. Wehrle, and Faiz Tuma. 2024. "Physiology, Liver." In *StatPearls*. Treasure Island (FL): StatPearls Publishing. https://www.ncbi.nlm.nih.gov/books/NBK535438/

Kim, Yoon, Jinserk Seo, So-Yeon An, Dong Hyun Sinn, and Ji Hye Hwang. 2020. "Efficacy and Safety of an mHealth App and Wearable Device in Physical Performance for Patients With Hepatocellular Carcinoma: Development and Usability Study." *JMIR mHealth and uHealth* 8 (3): e14435. https://doi.org/10.2196/14435

Laha, Bishal, Debopriya Basu, Souvik Biswas, Pallabi Gupta, and Bikash Sadhukhan. 2023. "Intrusion Detection in IoT Systems Using Ensemble Machine Learning Techniques." In *2023 IEEE 4th Annual Flagship India Council International Subsections Conference (INDISCON)*, 1–7. https://doi.org/10.1109/INDISCON58499.2023.10270505

Li, Xiao, Jessilyn Dunn, Denis Salins, Gao Zhou, Wenyu Zhou, Sophia Miryam Schüssler-Fiorenza Rose, Dalia Perelman, Elizabeth Colbert, Ryan Runge, and Shannon Rego. 2017. "Digital Health: Tracking Physiomes and Activity Using Wearable Biosensors Reveals Useful Health-Related Information." *PLoS Biology* 15 (1): e2001402.

Maurice, James, and Pinelopi Manousou. 2018. "Non-Alcoholic Fatty Liver Disease." *Clinical Medicine (London, England)* 18 (3): 245–50. https://doi.org/10.7861/clinmedicine.18-3-245

Mishra, Tejaswini, Meng Wang, Ahmed A. Metwally, Gireesh K. Bogu, Andrew W. Brooks, Amir Bahmani, Arash Alavi, et al. 2020. "Pre-Symptomatic Detection of COVID-19 from Smartwatch Data." *Nature Biomedical Engineering* 4 (12): 1208–20. https://doi.org/10.1038/s41551-020-00640-6

Naderi Yaghouti, Amir Reza, Hamed Zamanian, and Ahmad Shalbaf. 2024. "Machine Learning Approaches for Early Detection of Non-Alcoholic Steatohepatitis Based on Clinical and Blood Parameters." *Scientific Reports* 14 (1): 2442. https://doi.org/10.1038/s41598-024-51741-0

Neogi, Anandarupa, Anubhav Jaiswal, Ankush Kumar, Jyoti Anand, and Bikash Sadhukhan. 2024. "Predictive Modeling for Mortality Risk in Nonalcoholic Fatty Liver Disease Patients: A Machine Learning Approach." In *2024 Second International Conference on Data Science and Information System (ICDSIS)*, 1–6. https://doi.org/10.1109/ICDSIS61070.2024.10594545

Noble, William S. 2006. "What Is a Support Vector Machine?" *Nature Biotechnology* 24 (12): 1565–67. https://doi.org/10.1038/nbt1206-1565

Nusinovici, Simon, Yih Chung Tham, Marco Yu Chak Yan, Daniel Shu Wei Ting, Jialiang Li, Charumathi Sabanayagam, Tien Yin Wong, and Ching-Yu Cheng. 2020. "Logistic Regression Was as Good as Machine Learning for Predicting Major Chronic Diseases." *Journal of Clinical Epidemiology* 122 (June): 56–69. https://doi.org/10.1016/j.jclinepi.2020.03.002

Pan, Hong, Baocheng Liu, Xin Luo, Xinxin Shen, Jijia Sun, and An Zhang. 2023. "Non-Alcoholic Fatty Liver Disease Risk Prediction Model and Health Management Strategies for Older Chinese Adults: A Cross-Sectional Study." *Lipids in Health and Disease* 22. https://doi.org/10.1186/s12944-023-01966-1

Pathak, Tanusree, Susmit Bhakta, Arghya Das, and Bikash Sadhukhan. 2023. *Development of an Ensemble Machine Learning-Based Decision Support System for Patient Admission in Healthcare Unit.* https://doi.org/10.1109/ELEXCOM58812.2023.10370105

Razmpour, Farkhondeh, Reza Daryabeygi-Khotbehsara, Davood Soleimani, Hamzeh Asgharnezhad, Afshar Shamsi, Ghasem Sadeghi Bajestani, Mohsen Nematy, Mahdiyeh Razm Pour, Ralph Maddison, and Sheikh Mohammed Shariful Islam. 2023. "Application of Machine Learning in Predicting Non-Alcoholic Fatty Liver Disease Using Anthropometric and Body Composition Indices." *Scientific Reports* 13 (1): 4942. https://doi.org/10.1038/s41598-023-32129-y

Sabry, Farida, Tamer Eltaras, Wadha Labda, Khawla Alzoubi, and Qutaibah Malluhi. 2022. "Machine Learning for Healthcare Wearable Devices: The Big Picture." *Journal of Healthcare Engineering* 2022 (April): 4653923. https://doi.org/10.1155/2022/4653923

Schattenberg, Jörn M., Naga Chalasani, and Naim Alkhouri. 2023. "Artificial Intelligence Applications in Hepatology." *Clinical Gastroenterology and Hepatology* 21 (8): 2015–25. https://doi.org/10.1016/j.cgh.2023.04.007

Schneider, Carolin V., Inuk Zandvakili, Christoph A. Thaiss, and Kai Markus Schneider. 2021. "Physical Activity Is Associated with Reduced Risk of Liver Disease in the Prospective UK Biobank Cohort." *JHEP Reports* 3 (3). https://doi.org/10.1016/j.jhepr.2021.100263

Shmilovici, Armin. 2005. "Support Vector Machines." In *Data Mining and Knowledge Discovery Handbook*, edited by Oded Maimon and Lior Rokach, 257–76. Boston, MA: Springer US. https://doi.org/10.1007/0-387-25465-X_12

Sorino, Paolo, Angelo Campanella, Caterina Bonfiglio, Antonella Mirizzi, Isabella Franco, Antonella Bianco, Maria Gabriella Caruso, et al. 2021. "Development and Validation of a Neural Network for NAFLD Diagnosis." *Scientific Reports* 11 (October):20240. https://doi.org/10.1038/s41598-021-99400-y

Tang, Jianbin, Rima El Atrache, Shuang Yu, Umar Asif, Michele Jackson, Subhrajit Roy, Mahtab Mirmomeni, et al. 2021. "Seizure Detection Using Wearable Sensors and Machine Learning: Setting a Benchmark." *Epilepsia* 62 (8): 1807–19. https://doi.org/10.1111/epi.16967

Teng, Margaret Lp, Cheng Han Ng, Daniel Q. Huang, Kai En Chan, Darren Jh Tan, Wen Hui Lim, Ju Dong Yang, Eunice Tan, and Mark D. Muthiah. 2023. "Global Incidence and Prevalence of Nonalcoholic Fatty Liver Disease." *Clinical and Molecular Hepatology* 29 (Suppl): S32–42. https://doi.org/10.3350/cmh.2022.0365

Torres-Soto, Jessica, and Euan A. Ashley. 2020. "Multi-Task Deep Learning for Cardiac Rhythm Detection in Wearable Devices." *Npj Digital Medicine* 3 (1): 1–8. https://doi.org/10.1038/s41746-020-00320-4

Vijayan, Vini, James P. Connolly, Joan Condell, Nigel McKelvey, and Philip Gardiner. 2021. "Review of Wearable Devices and Data Collection Considerations for Connected Health." *Sensors* 21 (16): 5589. https://doi.org/10.3390/s21165589

Voss, Andreas, Rico Schroeder, Steffen Schulz, Jens Haueisen, Stefanie Vogler, Paul Horn, Andreas Stallmach, and Philipp Reuken. 2022. "Detection of Liver Dysfunction Using a Wearable Electronic Nose System Based on Semiconductor Metal Oxide Sensors." *Biosensors* 12 (2): 70. https://doi.org/10.3390/bios12020070

Wang, Yu-Chiang, Xiaobo Xu, Adrija Hajra, Samuel Apple, Amrin Kharawala, Gustavo Duarte, Wasla Liaqat, et al. 2022. "Current Advancement in Diagnosing Atrial Fibrillation by Utilizing Wearable Devices and Artificial Intelligence: A Review Study." *Diagnostics* 12 (3): 689. https://doi.org/10.3390/diagnostics12030689

Weng, Shuwei, Die Hu, Jin Chen, Yanyi Yang, and Daoquan Peng. 2023. "Prediction of Fatty Liver Disease in a Chinese Population Using Machine-Learning Algorithms." *Diagnostics* 13 (6): 1168. https://doi.org/10.3390/diagnostics13061168

Zhang, Chenmeng, Can Hu, Shijun Xie, and Shuping Cao. 2021. "Research on the Application of Decision Tree and Random Forest Algorithm in the Main Transformer Fault Evaluation." *Journal of Physics: Conference Series* 1732 (1): 012086. https://doi.org/10.1088/1742-6596/1732/1/012086

Zhao, Qi, Yadi Lan, Xunjun Yin, and Kai Wang. 2023. "Image-Based AI Diagnostic Performance for Fatty Liver: A Systematic Review and Meta-Analysis." *BMC Medical Imaging* 23 (1): 208. https://doi.org/10.1186/s12880-023-01172-6

8 Predicting Cognitive Impairment through Handwriting Analysis

A Machine Learning Framework for Enhanced Clinical Decision-Making

P. Swathypriyadharsini, and K. Premalatha

8.1 INTRODUCTION

Machine learning (ML) models allows machines to dynamically learn and perform a desired task with no intervention of explicit programming. The main objective of this technology is to replace the need for rule-based systems with more sophisticated statistical methods and algorithms. A key element in developing a good machine learning model is nothing by the underlying dataset. Consequently, if the dataset is more pertinent, then the prediction is more accurate. In several fields such as finance, retail, and health-care, has employed machine learning for various purposes (Dhillon and Singh 2019). Nowadays, Machine Learning algorithms are extensively applied in healthcare industry for diagnosing any disease at early stage and thereby enabling to provide the treatment (Sinha et al. 2020). Machine learning's capacity to continually improve data for precise prediction and categorization in disease diagnosis is one of its key features (Wuest et al. 2018). Machine learning techniques can be applied to extract relevant data from patient datasets contained in electronic health records (Chen et al. 2017). By evaluating data and applying disease-causing variables from electronic health records, machine learning algorithms can assist in the diagnosis of diseases and anticipate their underlying causes (Ngiam and Khor 2019). When it came to classification, prediction, and clustering tasks, machine learning became more popular than the conventional bio-statistical technique when it came to assessing and integrating massive volumes of complex healthcare data (Garg and Mago 2021). Reconstruction of medical images (Schlemper et al. 2017), segmentation of brain tumors (Mehta and Majumdar, 2017), classification of interstitial lung illnesses (Anthimopoulos et al. 2016), and identification of bodily organs from medical images (Yan et al. 2016) are only a few of the tasks in which machine learning has recently shown remarkable results.

8.1.1 ML in Medical Field

ML is a subset of AI where models are trained on data so they can predict future events or operate without explicit programming. Figure 8.1 illustrates how machine learning has the ability to completely change the pattern of disease identification, treatment, which in turn prevents the illnesses in the healthcare industry. The data may be collected from an existing database or it can be driven from the sensors of the patient monitoring devices. Initially, the data must be preprocessed before applying the machine learning model irrespective of its kind and type. Any machine learning techniques such as classification, clustering or simple mining techniques or a deep learning model can

DOI: 10.1201/9781003486640-8

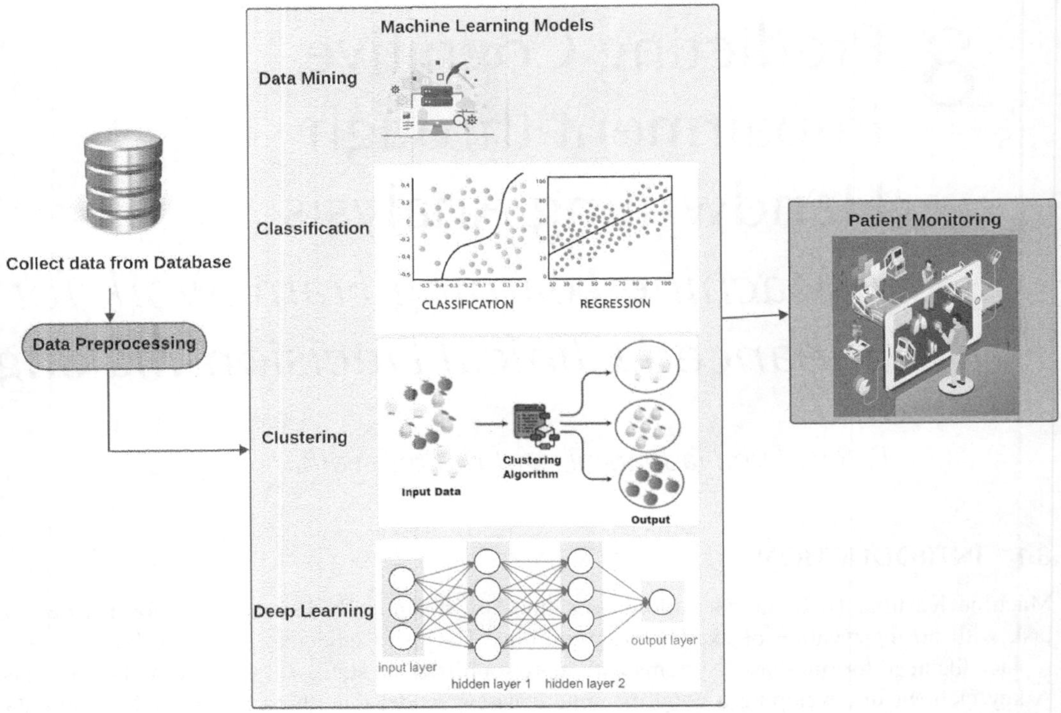

FIGURE 8.1 ML in medical industry.

then be constructed from a training data. After the system model is built, the model must be tested using test data before deployment. At last, the model can be deployed for monitoring the patient health condition and thereby help in early detection and identification of any kind of diseases which might help in the positive outcome for the patients.

Below are the predominant applications of ML in Medical industry:

- **Identifying Diseases and Diagnosis:**
  The primary use of ML within the medical industry are the identity and prognosis of illness and conditions that are normally thought to be hard to diagnose. This can encompass anything from hereditary illnesses to tumors that are difficult to detect in their early stages.
- **Drug Discovery and Manufacturing:**
  Early-stage drug development is one of the important clinical uses of machine learning. This also involves research and development tools that can aid in the discovery of alternate avenues for the treatment of multiple diseases, such as precision medicine and next-generation sequencing.
- **Medical Imaging Diagnosis:**
  The ML algorithm system employs a collection of input images for training purposes to determine which image features, when applied, would lead to the accurate classification of the image—that is, portraying a benign or malignant tumor.
- **Outbreak Prediction:**
  ML algorithms employ many data sources, including claims and digital health records, to predict the probability of particular fitness outcomes, such the onset of chronic illnesses or clinic readmissions. This can assist medical professionals in identifying high-risk patients and implementing preventative actions to avoid unfavorable consequences.

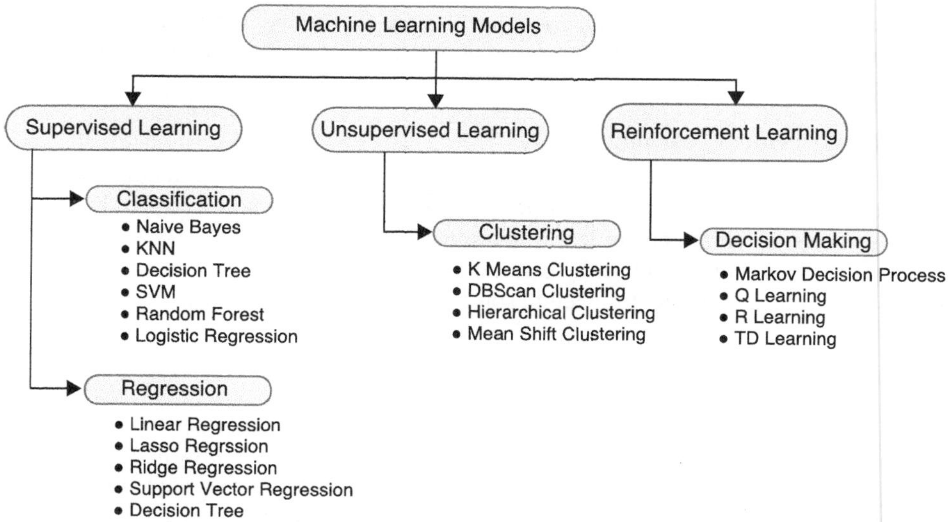

FIGURE 8.2 Types of ML models.

- **Clinical Trial and Research:**
  Clinical trials and research are two areas where machine learning may find various uses. Clinical trials are high priced in terms of both time and money, and they often take years to finish, as anyone in the pharmaceutical business will attest. Researchers can select participants for clinical trials by using machine learning based predictive analytics to combine data from social media, medical records, and other sources.

8.1.2 Types of ML Models

ML can be majorly categorized into three categories: supervised learning, unsupervised learning and reinforcement learning (Saravanan and Sujatha 2018). Different kinds of ML model types are shown in Figure 8.2 along with the techniques and algorithms applied to each category.

8.1.2.1 Supervised Machine Learning Model

One of the easiest ML models is the supervised learning model, where the output is a known label or result and the incoming data is referred to as training data (Jiang et al. 2020). Thus, supervised learning model works only with labeled datasets where it is trained with known input and output pair (Nasteski, 2017). Then, in order to perform some predictive analysis on unknown data, a function that can be trained using a training data set must be created. Task-based, labeled data sets are used to assess supervised learning. Classification and Regression are the two major widely used models in supervised learning (Hastie et al. 2009, Sen et al. 2020).

8.1.2.2 Unsupervised Machine Learning Model

Unsupervised machine learning is a type of machine learning methodology in which an algorithm looks for links and patterns in unlabeled data (Qian et al. 2019). Unsupervised learning does not require giving the algorithm labeled target outputs, in contrast to supervised learning. Finding underlying patterns, similarities, or clusters in the data is frequently the main objective of unsupervised learning. These findings can subsequently be applied to a variety of tasks, including dimensionality reduction, data exploration, and visualization (Li et al. 2020). Clustering is the majorly utilized unsupervised model for finding the relationships in the unlabeled dataset. It groups the similar data into clusters based on some similarity score (Serra and Tagliaferri 2019, Madhulatha 2012). It's particularly useful when there is need of obtaining labeled data costs a significant amount of money, time, or resources. (Reddy et al. 2018).

8.1.2.3 Reinforcement Learning

An approach to learning that engages with the environment by generating actions and identifying mistakes is the reinforcement machine learning algorithm (Qiang and Zhongli 2011). The most important features of reinforcement learning are trial and error and delay. With this method, the model learns the behavior or pattern by continuously improving its performance through Reward Feedback. These algorithms are designed to solve a specific issue (Nian et al. 2020).

8.2 LITERATURE REVIEW

In recent days, millions of individuals globally are impacted by diseases that cause cognitive impairments in which the diseases Alzheimer's and Parkinson's being the most prevalent (De Stefano et al. 2017). It is anticipated that in the coming decades, their incidence will rise due to the global average lifetime increment. Handwriting is one of the initial daily tasks that is impacted by cognitive deficits. Because of this, scientists have also started looking at the examination of changes in handwriting as diagnostic indicators for these kinds of illnesses.

To address cognitive impairments, it typically mean a broad range of neurological problems that affect particular populations of neurons in particular functional anatomic areas. These disorders begin for unknown reasons and proceed relentlessly (Przedborski et al. 2003). There is presently no cure for these diseases, despite the fact that therapies may help with some of the psychological or physical symptoms connected to them. Even if it's still a challenging task, an early detection greatly improves efficacy of the existing treatments. On the other hand, the action of Handwriting of a person results from a complex network composed by cognitive, kinesthetic, and perceptual-motor abilities (Tseng and Cermak 1993). In addition, there is a need for dexterity, manual abilities, visual-motor integration, eye-hand coordination, motor planning, and kinesthetic awareness. Both Parkinson's and Alzheimer's diseases are characterized by notable alterations in handwriting performance.

In order to distinguish Alzheimer patients from people with typical cognitive ability (accuracy of 0.924) and to forecast which mild cognitive impairment patients would progress to AD versus returning to typical cognition (area under the receiver operating characteristic curve/AUROC of 0.9708), (Hinrichs et al. 2011) employed machine learning to analyze a combination of imaging, biological, and cognitive assessment testing data. Their multi-kernel learning method served as the foundation for their ML model, limiting its overall complexity and facilitating the study of a broad scope of complicated and varied types of data. Using the findings of neuropsychological evaluations and Alzheimer biomarkers, (Massetti et al. 2022) used a random forest machine learning model to predict the transition from mild cognitive impairment to Alzheimer, and they were able to reach an accuracy of 0.86.

Key risk factors, such as demographics (education, venerable age, gender, etc.) (Perez et al. 2021), physical conditions (body mass index (BMI), hearing difficulty, etc.) (Ren et al. 2021, Chen 2021), lifestyle choices (drinking, smoking, and engaging in instrumental activities of daily living (IADL) (Katayama et al. 2020), low psychological wellbeing (depression, for example) (Fang et al. 2021, Costanza et al. 2015, 2020), and chronic illnesses (chronic lower back pain, for example), have all been successfully identified using conventional regression-based approaches. It was believed that long-term cognitive deterioration might be predicted by the RF model. Furthermore, compared to logistic regression, the random forest method may be able to predict long-term cognitive impairment outcomes more accurately. Additionally, the risk variables that have the most effects on cognitive impairment could be eliminated by an ML model (Abd-El Mohsen et al. 2021). Therefore, in our research work, we have applied ML models such as Decision Trees, Support Vector Machines, XGBoost, Random Forest and also neural networks are being utilized for the predictive analytics.

8.3 METHODOLOGY

This research study's main objective is to offer a coherent machine learning framework for selecting the optimum prediction model for every real-world data sample. In this research work, DARWIN handwriting dataset has been utilized for developing the machine learning model. Any real life handwriting dataset can also be applied for creating this prediction model. Preparing the data is an essential step that can improve the accuracy of the ML model. Data preprocessing methods include transformation, cleansing, and reduction; in the event that the dataset is extremely large, the dimension may be lowered. Subsequently, the prediction model is created by using various machine learning methods, including Decision Tree, Extreme Boost, Ada Boost, Random Forest, Linear Model, SVM, and Neural Networks. Finally, performance metrics including accuracy, precision, recall, specificity, and F1-score are used to assess each machine learning model's effectiveness. Figure 8.3 depicts the workflow of the developed framework.

8.3.1 Decision Tree

The Decision Tree (DT) is a popular ML technique used in regression and classification applications. It is a supervised learning method that iteratively separates the data into subsets based on the most significant characteristic at each step. Using a tree-like structure as a model, this technique creates internal nodes that represent tests on attributes, branches that indicate test results, and leaf nodes that represent numerical values or class labels. The decision tree model with a root node, branches, and leaf nodes is displayed in Figure 8.4.

8.3.1.1 Steps in Constructing DT

- Root node of the DT algorithm contains the complete dataset.
- It then determines which attribute will split the data the best for categorization based on information gain.

  Information Gain measures the estimated decrease in entropy, a metric that measures the impurity in the dataset. It evaluates the decrease in impurity in the data. The decision tree's root node is chosen based on the characteristic that has the least amount of impurity.

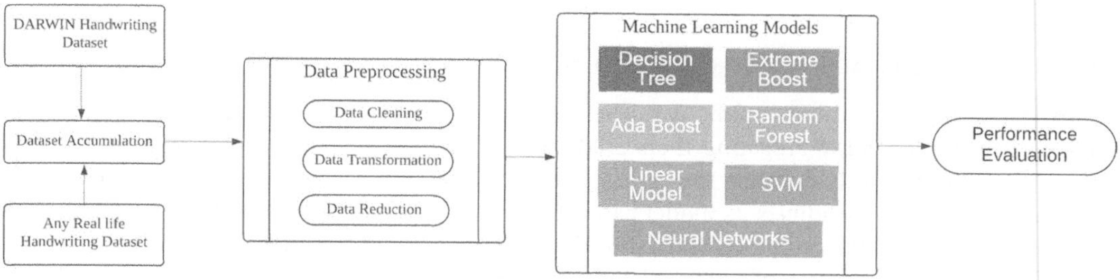

FIGURE 8.3 Proposed methodology framework.

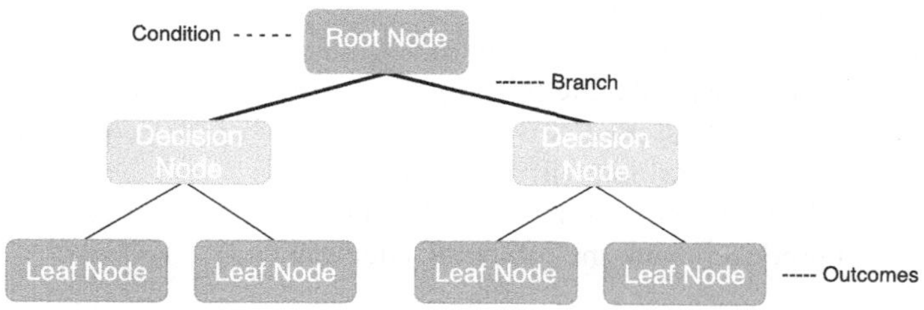

FIGURE 8.4 Decision tree model.

Every time the tree is built, it chooses which characteristic to split on. The generation of sub-nodes enhances homogeneity, thereby diminishing the entropy within these nodes. Greater homogeneity in the child nodes results in greater variance reduction following each split. Hence, information gain represents the variance reduction and can be computed by measuring the decrease in variance after each split, obtained by subtracting the entropy of the weighted mean of the child nodes from the entropy of the parent node.

The formula to find information gain is given in equation (8.1).

$$\text{Information}_{\text{gain}(D,A)} = \text{Entropy}(D) - \sum_{v \in \text{Values}(A)} \frac{D_v}{D} \text{Entropy}(D_v) \tag{8.1}$$

Where $\text{Values}(A)$ is the all potential values for attribute A and D_v is the subset of D for which the attribute A has value v.

Entropy provides impurity in the given dataset. The Entropy of the given dataset D is represented as in equation (8.2).

$$\text{Entropy}(D) = -\sum_{i=1}^{m} p_i \log_2 p_i \tag{8.2}$$

Where m – number of classes in the dataset and p_i – probability of choosing data from class i.

- The selected attribute is used to split the dataset into sub-sets. Each sub-set corresponds to a unique value of the selected attribute.
- For every subset generated in the preceding stage, the procedure is carried out recursively. Until one of the predefined thresholds is met—for example, a maximum tree depth is achieved, all instances in a node belong to the same class, or a node has a minimum number of instances—the loop never ends.

Constructing Tree: As the algorithm runs, a tree structure is created, with each internal node standing in for a choice made in response to an attribute and every leaf node for a number value or a class label.

8.3.2 Extreme Gradient Boost (XG Boost)

XGBoost constructs a robust predictive model by iteratively developing a number of weak learners- usually DT's, and aggregating their predictions. It employs boosting to create an ensemble model that progressively corrects the errors of its predecessors. The optimization process, based on gradients, iteratively adjusts its model parameters to reduce a cost function by responding to the errors' gradients. Additionally, XGBoost introduces the concept of "gradient boosting with decision trees," where the importance of each decision tree added to the ensemble is determined by reducing the objective function. Though XGBoost uses the same ensemble learning methodology, it differs from the traditional boosting algorithms by merging regularization, parallelization and inbuilt cross validation techniques in the algorithm.

Rather than carefully examining each potential split point, this approach employs weighted quantiles to rapidly identify the ideal node split. By estimating the ideal split, XGBoost significantly reduces the computational cost associated with assessing all possible splits, making the technique faster and more scalable when working with huge datasets.

If the dataset has m features and an n number of samples, then y will be the desired result of an ensemble tree method produced from the following equation (8.3)

$$A_i = \sum_{k=1}^{K} f_k(X_i) \tag{8.3}$$

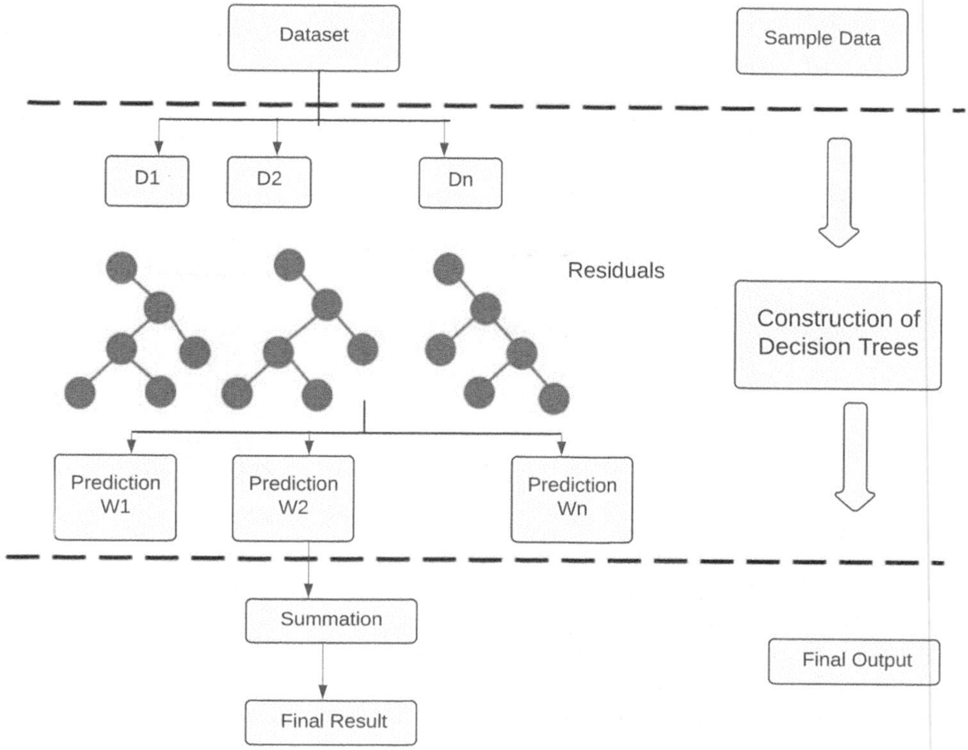

FIGURE 8.5 XG boost model.

Where K denotes number of trees constructed in the model, f_k represents the (k-th tree), to solve the above equation.

Building trees level by level, XGBoost determines if each level's objective function is improved overall by adding a new node (split). If not, the divide is trimmed. The trees are simpler to comprehend and make thanks to their level growth and trimming. The regularization terms are essential for reducing overfitting, enhancing generalization, and making XGBoost a strong and effective method for a range of ML problems. They work in tandem with other strategies like shrinkage and pruning. Figure 8.5 shows sample XGBoost model.

8.3.3 AdaBoost

The ML based meta-algorithm known as Adaptive Boosting, or AdaBoost, is mostly used for classification problems. It is a part of the ensemble learning techniques, which integrate several models to create a more robust composite model. AdaBoost generates a final strong classifier by integrating the predictions from number of weak classifier that have been iteratively trained on different subsections of the data.

The working principle of AdaBoost is given below:

1. **Initialize Sample Weights:** Assign equal weights to each sample in the dataset as shown in equation (8.4).

$$w(x_i, y_i) = \frac{1}{N}, \quad i = 1, 2, \ldots n \tag{8.4}$$

Where N is total number of data points.

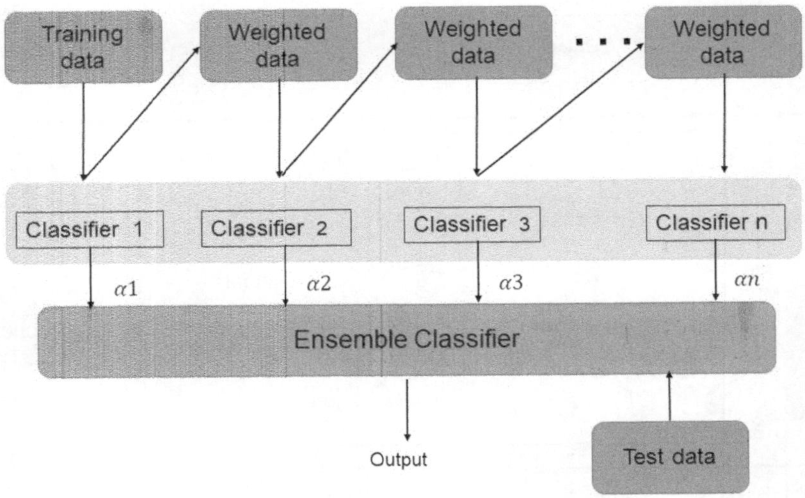

FIGURE 8.6 Adaptive boosting model.

2. **Training a Weak Classifier:** The term *M_k*, where *k* is the current iteration, refers to a weak classifier that has been trained on a dataset. A weak classifier, which is typically a decision tree, is a model that outperforms random chance by a tiny margin.
3. **Compute Error:** Calculate the error of the weak classifier as given in equation (8.5). This error is usually weighted by the sample weights, so misclassified samples contribute more to the error.

$$\text{Error} = \frac{1}{2}\log\frac{1-\text{Total Error}}{\text{Total Error}} \tag{8.5}$$

Update Weights: In order to increase the likelihood of the misclassified samples being sampled in the subsequent iteration, give them higher weights. Reduce the weights of the samples that were correctly classified by applying equation (8.6).

$$\text{New sample weight} = \text{old weight} * e^{\pm\propto} \tag{8.6}$$

When the sample is successfully identified, ∝, will be negative.
In the event that the sample is misclassified, the value of ∝ will be positive.

4. **Repeat:** Carry out again until a predetermined number of times or until the desired accuracy is attained.
5. **Combine Classifiers:** By combining all of the weak classifiers and giving each one a weight based on their performance, a strong classifier is ultimately produced. (better classifiers get higher weights).
6. **Prediction:** AdaBoost aggregates the predictions of all weak classifiers, weighted by their respective strengths, to generate predictions on new data.

Figure 8.6 shows the AdaBoost Model.

8.3.4 Random Forest

In ML, a Random Forest (RF) is analogous to a collaborative decision-making team. It creates an overall model that is more reliable and accurate by fusing the predictions from multiple trees. In the RF model, every decision tree is constructed with a subset of data points and features. To put it

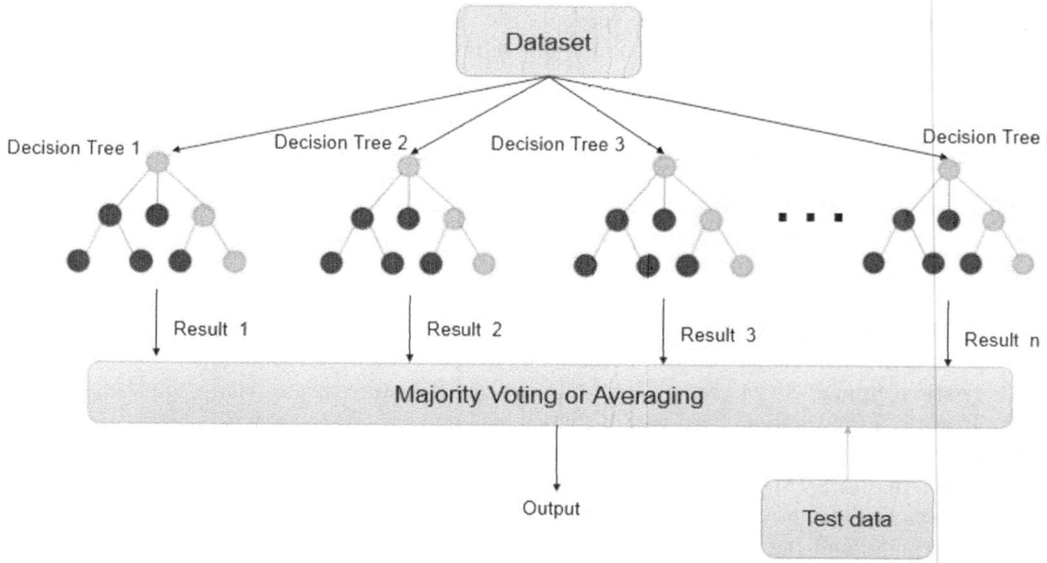

FIGURE 8.7 Random forest model.

simply, m features and n random records are selected from a data set containing k records. For every sample, a separate decision tree is built. Every decision tree will produce an output. The final product is evaluated using either regression or classification-based majority voting or averaging.

Algorithm

Input: *N, S*

for each $i = 1$ to *N*:

  create an empty vector – →RF.

  do

    Make a blank tree Ti

    Reproduce Sample *S* using Bootstrap sampling for all characteristics *F*.

    Make the *S* features into a vector

    Identify the Best Split Feature *B*

    Until there are no more instances to split on,

    create a new node using $B(\text{FS})$ in Ti. Then, add Ti to the RF

end

Output: A tree vector, RF

Figure 8.7 shows example random forest model. Random Forest include locating and using the dataset's most important features, or variables. The complexity of the model is decreased by eliminating unnecessary or redundant features, which lowers the possibility of overfitting. Data subset selection in Random Forest models is naturally accomplished through bootstrap sampling, where each DT receives training on a different random subset of the information. By introducing diversity among the trees, this technique lowers the probability of overfitting through reducing the trees' dependence on one another.

8.3.5 Support Vector Machine

A supervised ML method used for regressions and classification problems is called a Support Vector Machine (SVM). Finding the hyperplane in the feature space that best divides various classes is how it operates. The working principles of SVM is as given below:

1. **Data Representation:** SVM begins with a set of labeled training data, where each data point is divided into two classes based on its feature vector representation.
2. **Feature Space:** SVM creates a high-dimensional feature space from each data point. To put it simply, it looks for a way to change the input data such that it is simpler to identify the hyperplane that divides the classes.
3. **Hyperplane:** SVM searches the feature space for the hyperplane that best separates the classes. For this specific hyperplane, the largest margin, that is, the distance between the hyperplane and the nearest data point for each class is chosen. Increasing this margin contributes to the model's improved capacity for generalization.
4. **Support Vectors:** The nearest data points to the hyperplane and exert the greatest influence on its position are referred to as support vectors. These are the essential components for establishing the border of the choice.
5. **Kernel Trick:** By using the kernel trick, SVM can effectively handle nonlinear connections between features. SVM computes dot products between data points in the converted space without actually computing the transformation, as opposed to directly mapping the data into high-dimensional space. Sigmoid, polynomial, radial basis function (RBF), and linear kernels are common types of kernels.
6. **Optimization:** A convex optimization problem must be solved in order to determine the ideal hyperplane. The purpose is to increase the margin while minimizing the categorization mistake.
7. **Regularization:** To control the trade-off on the training data between minimizing the classification error and optimizing the margin, SVM has a regularization parameter (C). While a larger C value more severely penalizes misclassifications, a smaller C value permits a larger margin but may also result in more misclassifications. The SVM model is displayed in the ensuing Figure 8.8.

A linear decision boundary is a line that splits the data points into discrete classes (also known as a hyperplane in higher dimensions). In a two-dimensional space, this can be represented by in the form as given in equation (8.7).

$$w_1x_1 + w_2x_2 + b = 0 \tag{8.7}$$

Where w_1 and w_2 are the weights x_1 and x_2 are the feature values and b is the bias term. Sometimes a complex curve or other shape that divides the data samples into distinct classes is known as a non-linear decision boundary. When a straight line cannot divide classes, non-linear boundaries are required.

Kernels help transform the data into high-dimensional space such that a non-linear boundary in the original space becomes linear. Data that is not linearly separable in the original space can now be separated using linear classifiers (such as Support Vector Machines) in a higher-dimensional space thanks to this transformation.

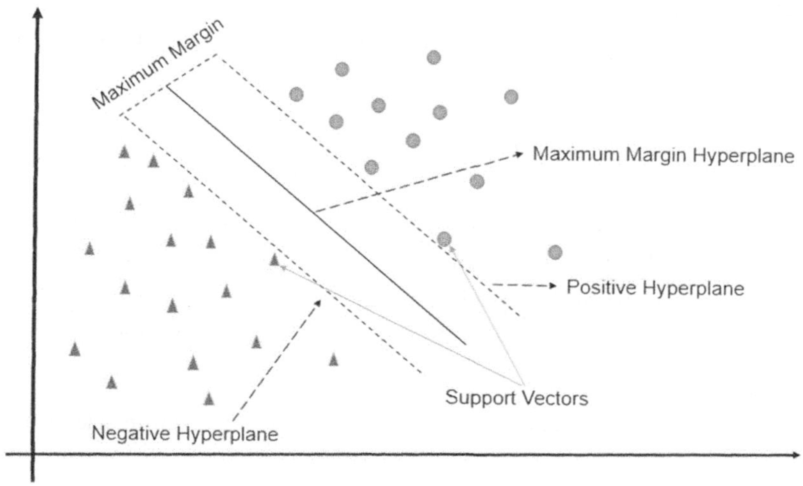

FIGURE 8.8 SVM model.

8.3.5.1 Types of SVM Kernel

Kernel method is a mathematical model which is used is machine learning. The Kernel function, which translates data from one space to another, is used in this method.

1. **Linear Kernel**

   When the data can be divided linearly, as in equation (8.8), it is employed.

$$k(x, y) = x.\ y \tag{8.8}$$

   Where x and y are input feature vectors.

2. **Polynomial Kernel**

   When the data cannot be separated linearly, as indicated by equation (8.9), it is employed.

$$k(x, y) = (x.\ y + c)^\wedge d \tag{8.9}$$

   Where x and y are the input feature vectors, c is a constant term, and d is the degree of the polynomial,

3. **Gaussian Kernel**

   When there is no prior knowledge about the data, as indicated by equation (8.10), the Gaussian kernel is utilized.

$$k(x, y) = \exp\left(\frac{\|x - y\|^2}{2\sigma^2}\right) \tag{8.10}$$

4. **Gaussian Radial Basis Function Kernel**

   One type of radial basis function kernel is the Gaussian kernel. It can be expressed using the equation (8.11) as provided.

$$k(x, y) = \exp\left(-\gamma * \|x - y\|^2\right) \tag{8.11}$$

   Where the input features are denoted by x and y, gamma (γ) is a parameter that controls the breadth of the Gaussian function, where > 0, and $\|x - y\|^2$ is the squared Euclidean distance between the input vectors.

5. **Laplacian Kernel**

Equation (8.12) illustrates how it has a sharper peak and a faster decay, just like the RBF Kernel.

$$k(x, y) = \exp\left(\frac{-\|x - y\|}{\sigma}\right) \tag{8.12}$$

The standard deviation is denoted by σ, the Manhattan distance or L1 norm between the input vectors is represented by $\|x - y\|$, and the input feature vectors are x and y.

where $\|x - y\|^2$ is the squared Euclidean distance between the input vectors, x and y are the input feature vectors, and gamma is a parameter that regulates the Gaussian function's breadth.

6. **ANOVA RBF**

It is a multiple-input kernel function that can be used for feature selection as given in equation (8.13).

$$k(x, y) = \sum_{k=1}^{n} \exp\left(-\sigma\left(x^2 - y^2\right)^2\right)^d \tag{8.13}$$

Here$x$ and y are the input feature vectors.

7. **Sigmoid Kernel**

It is used as the proxy of neural networks the equation (8.14).

$$k(x, y) = \tanh\left(\alpha x^T y + c\right) \tag{8.14}$$

8.3.6 Linear Model

A statistical technique called multiple Linear Regression (LR) is employed to investigate the linear relationship between 2 or more independent variables, often known as predictors, and a dependent variable. The idea of simple linear regression, which only considers one independent variable, is expanded upon by it.

Equation (8.15) illustrates the link between the independent variables X_1, X_2, ... X_p and the dependent variable Y in multiple linear regression.

$$Y = \beta_0 + \beta_1 X_1 + \beta_2 X_2 + \ldots + \beta_p X_p + \epsilon \tag{8.15}$$

The dependent variable is Y, the independent variables are X_1, X_2, ...X_p are, the intercept is β_0, the independent variable's coefficients are, β_1, β_2, ... β_p, and the error term is ε, which represents the difference between the observed and predicted values of Y, while all other variables are held constant.

Finding the coefficients (β_0, β_1, β_2, ... β_p) that best fit the data is the aim of multiple linear regression. This is often accomplished by reducing the sum of squared differences between the dependent variable's observed and predicted values.

8.3.7 Neural Networks

A neural network is a type of computing model that is based on the architecture and operation of the linked neurons seen in the human brain. This kind of machine learning technique is applied to learning tasks that are both supervised and unsupervised, including dimensionality reduction, clustering, regression, and classification.

The artificial neuron, often known as the perceptron, is the fundamental unit of a neural network. A perceptron multiplies each of its inputs by a weight before adding them all together and using

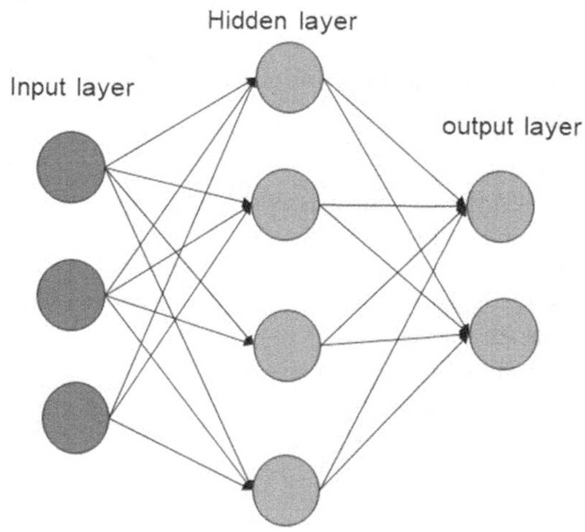

FIGURE 8.9 Neural network.

an activation function to generate an output. Other neurons may receive this output as an input. Multiple layers of neurons arranged hierarchically make up neural networks:

Input Layer: Neurons in this layer receive the initial input data.
Hidden Layers: These layers use weighted connections and activation functions to conduct intricate transformations on the input data. They are positioned between the input and output layers. There are several hidden layers in deep neural networks.
Output Layer: Neurons in this layer produce the final output, often after passing through an activation function appropriate for the specific task (e.g., softmax for classification, linear for regression).

Throughout a neural network's training phase, the weights of connections between neurons are changed using optimization algorithms like gradient descent to reduce the difference between the expected and actual outputs. In this process, the difference between the ground truth and the forecasts is often measured using a loss function. Figure 8.9 shows example neural network model.

The capacity of neural networks to comprehend complex patterns from data, adjust to different tasks, and achieve cutting-edge performance in domains like computer vision, natural language processing, and reinforcement learning is making them increasingly popular. But, they also need a lot of processing power to train and tune, and if they're not regularized properly, they might become overfit.

8.4 EXPERIMENT RESULT AND ANALYSIS

8.4.1 Dataset Description

The DARWIN dataset comprises handwriting data gathered following the acquisition protocol outlined by (Cilia et al. 2018). This dataset, consisting of 25 handwriting tasks, was specifically devised for early Alzheimer's disease (AD) detection. It encompasses information from 174 participants, comprising 89 AD patients and 85 healthy individuals. Table 8.1 (Cilia et al. 2022) shows the 25 handwriting tasks performed by the persons.

Contained within the file "DARWIN.csv," each participant is represented by a row, with the first row serving as the header. The subsequent 89 rows contain data from patients, while the remaining 84 rows pertain to healthy subjects. The file is structured with 452 columns. The first column

TABLE 8.1
Handwriting Tasks Performed by the Persons

Code	Description
1.	Put your signature in writing.
2.	Draw a horizontal line four times in a row to connect two spots.
3.	Draw a vertical line four times in a row to connect two locations.
4.	Draw a circle four times in a row, each time the diameter is equal to six centimeters.
5.	Draw a circle four times in a row, each time the diameter is equal to three centimeters.
6.	Copy characters like the "l," "m," and "p."
7.	Task 6's identical letters should be copied onto a nearby row.
8.	Write the letter "l" in cursive four times in a row.
9.	Write the bigram "le" in cursive four times in a series.
10.	Copy the exact word "foglio," which in Italian means "sheet."
11.	Copy the Italian word "foglio," which translates to "sheet," above a line.
12.	Copy the Italian word "mamma," which signifies "mom."
13.	Copy the word "mamma," which is Italian for "mom," above a line.
14.	Learn and rewrite the Italian terms for "telephone," "dog," and "store," which are "telefono," "cane," and "negozio."
15.	Replicating the Italian word "bottiglia," which means "bottle," backwards
16.	Replicating the Italian word "casa," which means "home," backwards
17.	Six regular, non-regular, and non-words should be copied and placed in the relevant boxes. In particular, "pane," "mela," and "apple," which are regular words; "prosciutto," and "ciliegia," which are non-regular words; and, lastly, "taganaccio" and "lonfo," which are non-words.
18.	Write the name of the thing (a chair, precisely) that is depicted in the photo.
19.	duplicating a postal order's fields
20.	Write the brief sentence that was given to you.
21.	redrawing a complicated diagram
22.	Copy and write phone number
23.	Record the transcribed phone number (24–25).
24.	In the clock drawing test, draw a complete clock with all of the hours and place the hands at 11:05.
25.	Make a copy of a paragraph in text. With regard to literature, the paragraph has 110 characters.

contains participant identifiers, and the last column indicates the participant's classification as either 'P' (Patient) or 'H' (Healthy) (Vandam et al. 2015, Cilia et al. 2018).

The intermediary columns contain features extracted from the 25 tasks. Each task contributes 18 features, identifiable by the feature name followed by a numeric task identifier. For example, the column labeled "total_time8" contains values for the "total time" feature extracted from task #8.

This study investigates the characteristics of handwriting tasks performed by subjects. Each participant completed 25 tasks involving drawing or writing given in Table 8.1. The tasks followed a protocol established by (Cilia et al. 2022). This protocol involved using a digital tablet to record data like pen coordinate (x and y), movements touching the paper (on-paper), and movement near surface without touching (in-air). Timestamps were also recorded. Written instructions were provided on the paper sheets and verbally by an instructor to ensure clear understanding of the tasks.

8.4.1.1 Feature Extraction

18 features (Cilia et al. 2022) were selected from 451 features that were recorded during the handwriting task based on how useful they would be for the analysis of cognitive impairment prediction. For every task in the raw data, there were eighteen features (x, y) points, pressures, and a time stamp. These features are detailed below.

Time:

- Entire amount of time needed to finish the task.
- The length of time an object is in flight.
- The duration of time devoted to written assignments.

Movement Characteristics:

- The average velocity of items on paper where speed represents the variance in displacement over time.
- The average velocity of atmospheric motions.
- The average acceleration of motions on paper is called mean acceleration on paper. The change in speed as a function of time is called acceleration.
- The mean acceleration of motions when in the air.
- The average movement jerk measured on paper. The acceleration variation in relation to time is referred to as a "jerk".

Pressure:

- The Pressure Mean (PM) is the average of the pressures that the pen tip applies.
- The term "Pressure Var" (PV) refers to the fluctuation in pressure that the pen tip applies.

Tremor:

- Mean Relative Tremor on-paper calculated for movements on paper is expanded upon.
- GMRT in-air is a generalized average Relative Tremor based on in-air movements.
- Mean GMRT is the average of previous two.

Handwriting Extent:

- The maximal extension along the *X* axis is called the Max *X* Extension. The greatest extension of a component along an axis is determined by measuring the distance between its farthest and nearest places to the origin on that axis.
- The maximal extension along the *Y* axis is known as the Max *Y* Extension.

Paper Coverage:

- The Dispersion Index determines how many fixed-size squares on the paper sheet the handwriting strokes covered relative to the overall number of squares.

This study essentially explores various aspects of handwriting behavior by analyzing the extracted features from a set of pre-defined tasks. In this work the Classifier Models Decision tree, Extreme Boost, Ada Boost, Random forest, Linear Model, SVM and Neural networks are applied as classifier models for the Darwin Dataset.

8.4.2 Confusion Matrix

A table used to evaluate a classification model's performance is termed a confusion matrix. It makes it possible to visualize how well an algorithm performs by contrasting expected and actual numbers. When examining the performance of binary classification algorithms which are algorithms with two possible outcomes, the confusion matrix is especially helpful. An illustration of a confusion matrix for a binary classification task is shown in Figure 8.10.

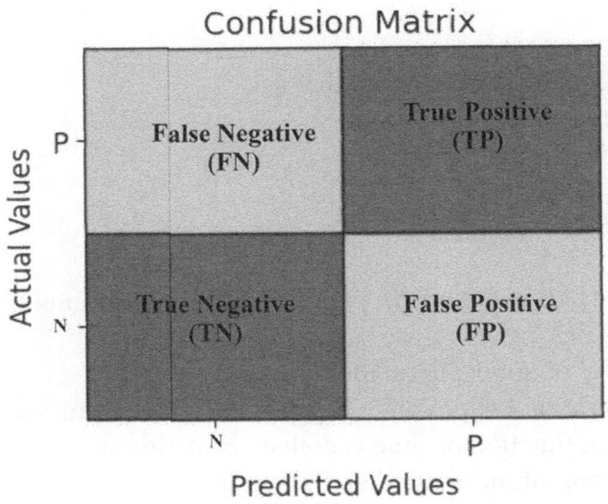

FIGURE 8.10 Confusion matrix.

In this matrix:

- **True Positive** (TP)**:** Instances where the model correctly predicts the positive class.
- **False Negative** (FN)**:** Instances where the model incorrectly predicts the negative class when it's actually positive.
- **False Positive** (FP)**:** Instances where the model incorrectly predicts the positive class when it's actually negative.
- **True Negative** (TN)**:** Instances where the model correctly predicts the negative class.

Confusion matrices can be generated using the predicted and actual labels from the classification model. They offer a thorough analysis of the model's performance, especially with regard to how well it can distinguish between positive and negative occurrences.

8.4.3 Performance Measures

From the confusion matrix, various performance metrics can be calculated, including:

- Accuracy
- Precision
- Recall (also called sensitivity or true positive rate)
- Specificity (also called true negative rate)
- F1 Score

8.4.3.1 Accuracy

One popular assessment criterion for evaluating a classification model's performance is accuracy. It calculates the percentage of cases that are correctly classified relative to the total number of instances. The formula for accuracy is given in equation (8.16).

$$\text{Accuracy} = \frac{\text{Number of corrected predictions}}{\text{Total Number of predictions}} = (\text{TP} + \text{TN})/(\text{TP} + \text{TN} + \text{FP} + \text{FN}) \tag{8.16}$$

Where TP (True Positives) denotes the proportion of correctly predicted positive instances; TN (True Negatives) the proportion of correctly predicted negative instances; FP (False Positives) the proportion of incorrectly predicted positive instances; and FN (False Negatives) the proportion of poorly predicted negative instances.

The value of accuracy is a number between 0 and 1, where 1 denotes perfect accuracy (all predictions are correct) and 0 denotes no accuracy (all predictions are erroneous). While accuracy is a useful criterion, datasets with a dominant class and imbalance may not be appropriate for its use. In such cases, additional metrics like recall, precision, area under the ROC curve (AUC-ROC), F1 score, or recall could provide a more in-depth evaluation of the model's effectiveness.

8.4.3.2 Precision

Precision is a performance indicator that is used to assess the percentage of correctly anticipated positive occurrences out of all positively predicted instances in classification tasks, especially binary classification. It assesses how well the model avoids producing false positive results. The precision is computed using the equation (8.17).

$$\text{Precision} = \frac{\text{True Positive}}{\text{Total Predicted Positive}} = \text{TP}/(\text{TP} + \text{FP}) \tag{8.17}$$

The model is good at identifying positive cases without incorrectly classifying negative instances as positive, as indicated by a high precision, which also suggests a low false positive rate.

8.4.3.3 Recall

Another crucial performance indicator in classification tasks is recall, which is often referred to as sensitivity or true positive rate, especially in binary classification. Out of all actual positive instances, it calculates the percentage of accurately anticipated positive instances. The calculation of the recall is presented in equation (8.18).

$$\text{Recall} = \frac{\text{True Positive}}{\text{Total Actual Positive}} = \text{TP}/(\text{TP} + \text{FN}) \tag{8.18}$$

A high recall suggests that the model minimizes false negatives by effectively capturing positive cases. It shows that the model can find every instance of the positive class that is pertinent.

8.4.3.4 Specificity

The ability of a test to identify real negatives, it is measured by its specificity or true negative rate as given in equation (8.19).

$$\text{Specificity} = \frac{\text{True Negative}}{\text{Total Actual negatives}} = \text{TN}/(\text{TN} + \text{FP}) \tag{8.19}$$

8.4.3.5 F1 Score

The mean of recall and precision is used to get the F1 score, which is equal to the relative contribution of these two metrics as shown in equation (8.20). The F1 score can have a minimum of 0 and a maximum of 1. A perfect model can be observed by an F1 score of 1, which shows that every prediction was made correctly. Since, recall and precision are both rates, the F1 score employs a harmonic mean in place of a standard arithmetic average.

$$\text{F1 Score} = \frac{2 \times \text{Precision} \times \text{Recall}}{\text{Precision} + \text{Recall}} \tag{8.20}$$

8.4.3.6 ROC Curve

A graph that shows a classification model's performance over all categorization levels is called a Receiver Operating Characteristic curve, or ROC curve. True Positives rate (TPR) and False Positives rate (FPR) are the two metrics that are shown as a curve.

A ROC curve is used to plot TPR versus FPR at different categorization criteria. Lowering the classification threshold causes more positive classifications, which in turn increases the quantity of False Positives and True Positives.

The acronym AUC represents "Area under the ROC Curve." Stated otherwise, the area under the complete ROC curve (AUC) in two dimensions, ranging from (0,0) to (1,1), is determined.

8.4.3.7 Precision/Recall Curve

The accuracy-recall curve shows the recall against precision trade-off at different thresholds. A low false positive rate is associated with good precision, whereas a low false negative rate is associated with strong recall. High precision and recall are both indicated by an area under the curve with a high value. High scores for both mean that the classifier is yielding largely positive (high recall) and accurate (high precision) results.

8.4.3.8 Sensitivity- Specificity Curve

It provides the tradeoff between True Positive and True Negative Rate.

8.4.3.9 H-Measure

Equation (8.21) provides the H-measure, sometimes referred to as the Matthews correlation coefficient (MCC), as a tool for assessing how well binary classification models work. Even in cases when the classes have varying sizes, it provides a balanced measure by accounting for true positives, true negatives, false positives, and false negatives. The H-measure has a range of –1 to 1, where a forecast is perfect, a prediction is random, and a prediction and observation are completely at odds.

$$\text{MCC} = \frac{\text{TP} \times \text{TN} - \text{FP} \times \text{FN}}{\sqrt{(\text{TP}+\text{TN})(\text{TP}+\text{FN})(\text{TN}+\text{FP})(\text{TN}+\text{FN})}} \tag{8.21}$$

The MCC ranges from –1 to 1, where 1 indicates perfect prediction, 0 indicates random prediction, and –1 indicates total disagreement between prediction and observation.

8.4.3.10 Smoothing Score Distribution

Smoothing score distribution refers to the process of applying techniques to make the distribution of scores produced by a classifier more regular or less noisy. This is often done to improve the interpretability of the scores or to enhance the performance of downstream tasks such as thresholding or ranking.

8.5 CLASSIFIER MODELS

8.5.1 Decision Tree

Figure 8.11 shows the decision tree constructed for the given dataset.

At the top, it is the overall probability of Healthy is 52% and Patient is 48%. This node asks total_time23<8505. If yes, then it goes down to the root's left child node (depth 2). And it identifies 89% Healthy and 11% are Patient. Otherwise it checks for mean_jerk_in_air3<0.22. It's keep on going like that to understand what features impact the likelihood of Healthy and Patient. The rules generated for the decision tree is given below:

```
1 root 121 58 H (0.5206612 0.4793388)
2 total_time23< 8505 55  6 H (0.8909091 0.1090909) *
3 total_time23>=8505 66 14 P (0.2121212 0.7878788)
6 mean_jerk_in_air3< 0.02155841 8  1 H (0.8750000 0.1250000) *
```

```
 7 mean_jerk_in_air3>=0.02155841 58  7 P (0.1206897 0.8793103)
14 pressure_mean5>=2004.784 23  7 P (0.3043478 0.6956522)
28 disp_index19< 3.305e-05 10  3 H (0.7000000 0.3000000) *
29 disp_index19>=3.305e-05 13  0 P (0.0000000 1.0000000) *
15 pressure_mean5< 2004.784 35  0 P (0.0000000 1.0000000) *
```

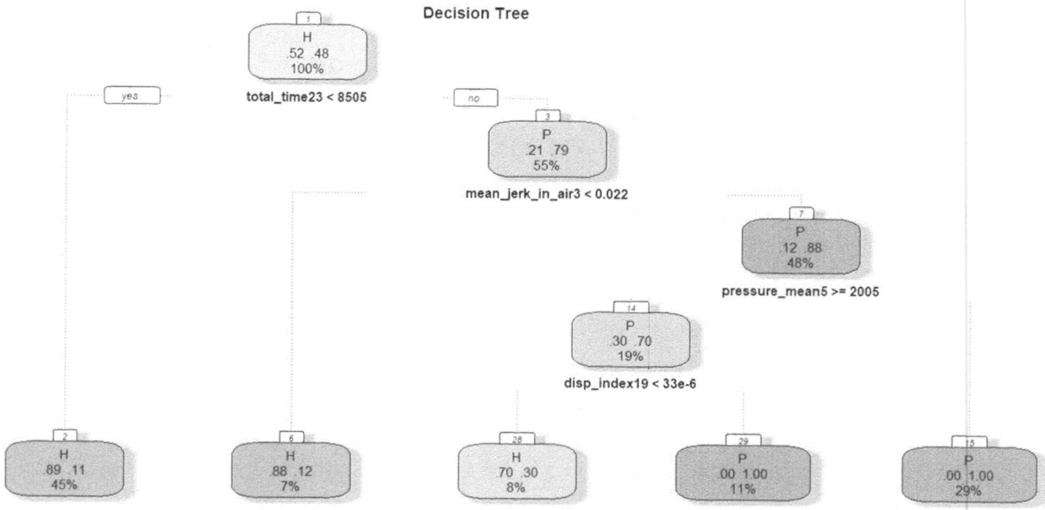

FIGURE 8.11 Constructed decision tree.

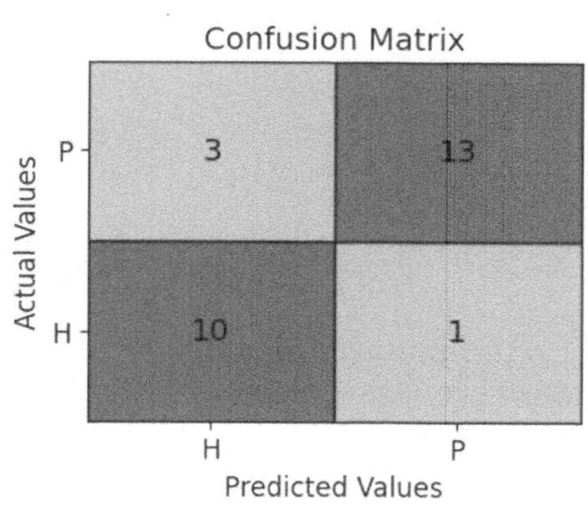

FIGURE 8.12 Confusion matrix obtained from decision tree.

The confusion matrix obtained for decision tree is given in Figure 8.12. Figure 8.13 shows ROC curve obtained from decision tree where the AUC is 0.92 indicating the better performance of the model. Figure 8.14 shows ROC, H measure, AUC, and smoothed score distribution of the dataset using Decision tree.

As per equations from (8.16) to (8.20), the calculation of the measures from the above confusion matrix is shown below.

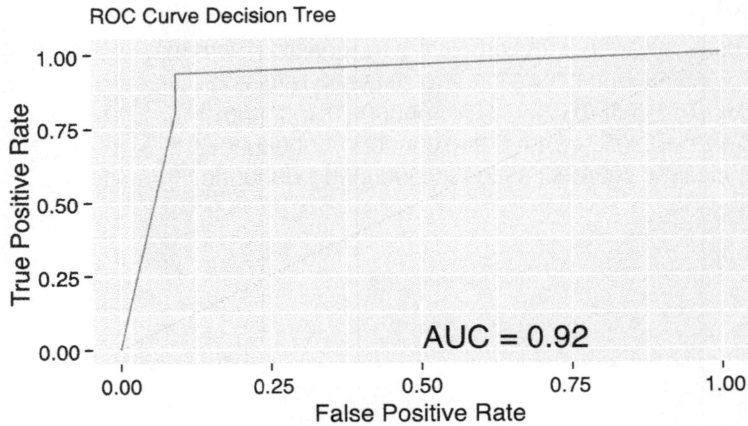

FIGURE 8.13 ROC curve obtained from decision tree.

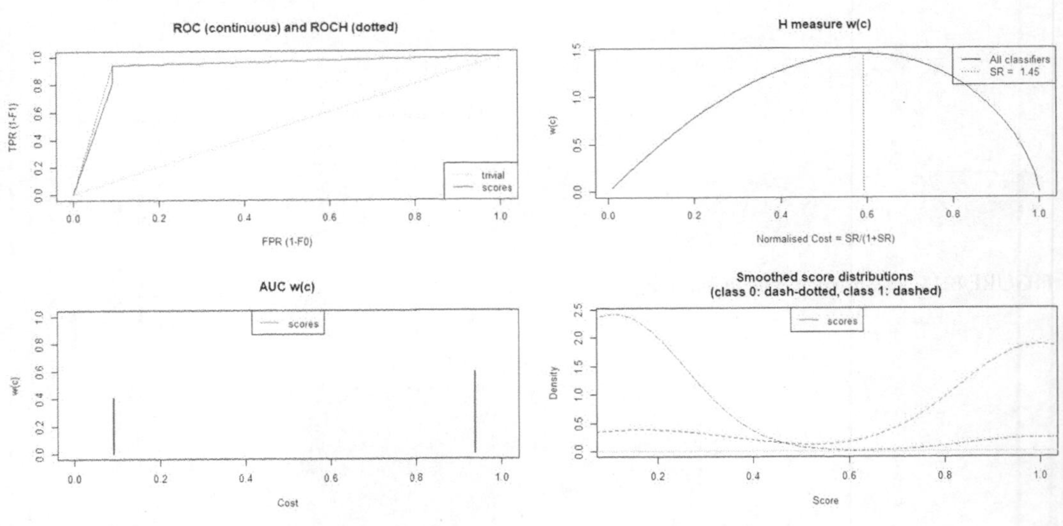

FIGURE 8.14 ROC, H measure, AUC, and smoothed score distribution.

Accuracy = (10 + 13)/(10 + 13 + 1 + 3) = 0.8519 = 85.19%
Precision = 10/(10 + 1) = 0.9091 = 90.91%
Recall = 10/(10 + 3) = 0.7692 = 76.92%
Specificity = 13/(13 + 1) = 0.9286 = 92.86%
F1 Score = 2*(0.9091*0.7692)/(0.9091 + 0.7692) = 0.8333 = 83.33%

8.5.1.1 Extreme Boost

Importance or frequency of the variable actually used is given in the Table 8.2. The Gain shows the relative contribution of the linked feature to the model by computing each feature's contribution for each tree in the model. A higher value for this metric means that it is more predictively significant when compared to another feature. The proportional number of observations pertaining to this feature is known as the Coverage measure. The percentage weight of a feature over the weights of all features is used to compute its frequency.

TABLE 8.2
Variable Frequency

Feature	Gain	Cover	Frequency
total_time23	0.2563299981	0.114730993	0.049019608
total_time17	0.1281243620	0.060266587	0.019607843
air_time17	0.0759290996	0.078589050	0.058823529
paper_time17	0.0687493258	0.062446926	0.049019608
mean_jerk_in_air3	0.0488874213	0.034345482	0.029411765
mean_acc_in_air3	0.0366894285	0.034900289	0.029411765
paper_time8	0.0359189865	0.032928485	0.019607843
mean_speed_in_air17	0.0307903582	0.029592695	0.019607843
pressure_var19	0.0290695092	0.026706890	0.029411765
air_time23	0.0255940880	0.029448191	0.029411765
num_of_pendown19	0.0246910218	0.042049147	0.049019608
mean_acc_on_paper1	0.0190986689	0.005684930	0.009803922
paper_time10	0.0160523142	0.014908818	0.009803922
max_y_extension2	0.0151969463	0.022358000	0.019607843
paper_time9	0.0130009223	0.016625188	0.009803922
pressure_mean10	0.0125050632	0.019738915	0.039215686
gmrt_in_air4	0.0120590800	0.015487353	0.009803922
mean_gmrt17	0.0103068445	0.014542766	0.009803922
mean_acc_in_air7	0.0094459451	0.018555150	0.009803922
mean_acc_in_air24	0.0086441256	0.015556124	0.009803922
air_time7	0.0082660381	0.004072634	0.009803922
total_time13	0.0076582172	0.012512425	0.009803922
mean_jerk_on_paper17	0.0076345926	0.012367104	0.009803922
pressure_mean1	0.0062158942	0.017141286	0.009803922
paper_time23	0.0060747039	0.012719307	0.019607843
max_y_extension7	0.0060513771	0.003690354	0.009803922
pressure_mean5	0.0059660118	0.013636685	0.029411765
pressure_mean19	0.0057257801	0.006706548	0.009803922
mean_acc_on_paper12	0.0051605319	0.014041730	0.009803922
air_time8	0.0051552159	0.010988037	0.009803922
total_time10	0.0045799156	0.003244378	0.009803922
total_time9	0.0043224205	0.009166869	0.009803922
pressure_mean8	0.0039823181	0.006391788	0.009803922
paper_time25	0.0039580860	0.008052034	0.009803922
total_time15	0.0038971400	0.010008926	0.019607843
max_y_extension8	0.0038311849	0.003276802	0.009803922
air_time6	0.0033749666	0.008237982	0.009803922
total_time3	0.0033577555	0.007219097	0.009803922
pressure_mean11	0.0031097827	0.017269672	0.019607843
pressure_var11	0.0031057634	0.002941484	0.009803922
max_x_extension15	0.0024892560	0.005373524	0.009803922
paper_time19	0.0021661573	0.010012623	0.029411765
total_time7	0.0020626761	0.010009008	0.029411765
air_time3	0.0019352964	0.006776509	0.019607843
total_time8	0.0015959592	0.007120774	0.019607843
gmrt_on_paper17	0.0013971968	0.004756528	0.009803922
disp_index20	0.0013569461	0.003238394	0.009803922
disp_index25	0.0013234695	0.006559586	0.019607843

(Continued)

TABLE 8.2 (*Continued*)
Variable Frequency

Feature	Gain	Cover	Frequency
mean_speed_on_paper1	0.0012302524	0.003798831	0.009803922
mean_speed_in_air21	0.0011313761	0.004762226	0.009803922
mean_acc_on_paper3	0.0008513207	0.003327803	0.009803922
gmrt_in_air12	0.0007192442	0.003449980	0.009803922
air_time5	0.0006661931	0.003302606	0.009803922
mean_acc_in_air18	0.0006005671	0.003006276	0.009803922
pressure_mean7	0.0005657891	0.013946953	0.009803922
total_time1	0.0004756642	0.017154761	0.009803922
gmrt_in_air1	0.0004756642	0.017154761	0.009803922
mean_gmrt8	0.0004457660	0.003101736	0.009803922

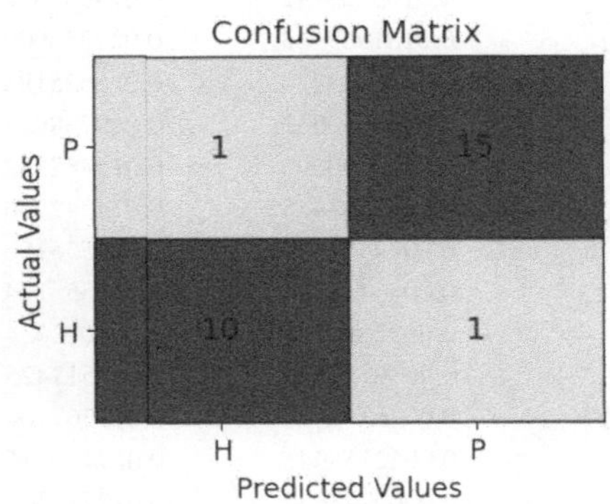

FIGURE 8.15 Confusion matrix obtained from extreme boost.

The confusion matrix of Extreme Boost is given in Figure 8.15. The ROC curve obtained from Extreme Boost is given in the Figure 8.16 where AUC is 0.99 and the curve shows the good trading off between sensitivity and specificity. Figure 8.17 shows ROC, H measure, AUC, and smoothed score distribution of the dataset using Extreme Boost.

8.5.2 AdaBoost

The frequency of variables actually used for AdaBoost is given below in Figure 8.18.

The confusion matrix obtained from AdaBoost is given in the Figure 8.19. The ROC curve obtained from AdaBoost is shown in Figure 8.20, where AUC is 1 indicating the best model performance correctly able to classify the data. Figure 8.21 shows ROC, H measure, AUC, and smoothed score distribution of the dataset using AdaBoost.

8.5.3 Random Forest

The variable importance given for Random Forest for top-10 is given in Table 8.3.

The amount of accuracy lost by the model when each variable is excluded is expressed by the Mean Decrease Accuracy. The variable is more crucial to the correct categorization the more precision it loses. The variables are arranged according to decreasing relevance. The mean decrease in the Gini coefficient indicates how much each variable helps to the homogeneity of the nodes and

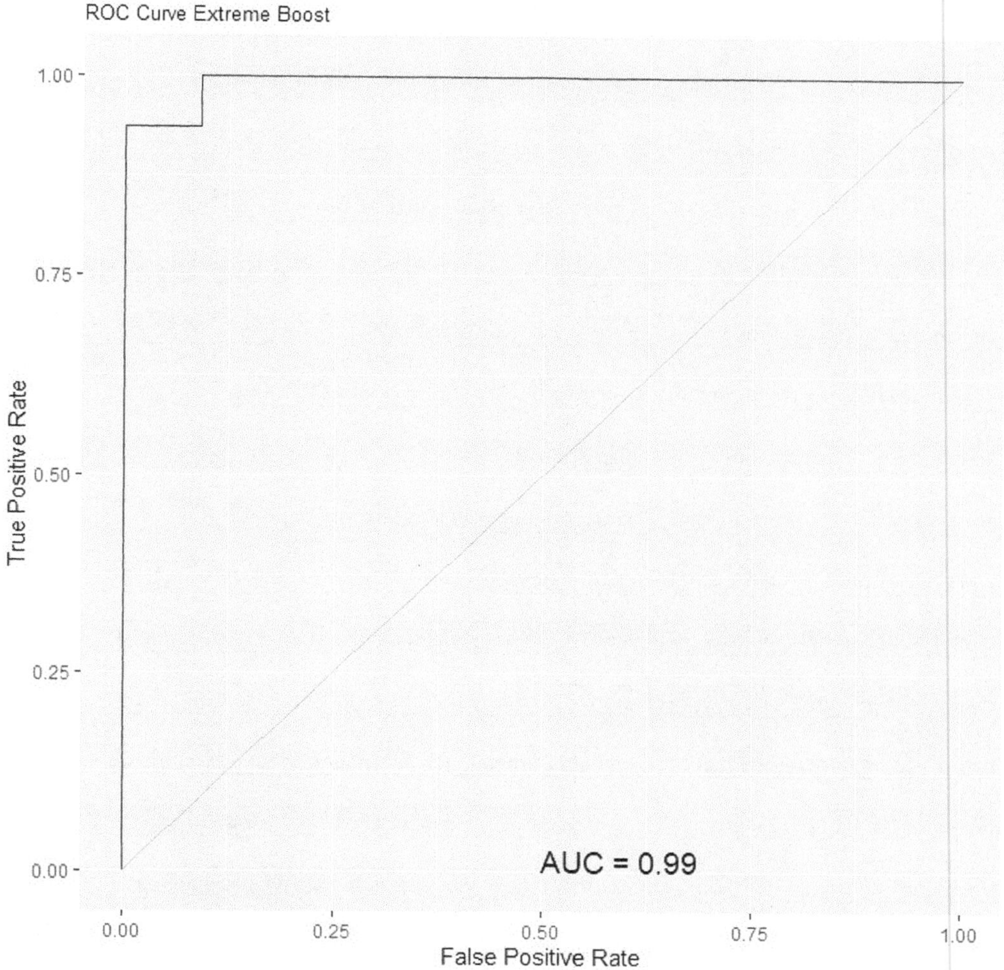

FIGURE 8.16 ROC curve obtained from extreme boost.

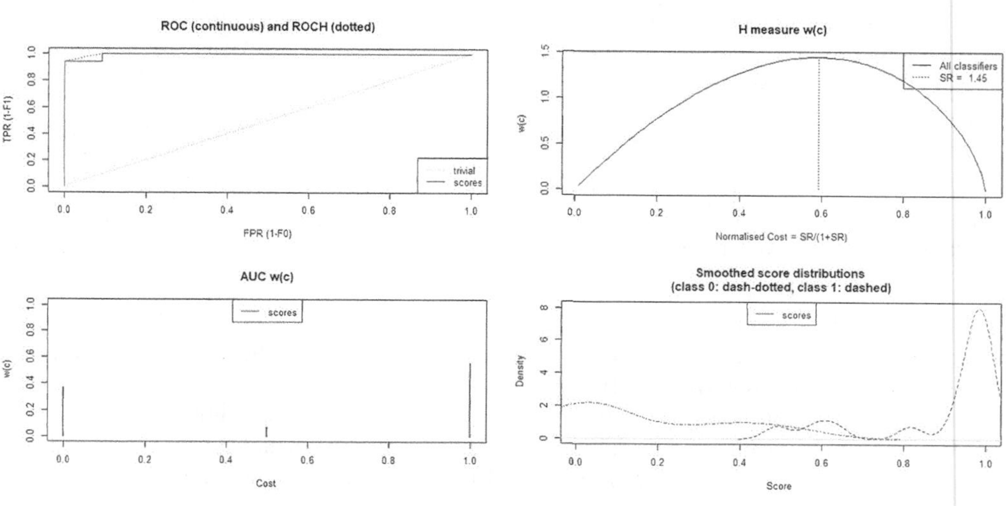

FIGURE 8.17 ROC, H measure, AUC, and smoothed score distribution.

total_time23	air_time17	num_of_pendown19	total_time17
12	5	5	5
paper_time19	mean_speed_in_air17	paper_time17	paper_time9
4	3	3	3
air_time7	disp_index10	mean_acc_in_air3	mean_jerk_in_air3
2	2	2	2
paper_time12	paper_time8	pressure_mean8	total_time15
2	2	2	2
air_time13	air_time20	air_time21	air_time22
1	1	1	1
air_time23	air_time3	air_time5	disp_index15
1	1	1	1
disp_index18	disp_index19	disp_index2	disp_index23
1	1	1	1
disp_index5	disp_index6	disp_index7	gmrt_in_air13
1	1	1	1
gmrt_in_air15	gmrt_in_air3	gmrt_on_paper13	gmrt_on_paper15
1	1	1	1
gmrt_on_paper17	gmrt_on_paper23	gmrt_on_paper25	max_x_extension1
1	1	1	1
max_x_extension10	max_x_extension17	max_y_extension2	max_y_extension20
1	1	1	1
max_y_extension21	max_y_extension23	max_y_extension3	mean_acc_in_air18
1	1	1	1
mean_acc_in_air21	mean_acc_on_paper17	mean_acc_on_paper2	mean_acc_on_paper20
1	1	1	1
mean_acc_on_paper21	mean_acc_on_paper6	mean_gmrt12	mean_gmrt17
1	1	1	1
mean_gmrt20	mean_jerk_on_paper21	mean_jerk_on_paper23	mean_speed_in_air25
1	1	1	1
mean_speed_on_paper5	mean_speed_on_paper8	paper_time1	paper_time16
1	1	1	1
paper_time18	paper_time23	paper_time24	pressure_mean17
1	1	1	1
pressure_mean3	pressure_mean5	pressure_var16	pressure_var19
1	1	1	1
pressure_var3	pressure_var4	total_time13	total_time20
1	1	1	1
total_time7	total_time8	total_time9	
1	1	1	

FIGURE 8.18 Variable frequency from AdaBoost.

leaves in the resulting random forest. A higher mean decrease accuracy or mean decrease Gini score for the variable raises its significance in the model. Figure 8.22 shows the Error rates obtained from Random for Out of Bag (OOB), Healthy and Patient classes.

A random sample of the observations, either a bootstrap sample or a subsample of the original data, is used to build each tree in an RF. Observations that are not included in the bootstrap sample or subsample are referred to as "out-of-bag" (OOB) observations as shown in Figure 8.23.

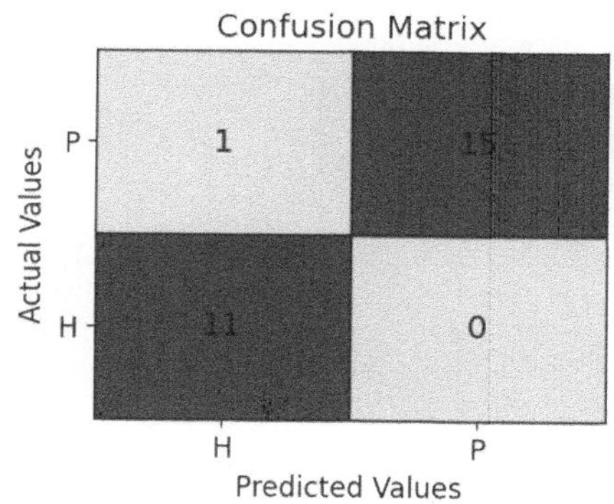

FIGURE 8.19 Confusion matrix obtained from AdaBoost.

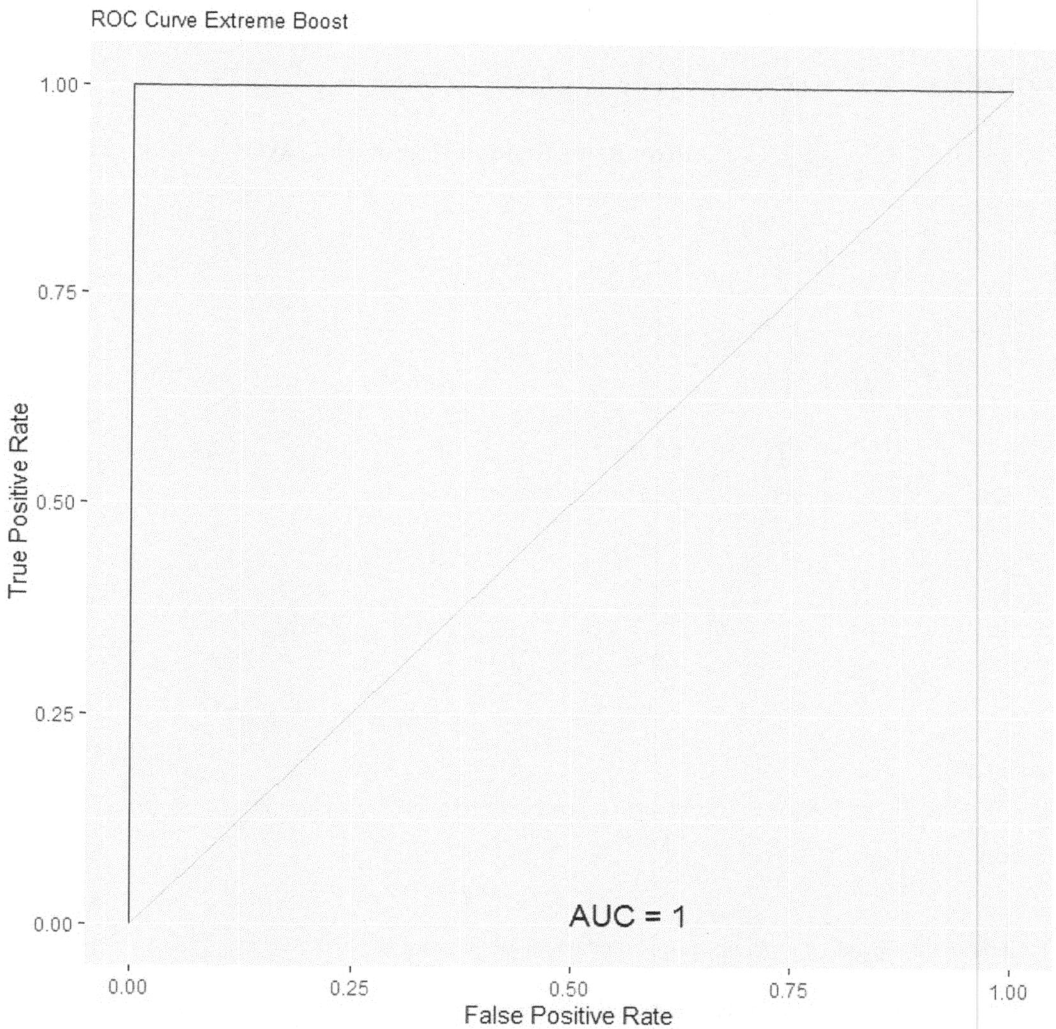

FIGURE 8.20 ROC curve obtained from AdaBoost.

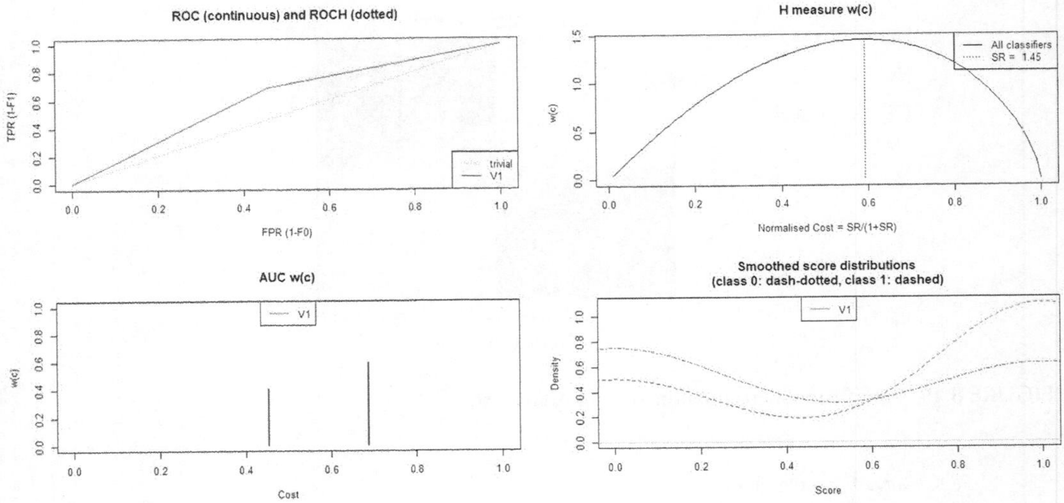

FIGURE 8.21 ROC, H measure, AUC, and smoothed score distribution.

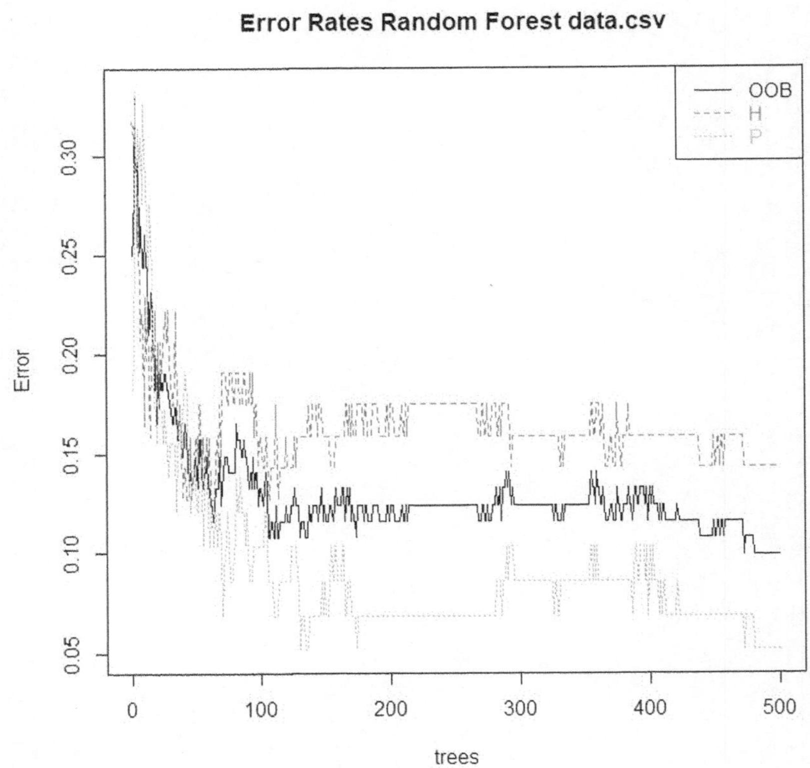

FIGURE 8.22 Error rates obtained from random for out of bag.

The confusion matrix for Random forest is given in the Figure 8.24. The ROC curve obtained from Random Forest is given in Figure 8.25, where AUC is 1 indicating the best model with 100% accuracy and able to correctly classify the complete data. Figure 8.26 shows ROC, H measure, AUC, and smoothed score distribution of the dataset using Random Forest.

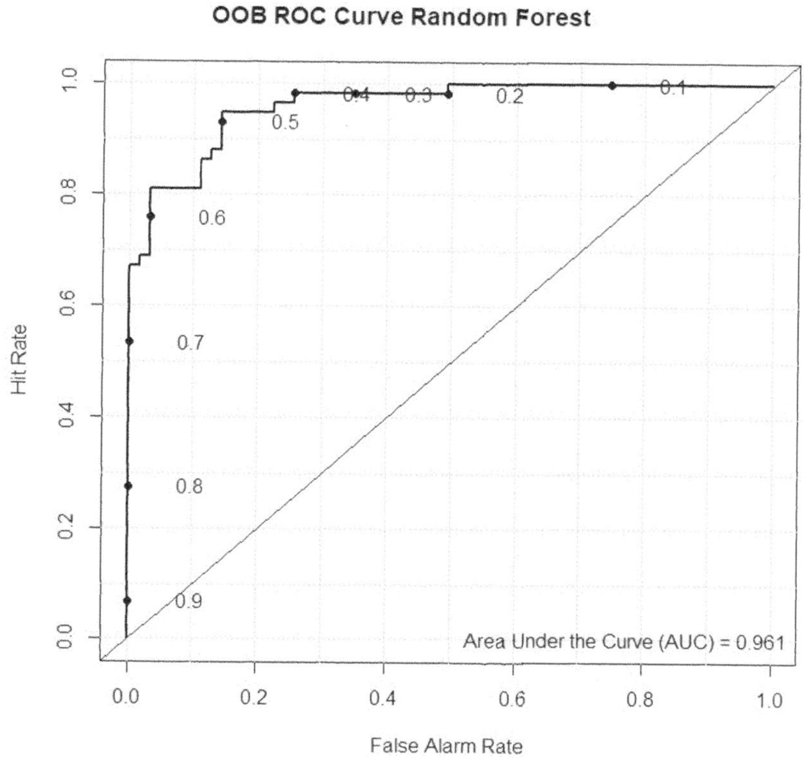

FIGURE 8.23 ROC of random for out of bag.

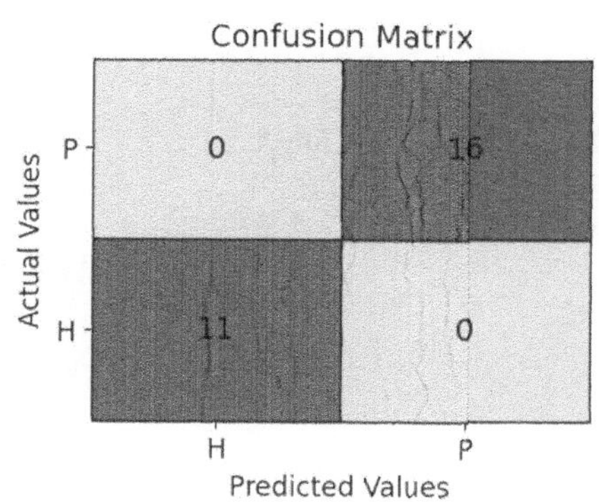

FIGURE 8.24 Confusion matrix obtained from random forest.

8.5.4 SVM RBF

In SVM, Gaussian Radial Basis kernel function is used, the hyper parameter: sigma= 0.00128276746783492 and number of support vectors generated is 89. Figure 8.27 depicts the confusion matrix obtained for SVM with RBF kernel. Figure 8.28 shows the ROC curve obtained from SVM is given below where AUC is 0.98. Figure 8.29 shows ROC, H measure, AUC, and smoothed score distribution of the dataset using SVM.

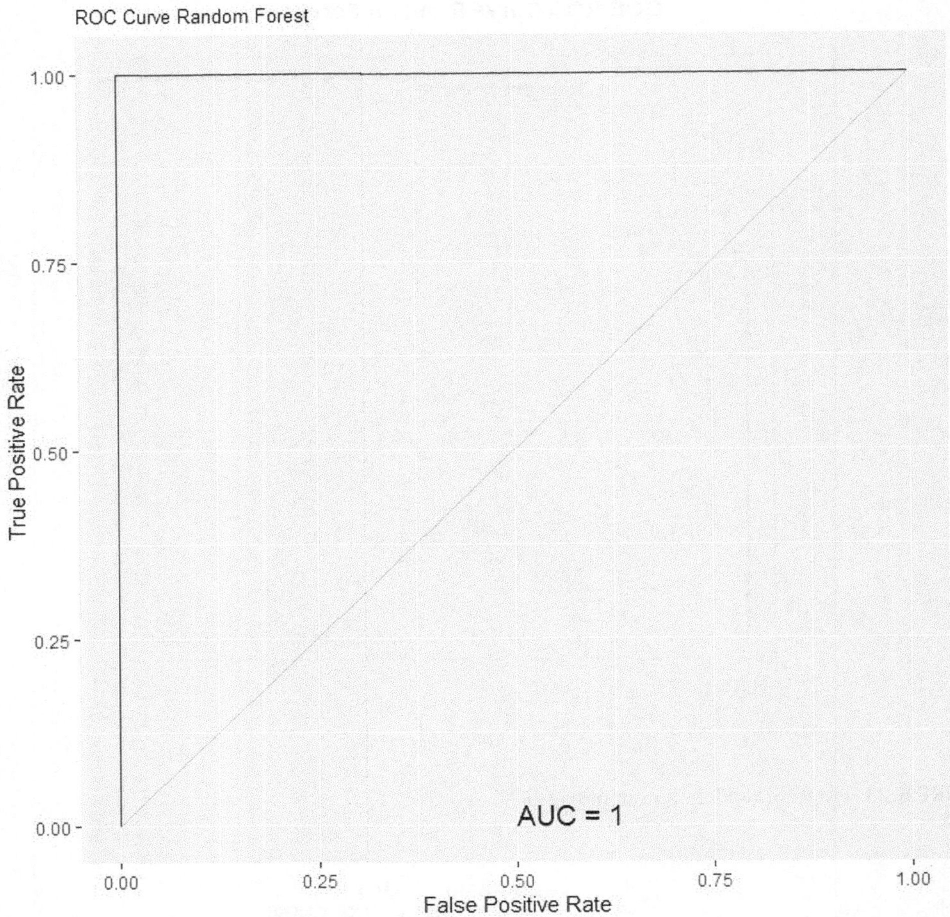

FIGURE 8.25 ROC curve obtained from random forest.

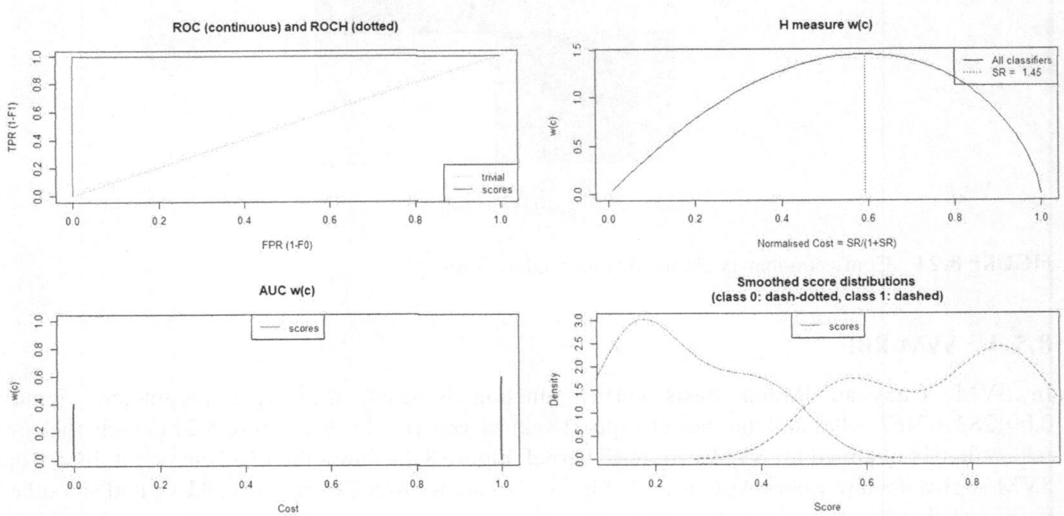

FIGURE 8.26 ROC, H measure, AUC, and smoothed score distribution.

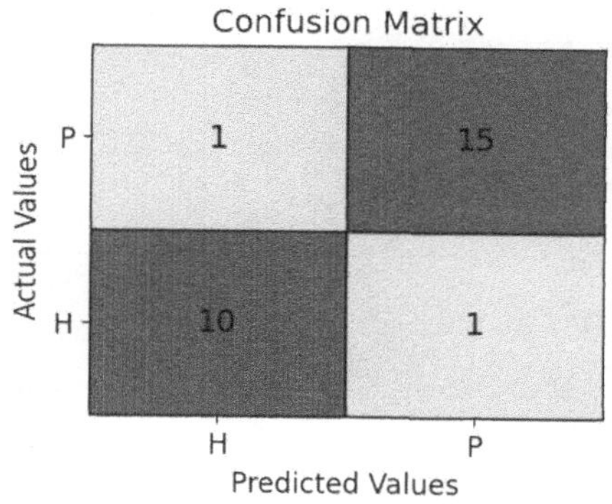

FIGURE 8.27 Confusion matrix obtained from SVM RBF.

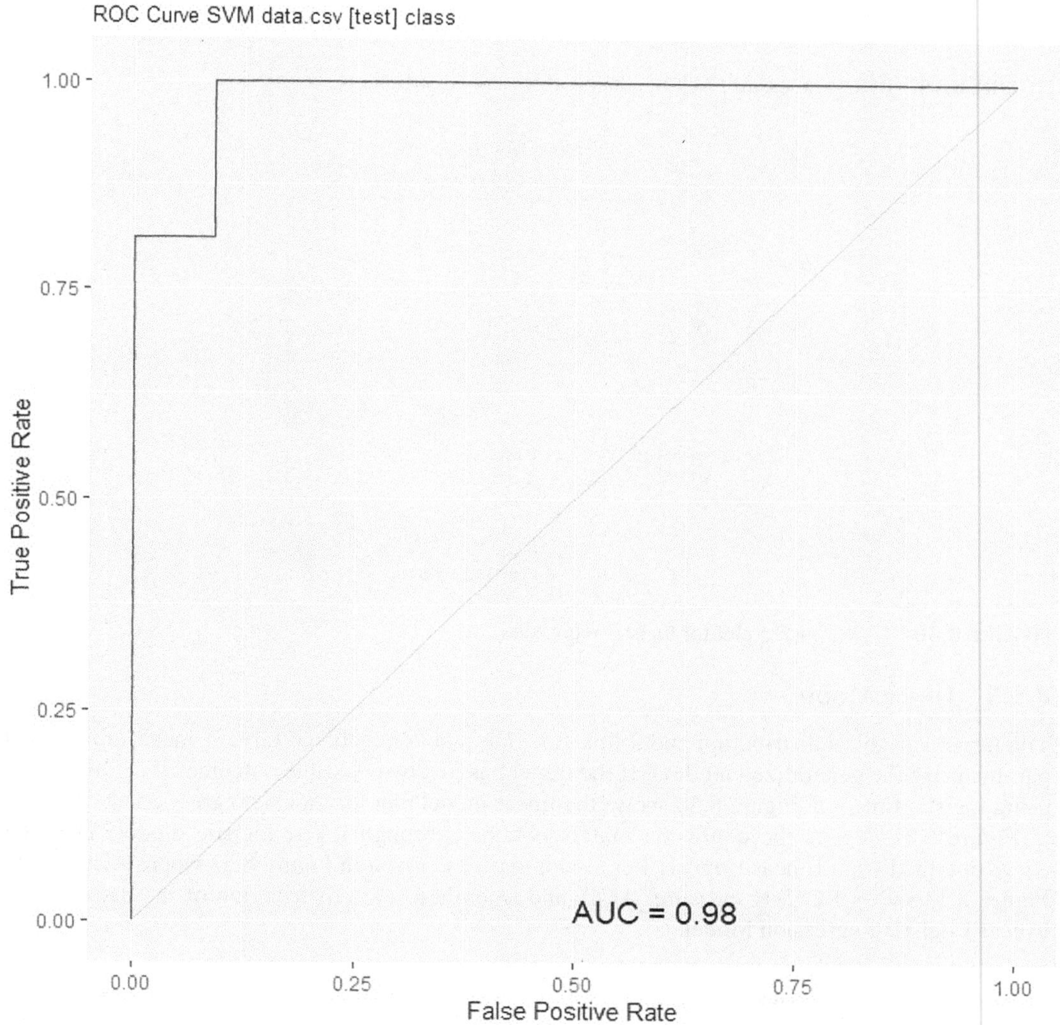

FIGURE 8.28 ROC curve obtained from SVM RBF.

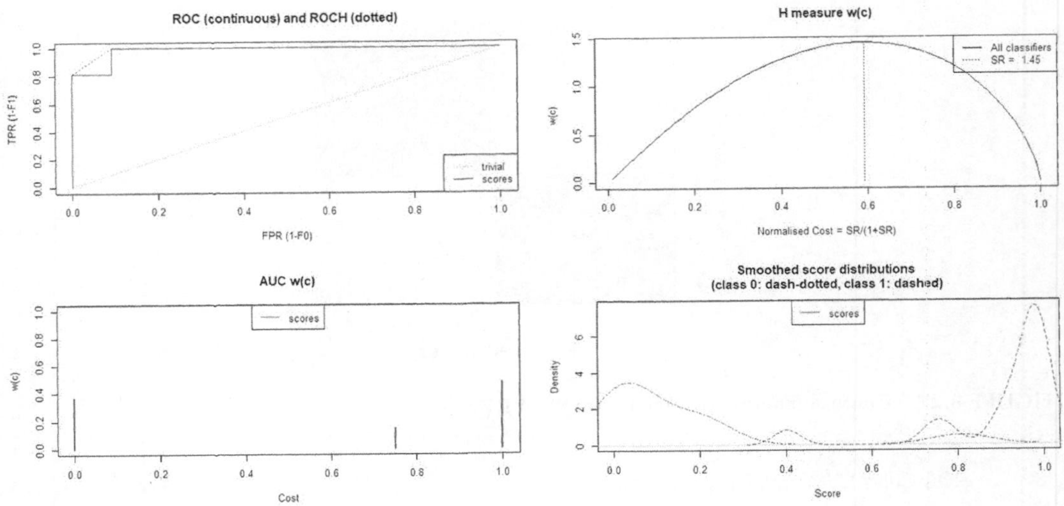

FIGURE 8.29 ROC, H measure, AUC, and smoothed score distribution.

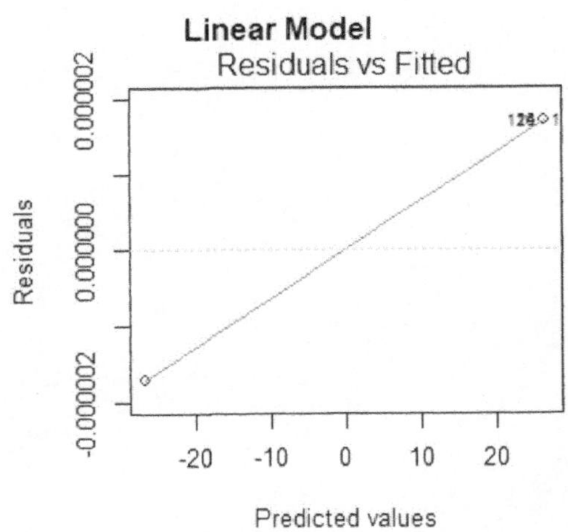

FIGURE 8.30 Linear model plot for logistic regression.

8.5.5 Linear Model

The target variable's distribution and a link function that connects the target's mean to the inputs parameterize the generalized method. If the target has just two possible outcomes it is transformed using logistic function. Figure 8.30 shows the linear model plot for logistic regression.

Figure 8.31 depicts the confusion matrix obtained through linear logistic model. The ROC curve obtained from Linear Logistic Regression model is given in Figure 8.32 where AUC is 0.65. Figure 8.33 shows ROC, H measure, AUC, and smoothed score distribution of the dataset using Linear Logistic Regression Model.

8.5.6 Neural Network

The construction of the Neural network is made with a 450 input nodes, 10 hidden layers and 1 output node network with 4,971 weights. The Sum of Squares Residuals: 34.00. Figure 8.34 shows the confusion matrix obtained through Neural Network. The ROC curve obtained from Neural

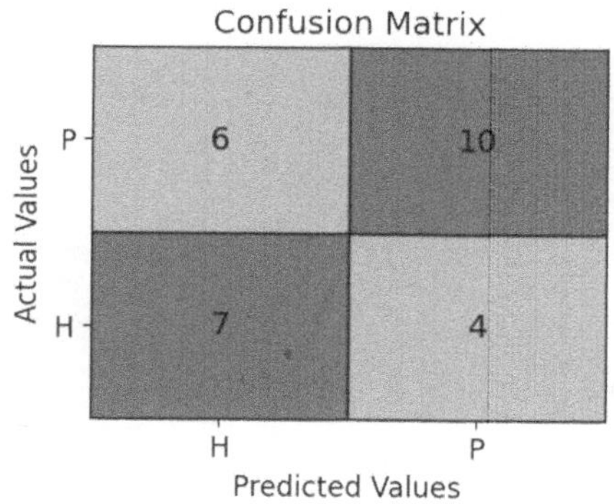

FIGURE 8.31 Confusion matrix obtained from linear model.

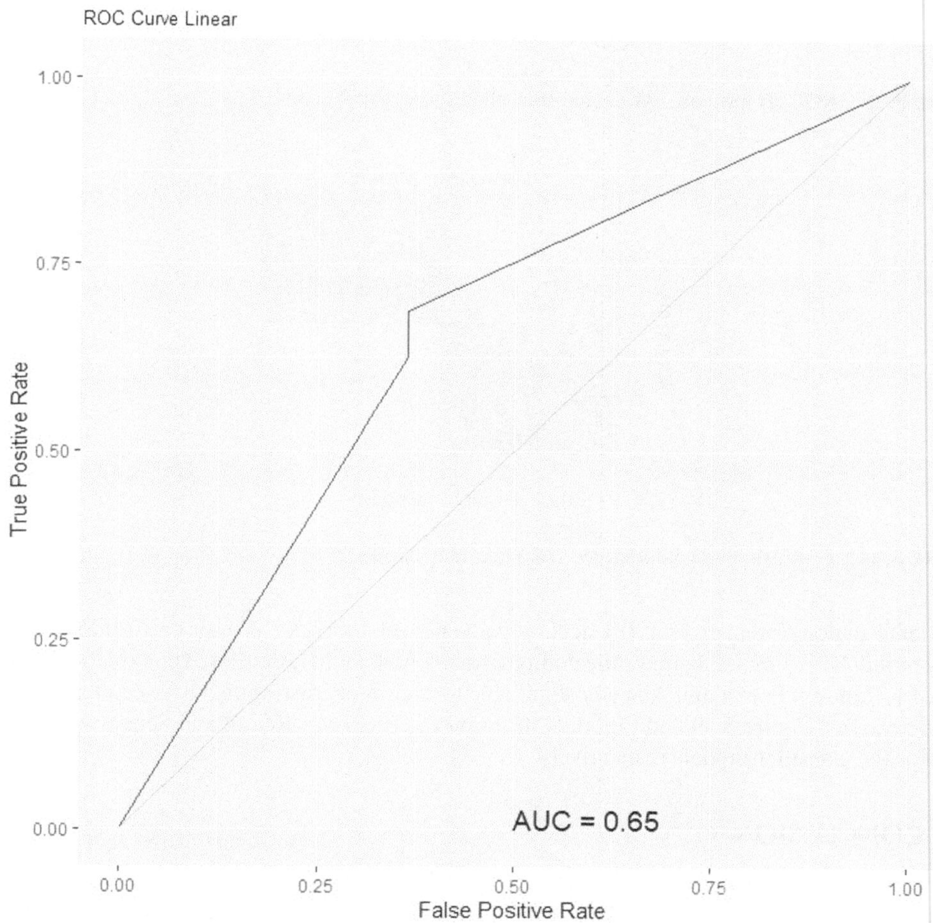

FIGURE 8.32 ROC curve obtained from linear model.

Network is given in Figure 8.35 where AUC is 0.62. Figure 8.36 shows ROC, H measure, AUC, and smoothed score distribution of the dataset using Neural Network.

Figure 8.37 shows the performance measures obtained from the classifiers Decision Tree, Extreme Boost, AdaBoost, Random forest, SVM, Linear Logistic model and Neural networks. Among these

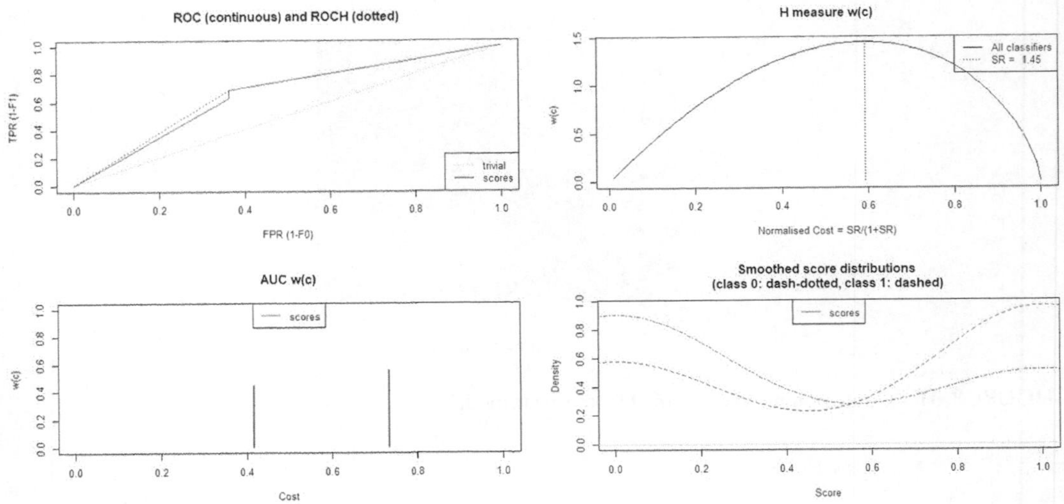

FIGURE 8.33 ROC, H measure, AUC, and smoothed score distribution.

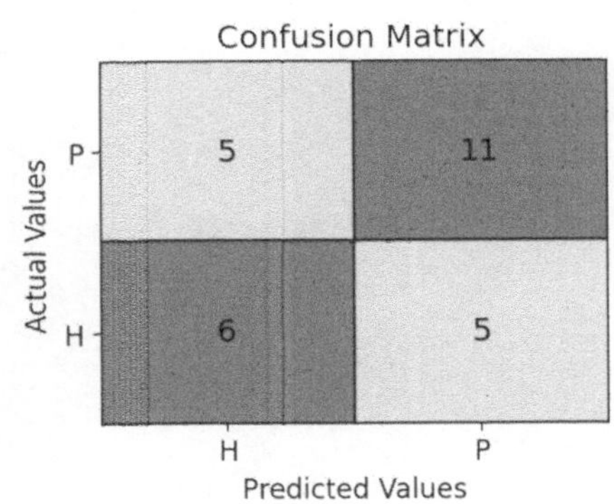

FIGURE 8.34 Confusion matrix obtained from neural network.

classifiers Random forest gives 100% accuracy and neural network has poor performance compared to other models. Figure 8.38 shows the comparison of AUC of ML models. Yet gain, by attaining an AUC of 1, Random Forest and Ada Boost are able to accurately distinguish between the positive and negative classes. Figure 8.39 and Figure 8.40 shows the Precision-Recall and Sensitivity-Specificity curve for the classifier models respectively.

8.6 CONCLUSION

Healthcare can be enhanced by utilizing the recent advancements in prediction modeling techniques which tends to improve the patient outcomes in a positive way. Cognitively-impairing diseases pose major challenges to both the individuals with the disease and the world's healthcare systems. Early diagnosis and prediction of certain conditions can lead to considerable improvements in treatment effectiveness and patient health condition. Online handwriting data that has been digitally gathered offers a novel means of continuously and painlessly evaluating cognitive function. In this work, we employ machine learning techniques to study the predictive power of online handwriting data for cognitive impairment diseases.

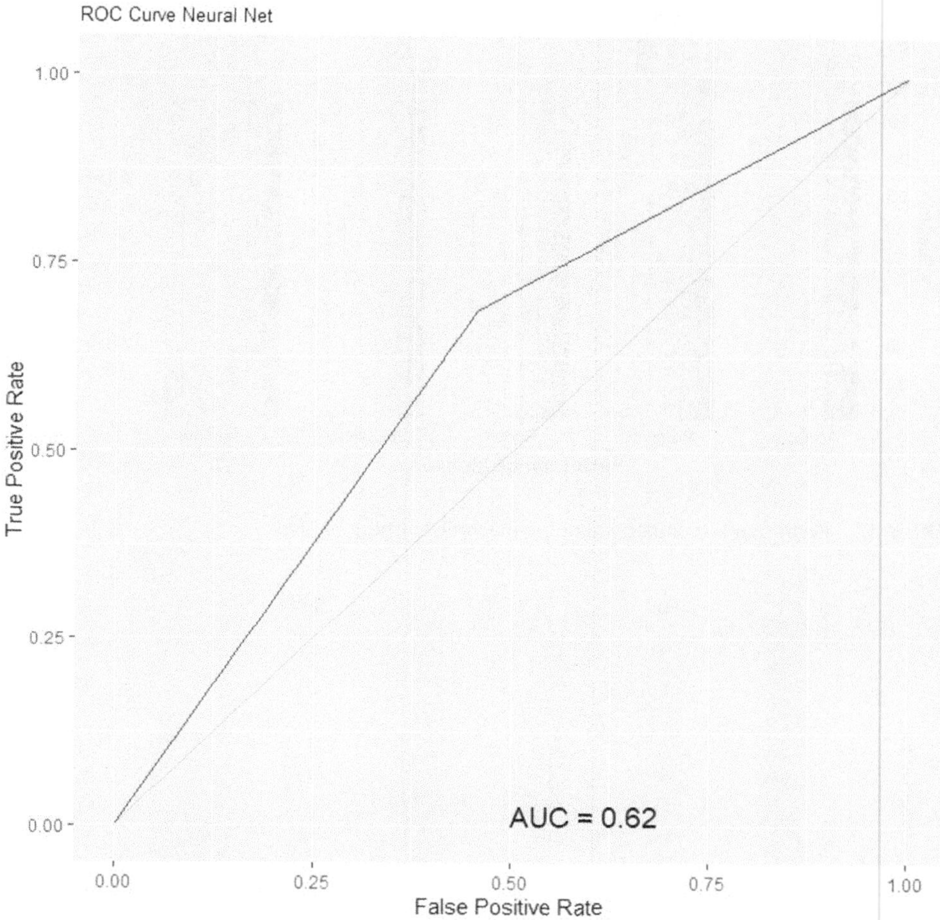

FIGURE 8.35 ROC curve obtained from neural network.

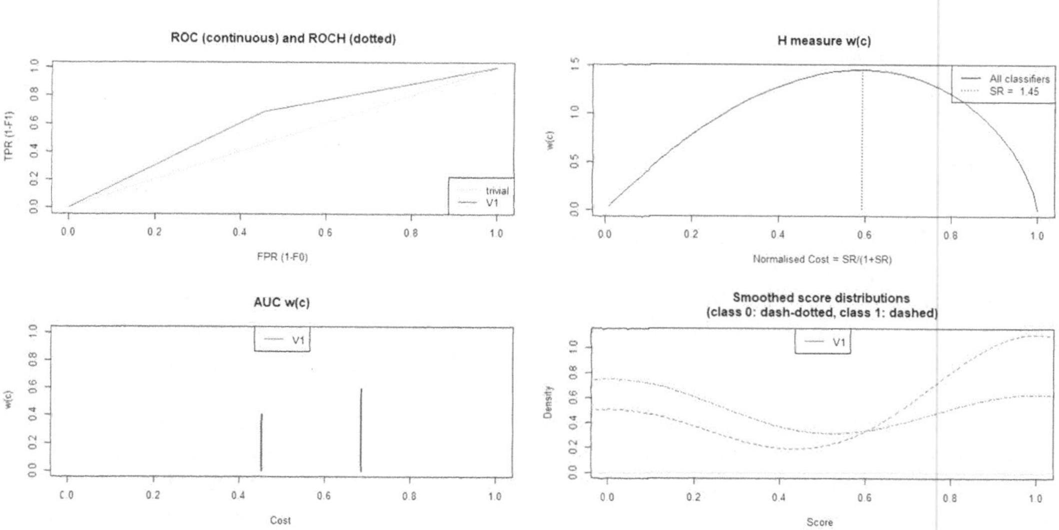

FIGURE 8.36 ROC, H measure, AUC, and smoothed score distribution.

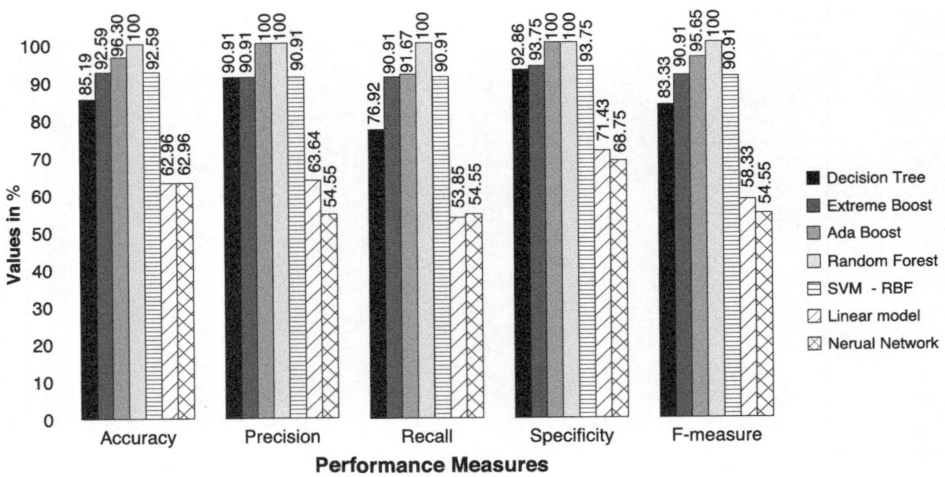

FIGURE 8.37 Performance comparison of the machine learning models.

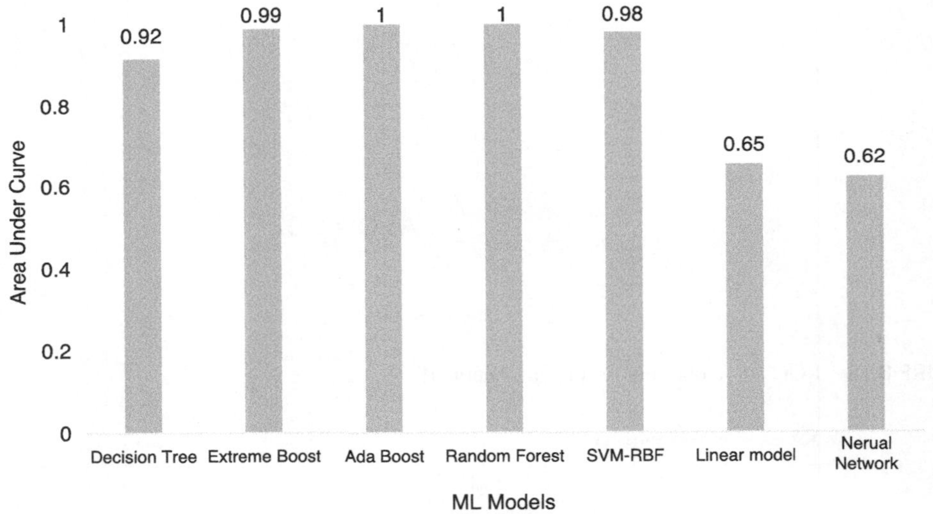

FIGURE 8.38 Comparison of AUC from machine learning models.

DARWIN dataset is a large collection of handwriting examples from the web annotated with the cognitive impairments P(Patient) and H(Healthy) is utilized for creating the predictive models. In particular, it contains data from 174 subjects, 85 of whom are healthy and 89 of whom are AD patients. In this research work, the different classifier models such as Decision Tree, Extreme Boost, Ada Boost, Random Forest, Linear Model, SVM, and Neural Networks are applied in order to perform the prediction task on the Darwin dataset.

Predictive Models built are analyzed with the standard performance measures such as accuracy, precision, recall, specificity and F1- score. Random forest outperforms all other machine learning models by achieving 100% accuracy. Also, Ada boost, Extreme boost and SVM –RBF provides a good accuracy of 96%, 92% and 92% respectively. The machine learning model's performance is also assessed using the AUC metric. Again, Random Forest and Ada Boost successfully discriminate the positive and negative classes, achieving an AUC of 1, signifying a flawless model.

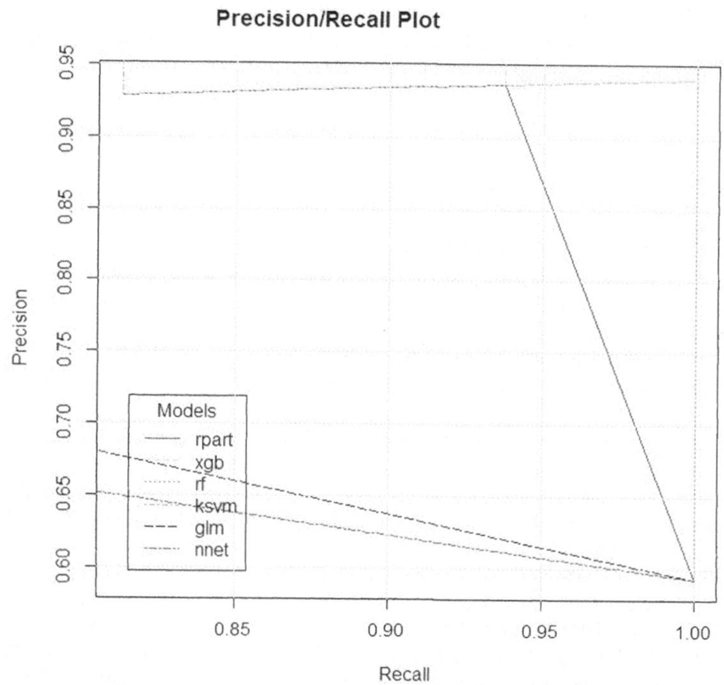

FIGURE 8.39 Precision-Recall curve for the classifier models.

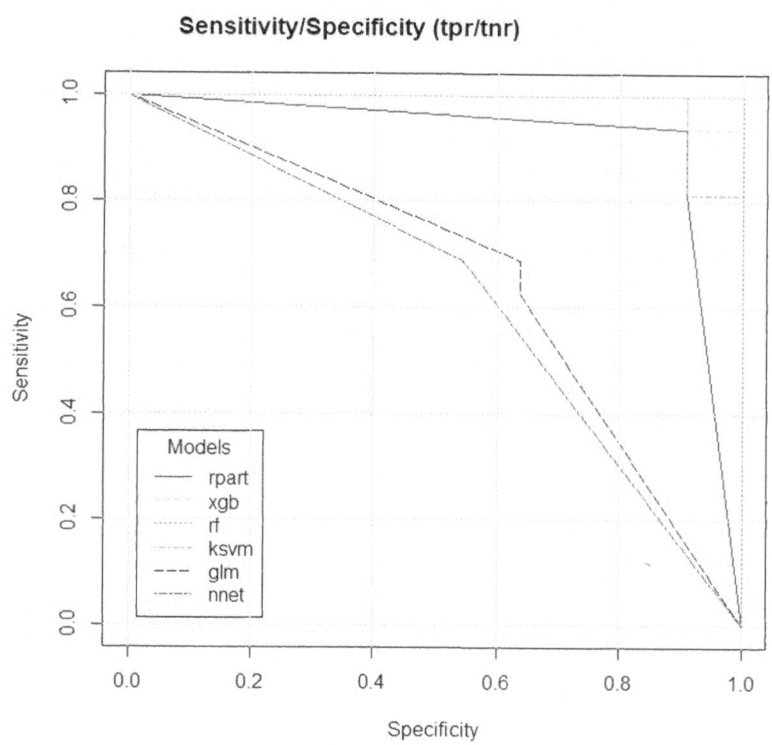

FIGURE 8.40 Sensitivity-Specificity curve for the classifier models.

Therefore, the proposed approach offers a framework and heuristics that clinician may apply to build numerous prediction models for binary outcomes and recommends the most accurate model outcome, which is intended to support clinical decision-making.

REFERENCES

Abd-El Mohsen, S. A., Algameel, M. M., Hawash, M., AbdElrahman, S., &Wafik, W. (2021). Predicting cognitive impairment among geriatric patients at Asir central Hospital, Saudi Arabia. *Saudi J. Biol. Sci.*, 28(10), 5781–5785. https://doi.org/10.1016/j.sjbs.2021.06.023

Anthimopoulos, M., Christodoulidis, S., Ebner, L.,Christe, A., & Mougiakakou, S. (2016). Lung pattern classification for interstitial lung diseases using a deep convolutional neural network. *IEEE Trans. Med. Imaging*, 35, 1207–1216.

Chen, L. (2021). Leisure activities and psychological wellbeing reduce the risk of cognitive impairment among older adults with hearing difficulty: a longitudinal study in China. *Maturitas*, 148, 7–13. https://doi.org/10.1016/j.maturitas.2021.03.011

Chen, M., Hao, Y., Hwang, K., Wang, L., & Wang, L. (2017). Disease prediction by machine learning over big data from healthcare communities. *IEEE Access*, 5, 8869–8879.

Cilia, N. D., De Stefano, C., Fontanella, F., & Di Freca, A. S. (2018). An experimental protocol to support cognitive impairment diagnosis by using handwriting analysis. *Proc. Computer Sci.*, 141, 466–471. https://doi.org/10.1016/j.procs.2018.10.141

Cilia, N. D., De Gregorio, G., De Stefano, C., Fontanella, F., Marcelli, A., & Parziale, A. (2022). Diagnosing Alzheimer's disease from online handwriting: a novel dataset and performance benchmarking. *Eng. Appl. Art. Intell.*, 111, 104822. https://doi.org/10.1016/j.engappai.2022.104822

Costanza, A., Amerio, A., Aguglia, A., Escelsior, A., Serafini, G., & Berardelli, I. (2020). When sick brain and hopelessness meet: some aspects of suicidality in the neurological patient. *CNS Neurol. Disord. Drug Targets*, 19(4), 257–263. https://doi.org/10.2174/1871527319666200611130804

Costanza, A., Baertschi, M., Weber, K., Canuto, A., & Canuto, A. (2015). Neurological diseases and suicide: from neurobiology to hopelessness. *Rev. Med. Suisse*, 11(461), 402–405.

De Stefano, C., Fontanella, F., Impedovo, D., Pirlo, G., & Scotto di Freca, A. (2017). A brief overview on handwriting analysis for neurodegenerative disease diagnosis. In: *Proceedings of the Workshop on Artificial Intelligence with Application in Health (WAIAH17)* (pp. 9–16), Bari, Italy.

Dhillon, A., & Singh, A. (2019). Machine learning in healthcare data analysis: a survey. *J. Biol. Today World*, 8, 1–10.

Fang, F., Gao, Y., Schulz, P. E., Selvaraj, S., & Zhang, Y. (2021). Brain controllability distinctiveness between depression and cognitive impairment. *J. Affect Disord.*, 294, 847–856. https://doi.org/10.1016/j.jad.2021.07.106

Garg, A., & Mago, V. (2021). Role of machine learning in medical research: a survey. *Comput. Sci. Rev.*, 40, 100370.

Hastie, T., Tibshirani, R., & Friedman, J. (2009). Overview of supervised learning. In The *Elements of Statistical Learning, Springer Series in Statistics* (pp. 9–41). New York: Springer.

Hinrichs, C., Singh, V., Xu, G., & Johnson, S. C. (2011). Predictive markers for AD in a multi-modality framework: an analysis of MCI progression in the ADNI population. *NeuroImage*, 55, 574–589.

Jiang, T., Gradus, J. L., & Rosellini, A. J. (2020). Supervised machine learning: a brief primer. *Behav. Ther.*, 51, 675–687.

Katayama, O., Lee, S., Bae, S., Makino, K., Shinkai, Y., & Chiba, I. (2020). Relationship between instrumental activities of daily living performance and incidence of mild cognitive impairment among older adults: a 48-month follow-up study. *Arch. Gerontol. Geriatr.*, 94, 104034. https://doi.org/10.1016/j.archger.2020.104034

Li, N., Shepperd, M., & Guo, Y. (2020). A systematic review of unsupervised learning techniques for software defect prediction. *Inf. Softw. Technol.*, 122, 106287.

Madhulatha, T. S. (2012). An overview on clustering methods. *IOSR J. Eng.*, 2, 719–725.

Massetti, N., Russo, M., Franciotti, R., Nardini, D., Mandolini, G. M., Granzotto, A., Bomba, M., DelliPizzi, S., Mosca, A., & Scherer, R. (2022). A machine learning-based holistic approach to predict the clinical course of patients within the Alzheimer's disease spectrum. *J. Alzheimers Dis.*, 85, 1639–1655.

Mehta, J., & Majumdar, A. (2017). Rodeo: robust de-aliasing autoencoder for real-time medical image reconstruction. *Pattern Recognit.*, 63, 499–510.

Nasteski, V. (2017). An overview of the supervised machine learning methods. *Horizons*, 4, 51–62.

Ngiam, K. Y., & Khor, W. (2019). Big data and machine learning algorithms for health-care delivery. *Lancet Oncol.*, 20, e262–e273.

Nian, R., Liu, J., & Huang, B. (2020). A review on reinforcement learning: introduction and applications in industrial process control. *Comput. Chem. Eng.*, 139, 106886.

Perez, A., Manning, K. J., Powell, W., & Barry, L. C. (2021). Cognitive impairment in older incarcerated males: education and race considerations. *Am. J. Geriatr. Psychiatry*, 29(10), 1062–1073. https://doi.org/10.1016/j.jagp.2021.05.014

Przedborski, S., Vila, M., & Jackson-Lewis, V. (2003). Series introduction: neurodegeneration: what is it and where are we? *J. Clin. Invest.*, 111, 3–10.

Qian, K. & Yu, Z. (2019). Domain adaptive dialog generation via meta learning. In *The Proceedings of the 57th Annual Meeting of the Association for Computational Linguistics* (pp. 2639–26490.

Qiang, W., & Zhongli, Z. (2011). Reinforcement learning model, algorithms and its application. *In Proceedings of the 2011 International Conference on Mechatronic Science, Electric Engineering and Computer (MEC 2011)*, Jilin, China, 19–22 August 2011 (pp. 1143–1146).

Reddy, Y. C. A. P., Viswanath, P., & Reddy, B. E. (2018). Semi-supervised learning: a brief review. *Int. J. Eng. Technol.*, 7, 81–85.

Ren, Z., Li, Y., Li, X., Shi, H., Zhao, H., & He, M. (2021). Associations of body mass index, waist circumference and waist-to-height ratio with cognitive impairment among Chinese older adults: based on the CLHLS. *J. Affect Disord.*, 295, 463–470. https://doi.org/10.1016/j.jad.2021.08.093

Saravanan, R., & Sujatha, P. (2018). A state of art techniques on machine learning algorithms: a perspective of supervised learning approaches in data classification. *In Proceedings of the 2018 Second International Conference on Intelligent Computing and Control Systems (ICICCS), Madurai, India,* 14–15 June 2018 (pp. 945–949).

Schlemper, J., Caballero, J., Hajnal, J. V., Price, A., & Rueckert, D. (2017). A deep cascade of convolutional neural networks for MR image reconstruction. *In Proceedings of the Information Processing in Medical Imaging: 25th International Conference, IPMI 2017, Boone, NC, USA, 25–30 June 2017* (pp. 647–658). Berlin/Heidelberg, Germany: Springer.

Sen, P. C., Hajra, M., & Ghosh, M. (2020). Supervised classification algorithms in machine learning: a survey and review. In Mandal, J. K., & Bhattacharya, D. (Eds.), *Emerging Technology in Modelling and Graphics. Advances in Intelligent Systems and Computing* (pp. 99–111). Singapore: Springer.

Serra, A., &Tagliaferri, R. (2019). Unsupervised learning: clustering. In *Encyclopedia of Bioinformatics and Computational Biology,* eds. Shoba Ranganathan, Michael Gribskov, and Kenta Nakai (pp. 350–357). Amsterdam, the Netherlands: Elsevier.

Sinha, U., Singh, A., & Sharma, D. K. (2020). Machine learning in the medical industry. In *Handbook of Research on Emerging Trends and Applications of Machine Learning*, eds. Arun Solanki, Sandeep Kumar, and Anand Nayyar (pp. 403–424).Hershey, PA: IGI Global.

Tseng, M. H., & Cermak, S. A. (1993). The influence of ergonomic factors and perceptual– motor abilities on handwriting performance. *Am. J. Occup. Therapy*, 47(10), 919–926.

Vandam, M., Oller, D. K., Ambrose, S., Gray, S., Richards, J., Gilkerson, J., Silbert, N. & Moeller, M. (2015). Automated vocal analysis of children with hearing loss and their typical and atypical peers. *Ear Hear.*, 36. https://doi.org/10.1097/AUD.0000000000000138

Wuest, T., Weimer, D., Irgens, C., &Thoben, K. D. (2016). Machine learning in manufacturing: advantages, challenges, and applications. *Prod. Manuf. Res.*, 4, 23–45.

Yan, Z., Zhan, Y., Peng, Z., Liao, S., Shinagawa, Y., Zhang, S., Metaxas, D. N., & Zhou, X. S. (2016). Multi-instance deep learning: discover discriminative local anatomies for bodypart recognition. *IEEE Trans. Med. Imaging*, 35, 1332–1343.

9 Optimizing Deep Learning for Pneumonia Diagnosis Using Chest X-Ray Data

Ramdas Kapila, Alluri Sai Sunanda, Sumalatha Saleti, and Elakkiya E

9.1 INTRODUCTION

Pneumonia is a lung infection that is defined by pus and fluids entering the air sacs. It can be painful and impair breathing. Various factors such as bacterial and viral infections, immunological problems, chemical exposure, and occasionally fungal causes contribute to its varied etiologic. Pneumonia is further classified into several groups, including Ventilator-Acquired Pneumonia (VAP), Hospital-Acquired Pneumonia (HAP), and Community-Acquired Pneumonia (CAP). What's noteworthy is how common CAP is—it's the most common type of pneumonia that gets reported—dominating the landscape. It is essential to comprehend the complex nature of this illness by employing Deep Learning (DL) applications for precise pneumonia prediction utilizing chest X-ray pictures (Bhatt and Shah 2023). There has been a sharp rise in respiratory illnesses and infections over time. Numerous lung-related contaminations have been made possible by the deterioration in air quality (Neupane et al. 2010). Acute lower respiratory infections such as pneumonia cause the alveoli to fill with pus and fluid, which lowers the lungs' ability to store oxygen. A shortage of oxygen has a direct effect on the body's normal functions. Lethargy and fatigue are only two of the numerous signs and symptoms of low oxygen levels. In extreme circumstances, the heart and brain may be deterred. Coughing, fever, and shallow breathing are signs of pneumonia (Ebell et al. 2020). In severe situations, coughing and inhaling produce stabbing chest pains. One of the numerous consequences of pneumonia is sepsis, which if ignored can cause organ failure, tissue damage, and even death. Research indicates that those with weakened immune systems are more vulnerable to pneumonia (Ramezani et al. 2015). Children mostly between the ages of one and five, whose immune systems are still developing from embryonic stages, are more vulnerable to this acute respiratory illness (Lee et al. 2010). Malnutrition, vomiting, and the inability to take in food or liquids are signs of severe pneumonia in children (Dean et al. 2018). Qualified medical personnel acquire and analyze X-rays of the thoracic cavity. White patches in the lungs can be used to detect infectious places. In addition, these pictures may be used to detect further issues such as pleural effusions or abscesses. Determining if a radiological scan is necessary after X-ray operations requires a great deal of experience (Wootton and Feldman 2014). The analysis of medical images and DL has come together in recent years to form a potent paradigm that is changing the diagnostic healthcare industry (Panayides et al. 2020, Wong et al. 2023). The classification problem of pneumonia detection requires that the given data be categorized as either normal or pneumonia (Mackenzie 2016). The medical diagnostics field has seen a rise in interest in pneumonia, a serious respiratory disease. The basic contributions of groundbreaking research must be acknowledged as a dive into the employment of Machine Learning (ML) and DL algorithms to forecast pneumonia (Bhattacharya et al. 2021). The combination of Support Vector Machines (SVM) with the RBF kernel and the VGG19 architecture produced remarkable (Chagas et al. 2021). A deep random forest ensemble model powered by Artificial Intelligence (AI) that uses essential DL components to detect

DOI: 10.1201/9781003486640-9

COVID-19 and other forms of pneumonia early on (Jothi Prabha et al. 2022). Accurate diagnosis is essential, and this work uses a variety of ML techniques to evaluate pneumonia (Akgundogdu et al. 2021). Although they have been remarkably successful in diagnosing pneumonia in adults, there are still difficulties in modifying these models for use in pediatric situations. Diagnosing pneumonia in children has distinct obstacles, such as overfitting and low generalizability in existing models, even though pediatric cases are comparable to adult instances. Some of the reasons for the restrictions are the way outliers are handled, training on unbalanced datasets unique to pediatric situations, and the complexity of model architectures meant for adult populations. To explore the complexities of pediatric pneumonia prediction, it is clear that solving these issues is critical to guaranteeing the useful use of reliable and broadly applicable models.

Identifying Pneumonia: The fundamental symptoms, causes, and medical features of pneumonia are covered in this chapter. After gaining a firm understanding of pneumonia, investigating the potential applications of ML in the diagnosis and management of the illness.

DL Place in Healthcare: Understanding DL's larger significance in healthcare is crucial before delving into pneumonia. DL has already shown promise in supporting precise diagnosis, prognoses, and decision-making in several medical domains.

Pneumonia DL Applications: The applications of DL to pneumonia-related problems are discussed in this section, including:

Early Diagnosis and Detection: DL uses wearable technology, clinical assessments, and patient data to help detect pneumonia symptoms early.

Symptom Monitoring: DL offers continuous observation of respiratory symptoms, improving the precision of tracking the development of pneumonia.

Treatment Personalization: DL generates tailored treatment regimens, figuring out the best dosages of medications and finding successful therapies based on patient-specific data.

Future Prospects: This chapter ends with a discussion of how DL could further the study of pneumonia, alter clinical procedures, and enhance patient outcomes while creating opportunities for more individualized treatment plans. Investigating DL's potential in pneumonia presents intriguing opportunities to change our knowledge of and approach to treating this respiratory illness.

9.1.1 Contributions

1. An evaluation of CNNs' performance in classifying pneumonia from chest X-rays.
2. Identifying and discussing particular difficulties in modifying CNN models to diagnose pneumonia.
3. Explored the most significant developments and unsolved requirements in employing DL algorithms for the prediction of pneumonia.
4. Analyzing the Inception, CNN, VGG16, ResNet50, Inception, MobileNetV2, DenseNet121, and LSTM for improved diagnostic precision.
5. A systematic strategy for hyperparameter tweaking that concentrates on important variables to enhance model performance.
6. Advancement in DL architectures for pneumonia forecasting.

In summary, DL has enormous potential to improve our understanding of and competence in the diagnosis and treatment of this complex neurological illness. Hyperparameter tuning allows us to improve DL models, which in turn opens doors for more tailored therapeutics, early detection, and ultimately improved quality of life for patients with pneumonia through the use of data-driven initiatives.

A review of the literature on pneumonia forecasting, an explanation of DL models, an assessment of the proposed framework and its findings, and a conclusion with recommendations for future research comprise the four components of this chapter.

9.2 RELATED WORK

To address the high mortality rate linked with pneumonia, it is imperative to enhance a DL approach to early pneumonia prediction to save lives through prompt treatment (Sharma et al. 2023). Chest X-ray images (CXR) are a vital diagnostic tool for pneumonia that is used in epidemiological research and medical settings. For this reason, it is still difficult to forecast pneumonia from CXR and needs the knowledge of qualified radiologists (Singh and Tripathi 2022). To forecast disease CXR is a powerful mechanism, which affects 7% of the world's population and causes 2 million juvenile deaths annually. To diagnose pneumonia, this study gives CNNs interpretability, and the results show that CNNs are better than benchmark models (Rajaraman et al. 2018). Gu et al. (2018) introduces a unique computer-aided diagnostic (CAD) method. The system can classify pneumonia and segment lung regions with accuracy by utilizing DL techniques. Employing deep CNN techniques with transfer learning, an assessment of the pediatric patient dataset shows increased accuracy and sensitivity. The combination of manual and DCNN capabilities improves classification performance even further. These results demonstrate the promise of CAD systems based on DL for the diagnosis of pneumonia. This work explores the automatic diagnosis of pneumonia using ML. RetinaNet and Mask R-CNN, an ensemble of two CNNs, are used in the proposed method to reliably diagnose pneumonia with a rate of recall of 0.793. A medical expert verified the solution's top 3% ranking using a sizable clinical database after it had been verified on 26,684 Kaggle Pneumonia Diagnosis Challenge images (Sirazitdinov et al. 2019). Xception and Vgg16 are employed in this study to examine their potential for diagnosing pneumonia by tuning and the results indicate that Xception outperformed Vgg16 in terms of pneumonia case detection accuracy (0.87%) (Ayan et al. 2019). Liang et al. (2020) suggests a DL framework for pediatric pneumonia diagnosis that combines dilated convolution with residual connections. The approach obtains an F1-score of 92.7% and a recall rate of 96.7% on the classification problem, overcoming overfitting and feature space information loss. This paper assesses the pneumonia detection and classification capabilities of two deep CNNs: mask-RCNN and residual network. The suggested strategy successfully detects pneumonia with a high recall rate of 96.7% and a F1-score of 92.7% (Al Mubarok et al. 2019). To diagnose pneumonia, this study suggests an improved CNN model. By deleting the pneumonia area, the technique concentrates on disease-specific areas and applies transfer learning to reduce background interference. When compared to the most advanced object detection models, experimental findings show that the suggested technique has reduced false positives and increased accuracy (Li et al. 2019).

To distinguish between lungs that have pneumonia and those that do not, this study investigates the use of Earth Mover's Distance (EMD). The approach involves transforming, normalizing intensity, and preparing the photos. The usefulness of the suggested method in differentiating between lungs afflicted with pneumonia is demonstrated by experimental data. EMD turns out to be a useful instrument for determining the degree of infection (Khatri et al. 2020). This paper suggests automated pneumonia diagnosis using deep CNN architectures. Training on both the original and enhanced datasets allows one to determine how much the work of CNN is impacted by the dataset's size (Sharma et al. 2020). Various architectures are trained and assessed, including models that have already been trained. 92.31% was the validation accuracy of the best model (Jain et al. 2020).

To identify pneumonia, this study created an automated method utilizing pre-trained models. An evaluation was conducted on four models: VGG19, DenseNet121, Xception, and ResNet50. Every model produced an accuracy of more than 83%; DenseNet121 had the greatest results, at 86.8%. Sensitivity exceeded 91% for all models, and the F1-score for DenseNet121 and Xception exceeded 89%. The range of the area under the curve was 0.78 to 0.86 (Salehi et al. 2021). To diagnose pneumonia, this study created a lightweight and precise model that used a CNN model. A weighted ensemble method was utilized to integrate three distinct approaches. The model showed little misclassification, with a F1-score of 88.56% and an impressive recall of 99.23%

(Bhatt and Shah 2023). This study employed CXRs to identify and categorize pneumonia using a DL model named VGG16 and it performed better and outperformed the others (Sharma et al. 2023).

9.3 GAPS IN THE RELATED WORK

1. **Investigation of Hyperparameter Tuning:** The impact of hyperparameter adjustment on the DL framework for pneumonia forecast is much less explored.
2. **Analysis of Model Foundations:** Not enough attention has been paid to the fundamentals of DL architectures, especially to the benefits and drawbacks they present for medical imaging.
3. **Complexities in Training Reportage:** Insufficient focus on the challenges associated with DL model training, such as approaches for preparing the dataset and augmentation.
4. The success rate of cutting-edge models is compared to the impact attained by adjusting hyperparameters in DL models are underrepresented.

9.4 EXPLORATION OF DEEP LEARNING ARCHITECTURES

An in-depth discussion of DL architectures used in pneumonia detection is provided in this section. Analyzing CNNs, Inception, ResNet50, VGG16, and MobileNetV2, DenseNet121, Recurrent Neural Networks (RNNs), among other models, examines their subtleties and efficiency. This chapter attempts to offer a thorough grasp of the advantages and disadvantages of different designs in improving pneumonia diagnosis accuracy by looking at their integration and performance subtleties. The knowledge gained from this investigation adds significantly to the field's continuing progress.

9.4.1 Deep Learning Architectures

Convolutional Neural Networks (CNNs): CNN are DL approaches, specifically designed for recognizing image activities like identifying objects and image classification. Important components include pooling layers for downsampling, convolutional layers for extraction of features, and fully connected layers for classification. Non-linear activation functions, such as ReLU, are used by CNNs to capture complex relationships. Their applications for facial recognition, object identification, and image grouping are their strongest points. Nevertheless, they have difficulties with interpretability and possible overfitting, which may be addressed using methods like transfer learning. Figure 9.1 and Algorithm 1 illustrates the model. Merits: CNNs are excellent at feature extraction using convolutional layers, which allows hierarchical representation learning. CNNs are designed for visual data. Drawbacks: Their "black box" nature makes them difficult to analyze, and huge datasets may cause overfitting issues (Krizhevsky et al. 2012).

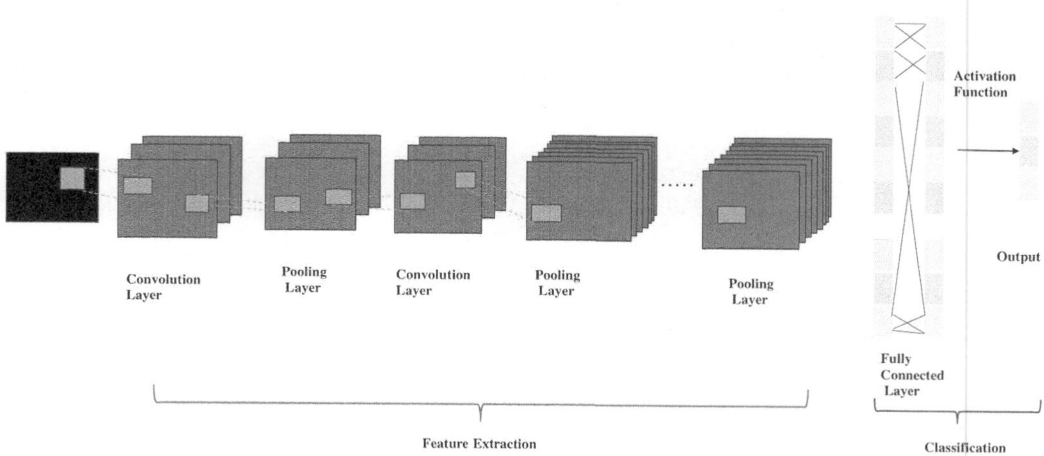

FIGURE 9.1 Convolutional neural networks.

Algorithm 1: CNN Architecture Algorithm

Step 1: Data from images is input.
Step 2: Convolutional Layers: Use filters and ReLU activation in conjunction with convolutional layers.
Step 3: Apply the max pooling layers.
Step 4: The feature map should be flattened.
Step 5: Fully Connected Layer: Use a dense layer that is activated by ReLU and contains neurons.
Step 6: Output Layer: Sigmoid activation, dense layer with a single neuron.

Inception: Inception, a neural network architecture crafted for image processing, is acclaimed for its computational efficiency. Notable features include Inception modules for multi-scale feature capture and global average pooling for reduced parameters. Although achieving high accuracy, its complexity may lead to longer training times. Suited for tasks prioritizing optimal resource utilization, Inception finds applications in image classification and competitions like the ImageNet Challenge. Figure 9.2 and Algorithm 2 illustrates the model. Benefits: The network's initiation modules, which let it collect data at several sizes and boost performance and efficiency, are well-known. Drawbacks: A more sophisticated model that might take longer to train (Szegedy et al. 2015).

Algorithm 2: Inception Algorithm:

Step 1: 224×224 RGB image entered.
Step 2: Use inception modules by applying various convolutions and pooling.
Step 3: Apply pooling and convolutional layers for reduction layers.
Step 4: The feature map should be flattened.
Step 5: Output Layer: Sigmoid activation, dense layer with a single neuron.

9.4.2 Residual Neural Network (ResNet50)

The innovative Residual Neural Network, or ResNet, architecture solves difficulties in deep network training. The resolution of the vanishing gradient issue, residual blocks, and skip connections for effective information flow are important characteristics. ResNet50 has shown promise in object identification, segmentation, and picture classification. It also makes training deep networks easier. Subsequent neural network topologies have been influenced by its significant impact on the field. Figure 9.3 and Algorithm 3 illustrates the model. Benefits: It addresses the problem of the vanishing gradient and facilitates the training of very deep networks through the use of skip connections. Drawbacks: A more sophisticated model might make interpretation more difficult (He et al. 2016).

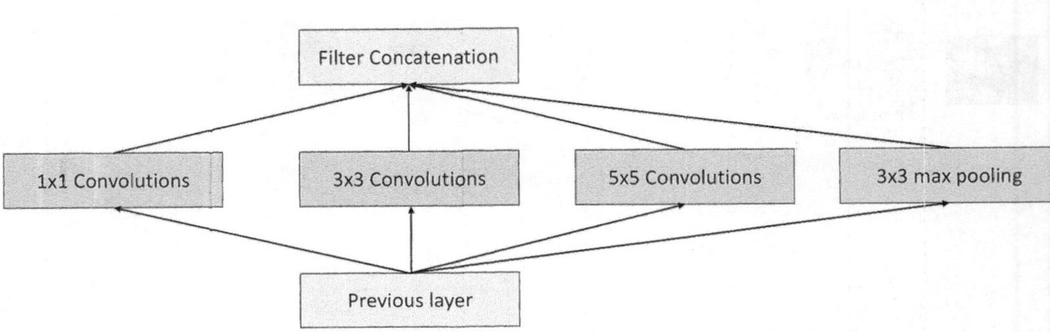

FIGURE 9.2 Inception.

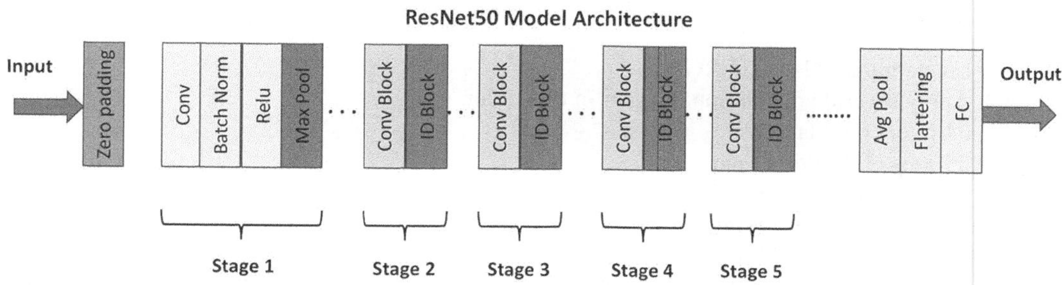

FIGURE 9.3 Residual neural network.

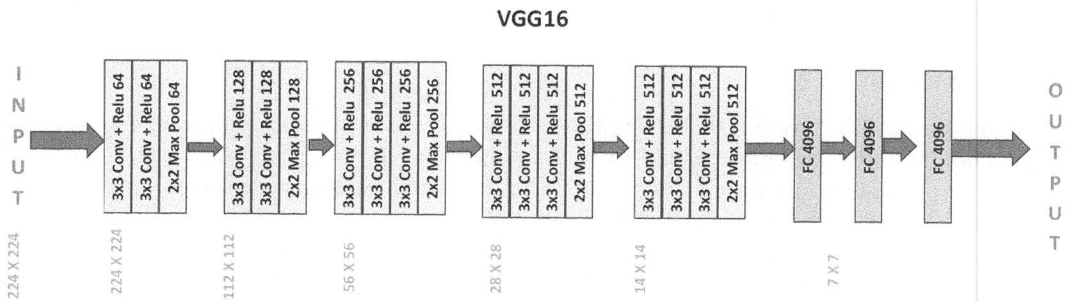

FIGURE 9.4 Visual geometry group16.

Algorithm 3: Residual Neural Network (ResNet50) Algorithm

Step 1: Image input: 224×224 RGB.
Step 2: Initial Convolution: Use max pooling and initial convolution.
Step 3: Utilize residual blocks:
- 64 filters spread across 3 blocks.
- 4 blocks, 128 filters each.
- 256 filters across 6 blocks.
- 512 filters across 3 blocks.

Step 4: Flatten: Make the feature map flat.
Step 5: Output Layer: Sigmoid activation, dense layer with a single neuron.

9.4.3 Visual Geometry Group (VGG16)

Convolutional neural networks, such as VGG16, are well known for being straightforward and efficient in classifying images. The feature extraction process is improved by its repeating blocks of small-sized filters; nonetheless, there are certain drawbacks, such as overfitting and increased processing requirements. Notwithstanding these drawbacks, VGG16 is still a well-liked option for benchmarking and baseline studies in image-related applications. Figure 9.4 and Algorithm 4 illustrates the model. Advantages: Repetitive blocks of tiny convolutional filters make the architecture simple and efficient for feature extraction. Drawbacks: It requires a lot of computation and is vulnerable to overfitting because of the abundance of parameters (Simonyan and Zisserman 2014).

Algorithm 4: Visual Geometry Group (VGG16) Algorithm:

Step 1: Image input: 224×224 RGB.
Step 2: Apply several convolutional layers in this order:
  64 filters on 2 layers.
  2 layers, 128 filters each.
  With 256 filters across 3 layers.
  512 filters across 3 layers.
  512 filters across 3 layers.
Step 3: Max Pooling: Following every convolutional layer set.
Step 4: The feature map should be flattened.
Step 5: Apply two dense layers, each with 4096 neurons, and activate ReLU to create fully connected layers.
Step 6: Output Layer: Sigmoid activation, dense layer with a single neuron.

9.4.4 MobileNetV2

The lightweight CNN MobileNetV2 emphasizes efficiency with a smaller memory footprint and computational cost, making it ideal for mobile and edge devices. It is the perfect option for on-device applications because of its adaptable design, which balances performance and resource limitations. Figure 9.5 and Algorithm 5 illustrates the model. Benefits: Designed with a smaller memory footprint and lower computational costs for mobile and edge devices. Drawbacks: Gives up some accuracy in comparison to bigger models, particularly for more difficult jobs (Tragoudaras et al. 2022).

Algorithm 5: MobileNetV2 Algorithm:

Step 1: Image input: 224×224 RGB.
Step 2: Apply the initial standard convolution.
Step 3: Implement depth-wise separable convolutions along with residual connections.
Step 4: The feature map has to be flattened.
Step 5: Output Layer: Sigmoid activation, dense layer with a single neuron.

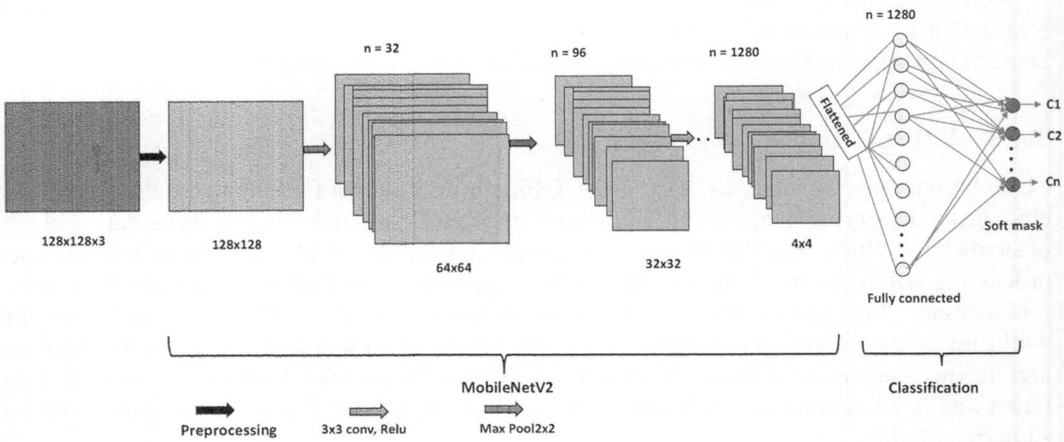

FIGURE 9.5 MobileNetV2.

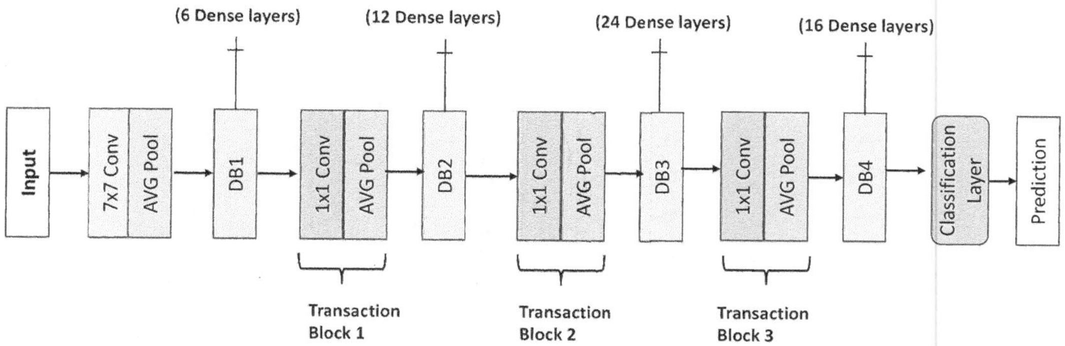

FIGURE 9.6 DenseNet121.

9.4.5 DenseNet121

DenseNet121 is a CNN that stands out for having many connections between layers, which encourages feature reuse and lessens training difficulties. It has demonstrated efficacy in computer vision applications such as object identification and picture classification, albeit with increased memory needs. Figure 9.6 and Algorithm 6 illustrates the model. Benefits: Dense layer connections encourage the reuse of features and solve vanishing gradient problems. Drawbacks: More memory use and computational expense in comparison to more straightforward designs (Huang et al. 2017).

Algorithm 6: DenseNet121 Algorithm:

Step 1: Image input: 224×224 RGB.
Step 2: Dense Blocks: Apply layers that receive input from all layers that came before them.
Step 3: Convolutional and pooling layers should be applied as transition layers in between dense blocks.
Step 4: The feature map should be flattened.
Step 5: Output Layer: Sigmoid activation, dense layer with a single neuron.

9.4.6 Recurrent Neural Networks (RNNs)

Naturally proficient at tasks like time-series analysis, RNNs are specialized in handling sequential input. They record temporal dynamics using memory cells for context retention. Although RNNs have drawbacks like the dilemma of the vanishing/exploding gradient and computing intensity, they are nonetheless useful for jobs that need sequential dependency comprehension. Technologies such as GRU and LSTM are attempting to tackle these issues. Figure 9.7 and Algorithm 7 illustrates the model. Advantages: RNNs are well-suited for jobs requiring time-series data because they can grasp temporal relationships in sequences. Cons: Hard to parallelize, computationally demanding, and prone to vanishing/exploding gradient issues.

Algorithm 7: Recurrent Neural Network (RNN) Algorithm:

Step 1: Source: Data in a sequence.
Step 2: Recurrent Layers: Use LSTM or GRU recurrent units.
Step 3: Fully Connected Layer: Use an activation function and a dense layer filled with neurons.
Step 4: Output Layer: Sigmoid activation and one neuron in a dense layer.

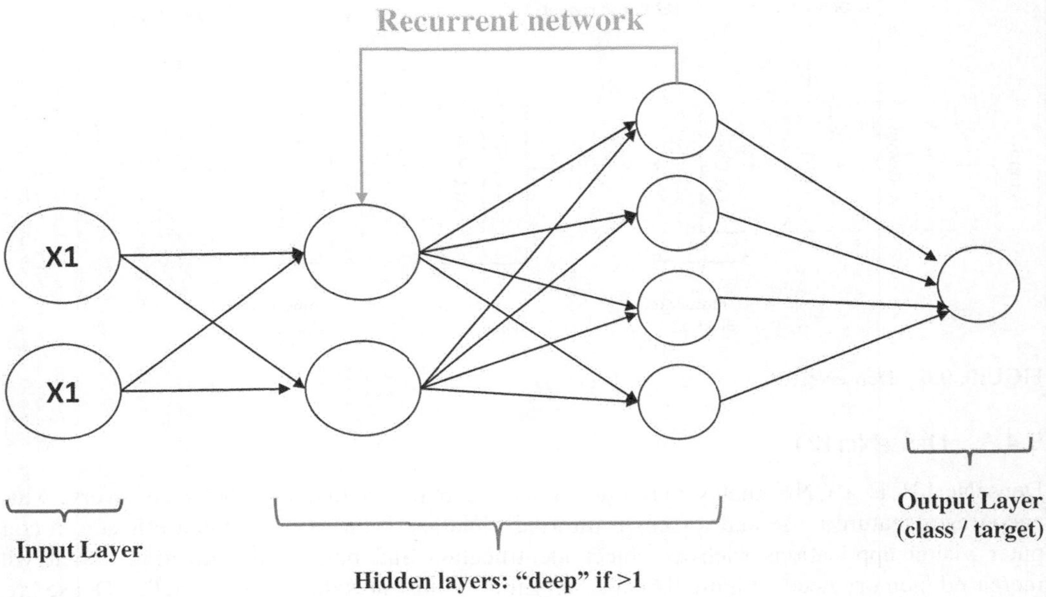

FIGURE 9.7 Recurrent neural network.

9.5 EXPERIMENTAL RESULTS AND DISCUSSION

The X-ray image dataset for pneumonia check, which is accessible through an open repository, was utilized in this work (Sharma et al. 2023). Figure 9.8 depicts the suggested architecture.

9.5.1 Image Dataset

The study relied on a dataset comprising images from chest X-rays specifically designed to identify and categorize pneumonia (Kermany et al. 2018).

9.5.2 Data Preprocessing

To improve it for DL tasks, the dataset in this work received extensive preprocessing. Important processes including image rescaling, brightness correction, vertical and horizontal altering, horizontal flipping, color mode transformation, batching and shuffling, and data transfer from the database are all part of the preprocessing pipeline. Standardizing image dimensions, adjusting the brightness, adding variability, improving dataset variety, lowering computing cost, and smoothly incorporating big datasets into the DL workflow all depended on these procedures. It is important to remember that all preprocessing steps are carried out by ethical standards to protect patient confidentiality and privacy.

Resizing Images: Resizing an image to a specific dimension is known as image rescaling.

$$\text{Image Resizing} = \text{Resize}\left(\text{original size},\, W_{\text{new}},\, H_{\text{new}}\right) \tag{9.1}$$

where W_{new}, H_{new} is the desired width and height of the image after resizing.
Brightness Adjustments: Modify the brightness of the images.

$$P_{\text{new}} - \text{clip}\left(P_{\text{original}} \times \alpha, 0, 255\right) \tag{8.2}$$

P_{original} is the image pixel original value of the grayscale, P_{new} is the image brightness modified pixel value, α is the factor used to regulate brightness.

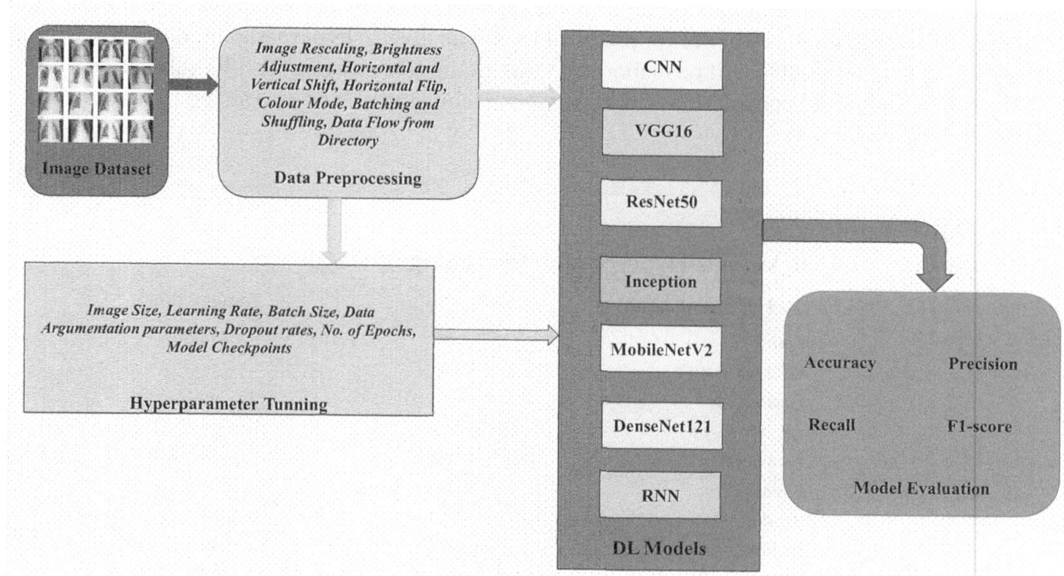

FIGURE 9.8 The architecture of the proposed methodology.

Images Shift/Flip: Apply both vertical and horizontal shifts as well as horizontal flips.

$$\text{Horizontal Shifted Image}(x, y) = \text{Original Image}(x - \Delta x, y) \tag{8.3}$$

The pixel shift in horizontal directions, expressed as Δx.

$$\text{Horizontal Flip Image}_{\text{flip}}(x, y) = I(W - x - 1, y) \tag{9.4}$$

Color Conversion: Make grayscale images using,

$$\text{Imagegray}(x, y) = \frac{1}{3}\sum I_{\text{orig}}(x, y, c) \tag{9.5}$$

I_{orig} (x,y,c): The pixel value in the original image at coordinates (x,y), (X,Y), and color channel (c).

I_{gray} (x,y): The grayscale image's pixel value at (x,y) coordinates (x,y).

Batching and Shuffling: Sort images into sets and then rearrange them.

Importing Data: Import pictures straight from the folder hierarchy.

9.6 HYPERPARAMETER TUNING

Hyperparameter adjustment is essential while trying to maximize the DL architecture's performance. A thorough hyperparameter on seven different architectures: CNN, ResNet50, RNN, Inception, VGG16, MobileNetV2, and DenseNet50. The following important hyperparameters have been investigated: number of epochs, dropout rates, picture size, learning rate, batch size, and model checkpoints, by carefully tweaking these hyperparameters through systematic testing and incremental improvement to determine the best combinations for every architecture. Throughout the process, which comprised rigorous training and assessment, noticed how adjustments to hyperparameters affected model performance measures. Through a methodical manipulation of hyperparameters and performance monitoring in various configurations, managed to obtain important insights into the subtleties of each architecture and how sensitive it is to different hyperparameter settings. In the end, this thorough hyperparameter tuning procedure helped us to improve our model's forecast accuracy and resilience for practical uses. The diverse hyperparameter tuning outcomes across the seven DL models will be elaborated upon in the forthcoming Results subsection.

Table 9.1 Comparing convolution neural network architectures with optimized hyperparameters for pneumonia prediction

TABLE 9.1
Illustrates all DL Models Hyperparameter Tuning in Detail

Model	Hyperparameter	Original Value	Tuned Value
CNN	optimizer	Adam	Adam
	Dropout Rate	0.2	0.2
	Batch Size	64	64
	Learning Rate	Not specified	Not specified
	Number of Filters	Not specified	Not specified
	Kernel Size	(3, 3)	(3, 3)
	Strides	1	1
	Padding	same'	same'
	Activation Function	ReLU	ReLU
	Number of Conv Layers	3	3
	Number of Dense Layers	1	1
	Dense Layer Units	128	128
	Pooling Size	(2, 2)	(2, 2)
	Pooling Type	MaxPool2D	MaxPool2D
	Regularization	None	None
	Data Augmentation	None	None
	Early Stopping	FALSE	Not specified
VGG16	Optimizer	Adam	RMSprop
	Dropout Rate	0.2	0.3
	Batch Size	32	64
	Learning Rate	0.001	0.01
	Number of Filters	32	64
	Kernel Size	(3,3)	(5,5)
	Strides	1	2
	Padding	same'	valid'
	Activation Function	ReLU	LeakyReLU
	Number of Conv Layers	3	4
	Number of Dense Layers	1	2
	Dense Layer Units	128	256
	Pooling Size	(2,2)	(3,3)
	Pooling Type	MaxPool2D	AveragePool2D
	Regularization	None	L2
	Data Augmentation	None	HorizontalFlip, RotationRange (20), ZoomRange (0.2)
	Early Stopping	FALSE	True, Patience(3)
RNN	Optimizer	Adam	RMSprop
	Dropout Rate	0.2	0.3
	Batch Size	32	64
	Learning Rate	0.001	0.01
	Number of Units	128	256
	Activation Function	Tanh	ReLU

(*Continued*)

TABLE 9.1 (*Continued*)
Illustrates all DL Models Hyperparameter Tuning in Detail

Model	Hyperparameter	Original Value	Tuned Value
ResNet50	Optimizer	Adam	RMSprop
	Dropout Rate	0.2	0.3
	Batch Size	32	64
	Learning Rate	0.001	0.01
	Number of Layers	50	100
	Activation Function	ReLU	LeakyReLU
Inception	Optimizer	Adam	RMSprop
	Dropout Rate	0.2	0.3
	Batch Size	32	64
	Learning Rate	0.001	0.01
	Number of Modules	3	5
	Pooling Size	(2,2)	(3,3)
MobileNetV2	Optimizer	Adam	RMSprop
	Dropout Rate	0.2	0.3
	Batch Size	32	64
	Learning Rate	0.001	0.01
	Alpha	1	0.5
	Pooling Type	MaxPooling2D	AveragePooling2D
DenseNet121	Optimizer	Adam	RMSprop
	Dropout Rate	0.2	0.3
	Batch Size	32	64
	Learning Rate	0.001	0.01
	Growth Rate	32	64
	Compression Factor	0.5	0.3

9.7 RESULTS AND DISCUSSION

The presentation of the experiment results and their comparison with the findings of relevant past research initiatives constitute this section of the work. This section emphasizes the value of Tables 9.1 and Table 9.3 comparative assessment, which offers a succinct yet insightful summary of the capabilities of various DL architectures. This tabular presentation serves as an invaluable point of reference, including measurements and performance indicators for each model.

As hyperparameters directly affect the model's computational efficiency, generalization, and performance, fine-tuning them is an essential part of developing DL architectures for medical imaging applications. By analyzing the hyperparameters of many CNN architectures, such as DenseNet121, RNN, ResNet50, VGG16, Inception, and MobileNetV2. Optimizer, activation function, number of convolutional layers, dropout rate, kernel size, padding, learning rate, number of dense layers, strides, batch size, pooling size, regularization, pooling type, number of filters, data augmentation techniques, number of dense layer units, and early stopping strategies are among the hyperparameters things are compared and taken into account.

Original vs. Tuned Hyperparameters: Here is a thorough examination of the initial and tuned values for the most important hyperparameters for each CNN architecture:

Optimizer Selection: Adam and RMSprop, two well-known optimizers, are frequently the default settings. Tuning each architecture's optimizer parameters to achieve a balance between model performance and convergence speed.

Dropout Rate and Regularization: Overfitting during training is minimized by setting the regularization settings and starting dropout rates. Assuring that the model behaves adequately on untested data and prevents underfitting, the ideal balance has to be achieved while tuning these variables.

Learning Rate and Batch Size: To increase training efficiency and accelerate convergence, changing the number of batches and learning rates. The tuned values are determined using empirical testing and validation outcomes.

Activation Functions: Many designs employ original activation functions, such as ReLU. To facilitate better capture of complex data patterns, tuning entailed investigating various parameters like Tanh or LeakyReLU.

Data Augmentation: Although the initial models may not have incorporated data augmentation, tuning is required using methods such as rotations, flips in the horizontal direction, and zoom ranges to improve model resilience and decrease overfitting.

Pooling Strategies: Standard techniques are usually used to determine the initial pooling sizes and varieties. Optimizing these parameters through tuning will enhance feature extraction and protect significant spatial information.

Early Stopping: Early stop tactics might not have been used in the original models. During tuning, early stop has been employed in conjunction with the right settings to determine the optimal training epochs and prevent overfitting.

9.8 METRICS FOR EVALUATING PERFORMANCE

An essential way to evaluate the effectiveness of categorization models is to look at metrics like precision, f1 score, accuracy, and recall. Accuracy, which gives an overall impression of the model's performance, is stated as the proportion of correctly anticipated cases among all instances. Precision addresses this by focusing on the exactness of positive forecasts and calculating the ratio of true positives to all positive expectations. On the other hand, recall also referred to as sensitivity measures the model's comprehensiveness by indicating its capacity to recognize every true positive. Table 9.2 displays the confusion matrix used to assess each model's success.

$$\text{Accuracy} = (\text{TP} + \text{TN})/(\text{TP} + \text{TN} + \text{FP} + \text{FN}) \tag{9.6}$$

$$\text{Precision} = \text{TP}/(\text{TP} + \text{FP}) \tag{9.7}$$

$$\text{Recall} = \text{TP}/(\text{TP} + \text{FN}) \tag{9.8}$$

$$\text{F1Score} = 2 \times (\text{Precision} + \text{Recall})/(\text{Precision} \times \text{Recall}) \tag{9.9}$$

TABLE 9.2
Confusion Matrix

	Actual Positive	Actual Negative
Predicted positive	True positive (TP)	False positive (FP) (Type -I error)
Predicted negative	False negative (FN) (Type -II error)	True negative (TN)

9.9 RESULTS OF DL MODEL WITHOUT HYPER TUNING AND WITH HYPER TUNING

The findings show how important hyperparameter adjustment is for the model's success in pneumonia prediction tasks. The model may be improved by carefully tweaking hyperparameters such as batch sizes, learning rates, optimizer settings, and dropout rates. Table 9.3 exhibits the results of the DL models both with and without hyper-tuning. Figure 9.9 illustrates the comparison of tuned DL models.

The results show that different DL designs perform differently in terms of pneumonia prediction. DenseNet121 and ResNet50 are two examples of models that demonstrate strong baseline performance and notable efficiency. In contrast, MobileNetV2 performs much worse, showing lower recall and accuracy, underscoring its limitations in identifying appropriate features for pneumonia prediction. The model's reliability is strongly impacted by the DL architecture selection, deeper models, such as VGG16, Inception, and ResNet50, frequently perform better than shallower architectures, such as CNN and MobileNetV2. ones that have been fine-tuned often perform surpassing ones that have not been fine-tuned, which emphasizes the importance of hyperparameter tuning when developing DL models. When choosing a DL model for pneumonia forecasting, baseline performance and the potential for improving results through hyperparameter adjustment must be considered. For this task, deeper architectures like ResNet50 and DenseNet121 that function well at baseline are excellent options. Shallower systems, like as CNN, may also be considered when computational resources are scarce. Hyperparameter tuning ought to be a vital aspect of building DL models since it optimizes the model's effectiveness and generalizability. The best method for hyperparameter tuning will rely on the time and computer resources available. Some possible methods for hyperparameter tuning are grid search, random search, and Bayesian optimization. Choosing the appropriate architecture and optimizing model parameters are critical to accurately forecast pneumonia, as the comparative analysis of DL algorithms and hyperparameter tweaking highlights. Hyperparameter tuning proved to be useful in developing DL models as it leads to considerable performance improvements when pre-trained models are fine-tuned. Further investigations to enhance the reliability of models in pneumonia prediction might involve the use of ensemble approaches or sophisticated hyperparameter tuning techniques. All other models in the research, including those in Table 9.4 and existing

TABLE 9.3
Comparison of Optimized Convolution Neural Network Architectures Performance

	Accuracy	Precision	Recall	F1-score
CNN	89.59	85.72	93.86	88.71
Tuned-CNN	91.43	93.4	92.22	91.96
VGG16	86.86	88.47	89.57	87.57
Tuned-VGG16	88.88	90.14	88.52	91.42
Inception	86.88	97.14	82.92	89.47
Tuned-Inception	89.91	88.18	92.56	90.32
RNN	92.01	90.55	94.26	92.36
Tuned-RNN	93.69	92.12	95.9	93.97
MobileNetV2	88.49	85.87	82.72	83.85
Tuned-MobileNetV2	90.55	94.26	86.88	88.52
ResNet50	93.01	92.55	94.35	93.36
Tuned-ResNet50	**96.63**	**96.85**	**96.85**	**96.85**
DenseNet121	92.56	89.91	90.32	89.36
Tuned-DenseNet121	94.26	95.9	93.69	92.36

Bold values indicate the superior performance of the Tuned-RestNet50.

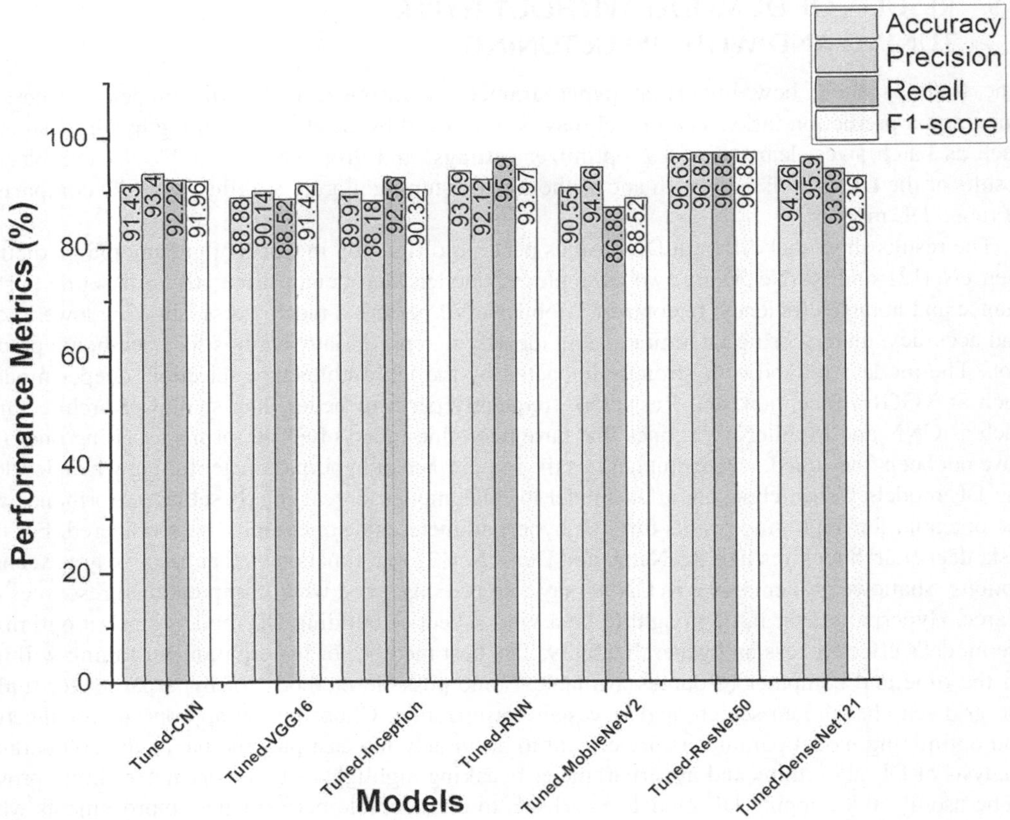

FIGURE 9.9 Comparison of tuned deep learning models.

TABLE 9.4
Comparison of Existing Models with Proposed Methodology

Author (s)	Year	Best Model	Accuracy	Precision	Recall	F1-Score
Gu et al.	2018	Deep Convolutional neural network	80.4	88.86	77.55	–
Sirazitdinov et al.	2019	Ensemble of RetinaNet and Mask R-CNN	–	75.8	79.3	77.5
Ayan et al.	2019	Vgg16	87	91	89	90
Liang.G et al.	2019	CNN	90.5	89.1	96.7	92.7
Al Mubarok et al.	2019	mask-RCNN	85.6	–	51.52	–
Li.B et al.	2019	CNN	26.2	61.1	83.5	–
Khatri et al.	2020	Earth Mover's Distance (EMD) approach	83.3	80	89.5	–
Sharma.H et al.	2020	CNN	90.68	–	–	–
Jain.R et al.	2020	VGG16	87.28	–	95	94
Salehi et al.	2021	DenseNet121	86.8	87	92.8	89.8
Bhatt and Shah	2023	A novel weighted ensemble approach	84.12	80.04	99.23	88.56
Sharma et al.	2023	NN with VGG 16	92.15	94.23	93.08	93.7
Proposed Methodology		**Tuned-ResNet50**	**96.63**	**96.85**	**96.85**	**96.85**

Bold values indicate the superior performance of the Tuned-RestNet50.

benchmarks, are surpassed by ResNet50 with hyperparameter tuning. This outstanding result highlights the effectiveness of the ResNet50 architecture with meticulous fine-tuning.

9.10 CONCLUSION

This chapter has examined the application of DL models in medical image analysis, with a focus on predicting the occurrence of pneumonia using chest X-ray images. Through analysis of Inception, ResNet50, CNN, RNN, VGG16, MobileNetV2, and DenseNet121 have emphasized how crucial it is to optimize hyperparameters to get the best possible model performance. It has shown that hyperparameter tweaking may effectively increase pneumonia prediction accuracy through thorough study and testing. According to the findings, tuned ResNet50 obtained a maximum accuracy of 96.63%, highlighting the substantial influence of fine-tuning on predicting effectiveness. The significance of image-specific augmentation techniques and dataset preparation, as well as the difficulties and factors to be taken into account while training DL models on medical imaging datasets. All things considered, this chapter advances the knowledge of DL in the context of medical image processing and emphasizes how crucial hyperparameter tweaking is to maximizing model performance for practical uses. There are plenty of interesting prospects for future development. By investigating more intelligent methods of fine-tuning model parameters to improve performance and speed. It's also critical to investigate the potential use of these improved models for various medical datasets and jobs. Integrating disparate data sets, for example, X-ray images and medical records may improve the precision of our forecasts. To gain doctor's trust also need to find more straightforward explanations for our models' decision-making processes. Future paths include investigating state-of-the-art DL architectures, optimizing feature extraction techniques, and creating more resilient models via ensemble approaches. These methods seek to improve the reliability as well as the efficiency of the model.

REFERENCES

Akgundogdu, Abdurrahim. "Detection of pneumonia in chest X-ray images by using 2D discrete wavelet feature extraction with random forest." *International Journal of Imaging Systems and Technology* 31, no. 1 (2021): 82–93.

Al Mubarok, Abdullah Faqih, Jeffrey AM Dominique, and Ahmad Habbie Thias. "Pneumonia detection with deep convolutional architecture." In *2019 International Conference of Artificial Intelligence and Information Technology (ICAIIT)*, pp. 486–489. IEEE, Yogyakarta, Indonesia, 2019.

Ayan, Enes, and Halil Murat Ünver. "Diagnosis of pneumonia from chest X-ray images using deep learning." In *2019 Scientific Meeting on Electrical-Electronics & Biomedical Engineering and Computer Science (EBBT)*, pp. 1–5. IEEE, Istanbul, Turkey, 2019.

Bhatt, Harsh, and Manan Shah. "A convolutional neural network ensemble model for Pneumonia detection using chest X-ray images." *Healthcare Analytics* 3 (2023): 100176.

Bhattacharya, Sweta, Praveen Kumar Reddy Maddikunta, Quoc-Viet Pham, Thippa Reddy Gadekallu, Chiranji Lal Chowdhary, Mamoun Alazab, and Md Jalil Piran. "Deep learning and medical image processing for coronavirus (COVID-19) pandemic: A survey." *Sustainable Cities and Society* 65 (2021): 102589.

Chagas, João Victor S. das, Douglas de A. Rodrigues, Roberto F. Ivo, Mohammad Mehedi Hassan, Victor Hugo C. de Albuquerque, and Pedro P. Rebouças Filho. "A new approach for the detection of pneumonia in children using CXR images based on an real-time IoT system." *Journal of Real-Time Image Processing* 18, no. 4 (2021): 1099–1114.

Dean, Preston, and Todd A. Florin. "Factors associated with pneumonia severity in children: a systematic review." *Journal of the Pediatric Infectious Diseases Society* 7, no. 4 (2018): 323–334.

Ebell, Mark H., Hulme Chupp, Xinyan Cai, Michelle Bentivegna, and Maggie Kearney. "Accuracy of signs and symptoms for the diagnosis of community-acquired pneumonia: a meta-analysis." *Academic Emergency Medicine* 27, no. 7 (2020): 541–553.

Gu, Xianghong, Liyan Pan, Huiying Liang, and Ran Yang. "Classification of bacterial and viral childhood pneumonia using deep learning in chest radiography." In *Proceedings of the 3rd International Conference on Multimedia and Image Processing*, pp. 88–93, Guiyang, China, 2018.

He, Kaiming, Xiangyu Zhang, Shaoqing Ren, and Jian Sun. "Deep residual learning for image recognition." In *Proceedings of the IEEE Conference on Computer Vision and Pattern Recognition*, pp. 770–778. 2016.

Huang, Gao, Zhuang Liu, Laurens van der Maaten, and Kilian Q. Weinberger. "Densely Connected Convolutional Networks." In *2017 IEEE Conference on Computer Vision and Pattern Recognition (CVPR)*, pp. 2261-2269. IEEE, Honolulu, HI, USA, 2017. doi: 10.1109/CVPR.2017.243.

Jain, Rachna, Preeti Nagrath, Gaurav Kataria, V. Sirish Kaushik, and D. Jude Hemanth. "Pneumonia detection in chest X-ray images using convolutional neural networks and transfer learning." *Measurement* 165 (2020): 108046.

Jothi Prabha, A., N. Venkateswaran, and Prabaharan Sengodan. "AI-based deep random forest ensemble model for prediction of COVID-19 and pneumonia from chest X-ray images." In *Artificial Intelligence for Innovative Healthcare Informatics*, eds, Shabir Ahmad Parah, Mamoon Rashid, and Vijayakumar Varadarajan, pp. 133–149. Cham: Springer International Publishing, 2022.

Kermany, Daniel S., Michael Goldbaum, Wenjia Cai, Carolina CS Valentim, Huiying Liang, Sally L. Baxter, Alex McKeown et al. "Identifying medical diagnoses and treatable diseases by image-based deep learning." *Cell* 172, no. 5 (2018): 1122–1131.

Khatri, Archit, Rishabh Jain, Hariom Vashista, Nityam Mittal, Priya Ranjan, and Rajiv Janardhanan. "Pneumonia identification in chest X-ray images using EMD." In *Trends in Communication, Cloud, and Big Data: Proceedings of 3rd National Conference on CCB*, 2018, pp. 87–98. Springer Singapore, Sikkim, India, 2020.

Krizhevsky, Alex, Ilya Sutskever, and Geoffrey E. Hinton. "Imagenet classification with deep convolutional neural networks." *Advances in Neural Information Processing Systems* 25 (2012): 84–90

Lee, Grace E., Scott A. Lorch, Seth Sheffler-Collins, Matthew P. Kronman, and Samir S. Shah. "National hospitalization trends for pediatric pneumonia and associated complications." *Pediatrics* 126, no. 2 (2010): 204–213.

Li, Bingchuan, Guixia Kang, Kai Cheng, and Ningbo Zhang. "Attention-guided convolutional neural network for detecting pneumonia on chest x-rays." In *2019 41st Annual International Conference of the IEEE Engineering in Medicine and Biology Society (EMBC)*, pp. 4851–4854. IEEE, Berlin, Germany, 2019.

Liang, Gaobo, and Lixin Zheng. "A transfer learning method with deep residual network for pediatric pneumonia diagnosis." *Computer Methods and Programs in Biomedicine* 187 (2020): 104964.

Mackenzie, Grant. "The definition and classification of pneumonia." *Pneumonia* 8, no. 1 (2016): 14.

Neupane, Binod, Michael Jerrett, Richard T. Burnett, Thomas Marrie, Altaf Arain, and Mark Loeb. "Long-term exposure to ambient air pollution and risk of hospitalization with community-acquired pneumonia in older adults." *American Journal of Respiratory and Critical Care Medicine* 181, no. 1 (2010): 47–53.

Panayides, Andreas S., Amir Amini, Nenad D. Filipovic, Ashish Sharma, Sotirios A. Tsaftaris, Alistair Young, David Foran et al. "AI in medical imaging informatics: current challenges and future directions." *IEEE Journal of Biomedical and Health Informatics* 24, no. 7 (2020): 1837–1857.

Rajaraman, Sivaramakrishnan, Sema Candemir, Incheol Kim, George Thoma, and Sameer Antani. "Visualization and interpretation of convolutional neural network predictions in detecting pneumonia in pediatric chest radiographs." *Applied Sciences* 8, no. 10 (2018): 1715.

Ramezani, Monir, Seyedeh Zahra Aemmi, and Zahra Emami Moghadam. "Factors affecting the rate of pediatric pneumonia in developing countries: a review and literature study." *International Journal of Pediatrics* 3, no. 6.2 (2015): 1173–1181.

Salehi, Mohammad, Reza Mohammadi, Hamed Ghaffari, Nahid Sadighi, and Reza Reiazi. "Automated detection of pneumonia cases using deep transfer learning with paediatric chest X-ray images." *The British Journal of Radiology* 94, no. 1121 (2021): 20201263.

Sharma, Harsh, Jai Sethia Jain, Priti Bansal, and Sumit Gupta. "Feature extraction and classification of chest x-ray images using CNN to detect pneumonia." In *2020 10th International Conference on Cloud Computing, Data Science & Engineering (Confluence)*, pp. 227–231, IEEE, Noida, India 2020.

Sharma, Shagun, and Kalpna Guleria. "A deep learning based model for the detection of pneumonia from chest X-ray images using VGG-16 and neural networks." *Procedia Computer Science* 218 (2023): 357–366.

Simonyan, Karen, and Andrew Zisserman. "Very deep convolutional networks for large-scale image recognition." arXiv preprint arXiv:1409.1556 (2014).

Singh, Sukhendra, and B. K. Tripathi. "Pneumonia classification using quaternion deep learning." *Multimedia Tools and Applications* 81, no. 2 (2022): 1743–1764.

Sirazitdinov, Ilyas, Maksym Kholiavchenko, Tamerlan Mustafaev, Yuan Yixuan, Ramil Kuleev, and Bulat Ibragimov. "Deep neural network ensemble for pneumonia localization from a large-scale chest x-ray database." *Computers & Electrical Engineering* 78 (2019): 388–399.

Szegedy, Christian, Wei Liu, Yangqing Jia, Pierre Sermanet, Scott Reed, Dragomir Anguelov, Dumitru Erhan, Vincent Vanhoucke, and Andrew Rabinovich. "Going deeper with convolutions." In *Proceedings of the IEEE Conference on Computer Vision and Pattern Recognition*, pp. 1–9. IEEE, Boston, MA, USA, 2015.

Tragoudaras, Antonios, Pavlos Stoikos, Konstantinos Fanaras, Athanasios Tziouvaras, George Floros, Georgios Dimitriou, Kostas Kolomvatsos, and Georgios Stamoulis. "Design space exploration of a sparse mobile-netv2 using high-level synthesis and sparse matrix techniques on FPGAs." *Sensors* 22, no. 12 (2022): 4318.

Wong, Kelvin KL, Muhammad Ayoub, Zaijie Cao, Cang Chen, Weimin Chen, Dhanjoo N. Ghista, and Chris WJ Zhang. "The synergy of cybernetical intelligence with medical image analysis for deep medicine: a methodological perspective." *Computer Methods and Programs in Biomedicine* 240 (2023): 107677.

Wootton, Dan, and Charles Feldman. "The diagnosis of pneumonia requires a chest radiograph (x-ray) – yes, no or sometimes?." *Pneumonia* 5, no. 1 (2014): 1–7.

10 Melanoma Detection Using Deep Convolutional Neural Networks

A High-Resolution Image-Based Approach

Anitha B, Umapathi K, and Jayasheela M

10.1 INTRODUCTION

Skin cancer, defined as abnormal growth of skin cells, is categorized into three major types based on the type of skin cell that is cancerous. When skin coloring cells, say melanocytes, grow rapidly, it leads to melanoma. According to World Health Organization (WHO) report, the major cause for skin cancer is unprotected exposure to solar Ultraviolet (UV) radiations. As with any type of cancer, even melanoma is benign or malignant, and if detected early, is highly treatable. Conventional melanoma diagnosis starts with visual inspection of the affected area followed by dermoscopy, in order to understand the lesion better. Finally, biopsy is done to confirm cancerous growth of skin cells. Conventional diagnosis is time-consuming and labor-intensive. In addition, it is tedious to make a diagnosis in early stages of the disease. Non-invasive melanoma diagnosis is made feasible with the advent of advanced image processing algorithms. Whereas, Artificial Intelligence (AI) tools aid in advancing melanoma diagnosis towards early disease prediction (Wu et al. 2022).

AI tools mimic human intelligence in executing a task. Machine learning (ML) and deep learning (DL) are the two broad classifications of AI techniques. Deep learning tools are built over Deep Neural Networks (DNN) models such as Convolutional Neural Networks (CNN), which are trained to learn inherent patterns present in input training data and make predictions with test data. Such DNN models become capable of diagnosing melanoma in early stages when trained with dermoscopy images obtained from different stages of the disease. But technologies are born with limitations. A major limitation that affects the efficiency of an AI model in biomedical applications is the unavailability of required datasets for training. Specific to skin cancer diagnosis, class imbalance and images of different resolution are the major limitations that hurdle the effective implementation of AI-based melanoma classification. Whereas, the implementation of an AI model is hurdled by ethical considerations and the black box nature of AI models (Naeem et al. 2020). Motivated towards devising an AI solution for the early diagnosis of melanoma, the objective of this work is

1. To conduct a detailed study of the recent techniques adapted for melanoma classification and present a brief review of the state-of-the-art techniques in early detection and classification of melanoma
2. To develop a novel deep convolutional neural network model specifically tailored for early detection and classification of melanoma by addressing the limitations in each stage of the dermoscopic image processing.
3. To demonstrate efficiency of the developed framework on different performance metrices accuracy, sensitivity and specificity.

DOI: 10.1201/9781003486640-10

10.2 RELATED WORKS

Early detection is the only known solution for survival from cancer. With the advent of artificial intelligence algorithm, a number of researches have been initiated towards the automatic detection and classification of melanoma (Dildar et al. 2021, Saeed and Zeebaree 2021). Even conventional image processing techniques have been used rigorously for the early detection of melanoma from dermoscopic images (Keerthan et al. 2020). But simple image processing methods were not as effective as deep neural network models. Various ML and DL techniques adapted for melanoma detection and classification is presented in Figure 10.1. The steps involved and frequently used methods are also presented in Figure 10.1.

As AI models learn from the training data, their prediction accuracy is highly dependent on the quality and quantity of input data. Especially, in the context of melanoma classification task, image pre-processing and data augmentation plays a major role in deciding model accuracy. Dermoscopic images often include gel bubbles, clinical markings, ruler marks, hair and uneven illumination which necessitates pre-processing. Methods such as thresholding, filtering and morphological processing are frequently adapted for removing artifacts from dermoscopic images. Whereas, image enhancement is carried out by using histogram equalization, contrast adjustment, filtering and contrast limited adaptive histogram equalization (CLAHE) techniques. In addition, deep learning, adaptive gamma correction, multi-scale decomposition was also used for image enhancement. For instance, image enhancement by adaptive sigmoid function followed by segmentation was proposed (Jamil et al. 2016). Image super resolution techniques (ISR) were adapted to improve dermoscopic image resolution and the impact of image quality on melanoma classification task was demonstrated (Ashutosh et al. 2023). A probabilistic estimation method combined with supervised learning was used for the effective segmentation of lesion in order to achieve greater classification accuracies (Wighton et al. 2011).

In addition, limited data availability and data imbalances in dermoscopic datasets leads to model overfitting and hence should be addressed for improving the classification efficiency of DNN models. Data augmentation by employing geometric transformations, color transformations and image

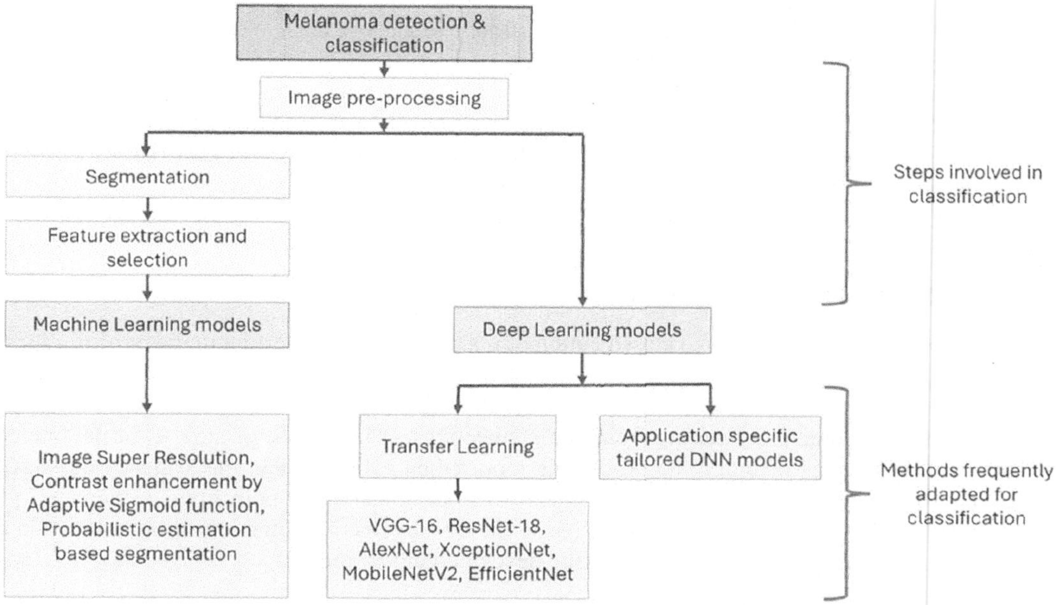

FIGURE 10.1 Melanoma detection and classification by ML and DL models (Steps involved and methods adapted).

mixing could generate new images from existing images and aid in addressing the limited data availability problem. Multi-layer augmentations were also employed for increasing the data samples. Further, generation of synthetic data by generative adversarial networks (GANs) was demonstrated to improve accuracy in melanoma classification task (Li et al. 2016).

Transfer learning approach have been utilized exhaustively in melanoma detection and classification task. For instance, (i) a light-weight framework based on MobileNetV2 is proposed for melanoma detection (Indraswari et al. 2022), (ii) an improved XceptionNet activated by swish function is utilized for classification tasks (Lu and Firoozeh Abolhasani Zadeh 2022), (iii) an EfficientNet architecture is adapted for learning fine-grained patterns from lesion images (Jaisakthi et al. 2023). In addition, a hybrid approach that uses pre-trained CNN, Visual Geometry Group-16 (VGG-16) for feature extraction and XGBoost for classification task was demonstrated (Thanka et al. 2023). Adding to the use of transfer learning technique modified VGG16 and Inception V3 nets are used for Melanoma classification into benign and malignant classes. The modified nets were demonstrated to produce a classification accuracy of 79% (Kahia et al. 2022). Attempts to compare the classification efficiency of CNN with Naïve bayes and Random Forest algorithms demonstrated that CNN based classifications achieve good results (Civelek and Kfashi 2022). Optimized deep features extracted using well established VGG-16, ResNet-18 and AlexNet are used to train a Support Vector Machine (SVM) classifier and the model so developed was able to achieve a classification accuracy of 97% (Mahbod et al. 2019).

Compared to generic models, specifically trained models could give excellent prediction accuracy. A hybrid framework that uses morphological filtering, Grab-cut segmentation, detection based on conventional diagnostic rule and classification by ResNET-50 is proposed and results were produced (Salma and Eltrass 2022). Dermoscopic images obtained from datastore say International Skin Imaging Collaboration were used by a light-weight and less complex DCNN for melanoma classification (Kaur et al. 2022). Even ground truth images retrieved from confirmed melanoma cases were used to train CNN model in order to provide efficient results (Esteva et al. 2017) (Brinker et al. 2019). In an experiment to classify melanoma types, images pre-processed by conventional image processing techniques were augmented and used to training a CNN. The so trained CNN was able to classify the given dataset with an accuracy of 79.45% (Rezaoana and Hossain. 2020).

A CNN image processing pipeline WonDerM based on image pre-processing followed by CNN based segmentation and classification is demonstrated to achieve 89% classification accuracy in classifying the input into seven different classes (Lee et al. 2018). Classification of melanoma by using features extracted by following (Asymmetry, Border irregularity, Color, Diameter and Evolution (ABCDE) rule, Histogram of Oriented Gradients (HOG) and Gray-Level Co-occurrence Matrix (GLCM) method have demonstrated to achieve an accuracy of 97% (Vidya and Karki 2020). In conclusion, CNNs were demonstrated to achieve good classification accuracy in melanoma classification task (Nahata and Singh 2020).

10.3 PROPOSED METHODOLOGY

Rapid detection, identification and classification of malignancy are important in diagnosing cancer. Thus, a tool that could identify and classify the skin lesions effectively is the need of the hour. In spite of their reasonably accurate prediction, pre-trained Dense CNN models showcase limitations in the form of (i) complexity arising from hop connections, (ii) presence of number of parameters which demands a huge memory and processing requirements. In addition, the tendency of overfitting leads to poor object recognition performance. Considering all these points into account, a CNN model based on an all-inclusive approach is proposed for the effective detection and classification of melanoma in this article. The highlights of the developed model include,

i. Capable of predicting the malignancy accurately even with limited dataset training
ii. Uses only CNN layers – the model is light-weight and thus associated computational complexity is less

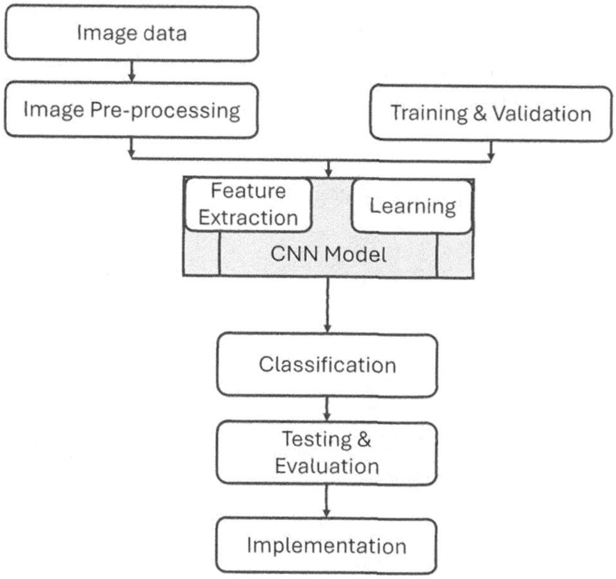

FIGURE 10.2 Architecture of melanoma detection using deep convolutional neural networks.

The architecture of melanoma detection using deep convolutional neural networks is presented in Figure 10.2. As enhancing image quality and diversifying the dataset play a major role in deciding the efficiency of the model, an exclusive image pre-processing step is adapted in the proposed model. The primary objective of producing accurate classification with limited input dataset is achieved by a set of data augmentation techniques and the limitation due to class imbalance is corrected by using class-weighted training method. The proposed model is computationally less complex as it uses light-weight CNN layers however, accuracy is ensured by efficient data augmentation and class-balancing.

10.3.1 Model Workflow

10.3.1.1 Image Pre – Processing

Image pre-processing techniques strives to improve the quality of input images in order to facilitate efficient training of the model. Typical image pre-processing for melanoma classification with deep learning models include resizing and normalization. In addition to enhancing image quality, imbalances and limitations in data quantity is also addressed in the pre-processing state. For instance, major challenges in image-based skin cancer classification task are limited data availability and imbalanced nature of the available dataset. In order to achieve better results with AI model these two limitations should be addressed effectively. Training data is increase by adapting augmentation techniques. Methods adapted for increasing and balancing training data are discussed individually in below topics.

Image Resizing: Images obtained are cropped in order to obtain square image of the skin lesion. All images were resized to 224×224 pixels in order to achieve a consistent resolution and thus facilitate efficient CNN training. This resizing is carried out by using bilinear interpolation in order to preserve the aspect ratio.

Data Normalization: Skin image datasets often have similar images with different labels. Such images reduce the prediction capability and thus needs to be removed. This issue is addressed by using data normalization. By comparing the correlation index between the similar images enable detection of redundancy. Initially, images were converted to greyscale and their histogram is calculated using equation (10.1) then mean of image histogram is found by equation (10.2). Correlation between them is found using equation (10.3) and a correlation above 0.99 is used to confirm redundancy.

$$h = \text{histogram}\left(I\left(x, y\right)\right) \tag{10.1}$$

$$X_h = \text{mean}\left(h\right) \tag{10.2}$$

$$\text{Correlation index} = \frac{\sum_x \sum_y \left(I_1\left(x, y\right) - h_1\right)\left(I_2\left(x, y\right) - h_2\right)}{\sqrt{\left(\sum_x \sum_y \left(I_1\left(x, y\right) - h_1\right)^2\right)\left(\sum_x \sum_y \left(I_2\left(x, y\right) - h_2\right)^2\right)}} \tag{10.3}$$

Data Augmentation: Data augmentation is defined as the process of extending a dataset, by introducing various transformations and operations. Such a diversification of available inputs results in achieving accurate predictions and classifications. Generative Adversarial Networks (GANs) are a boon to such data limitation problem. GANs generated synthetic data are good alternatives to address data limitation and imbalances. Different variants of GAN models were used achieve good quality training data. Meanwhile, applying geometric transformations, image mixing, color space transformation, are the common methods used for augmenting skin datasets. Augmentation models developed for increasing datasets often address imbalance issues together. Scaling the images by rotation, flipping, zooming and light alterations is the frequently used method to broaden the initial dataset inclusion. These methods guarantee that the prediction generalizes effectively to new data and overfitting is avoided. In this work, augmentation of data is carried out by rotating the images by 30°, flipping, zooming and shifting. Such an augmentation could produce different data for training in each epoch at the same time ensures the same quantity of data for training.

Handling Class Imbalance: Class imbalances are inherent to skin cancer datasets and if not addressed may lead to a biased prediction. In addition, evolutionary algorithms based on interpolate data sets are used for balancing training data. Data augmentation that oversamples minority classes were used to address imbalances. GAN based data balancing methods are capable of addressing both data imbalances and limitations together. One of the significant methods used for addressing data imbalances is weighted-class based model training. Different weights are assigned to different lesion classes while computing the associated losses. The majority class is assigned a smaller weight and the minority class is assigned with a larger weight. Such a class-weighted training reduces bias due to class imbalance and improves accuracy of prediction. Due to its reduced complexity and efficiency, weighted-class method is used in this model.

10.3.1.2 Model Training and Validation

The pre-processed images are fed to the CNN model for training. During model training the network learns from the input data. Model parameters say network weights; biases are updated based on a loss function during learning. These parameters can be updated optimally by using optimization algorithms like gradient descent, Adam, Adagrad. The CNN model proposed uses a class-weighted learning in order to address class imbalance. A class-entropy loss function and probabilistic estimation method are employed in order to keep an eye on the model development.

Once trained a validation set is used to validate the predictions. In the validation phase, the model is evaluated for its performance against new unseen data by various cross validation techniques. Based on the evaluations, model hyperparameters can be updated. These hyperparameters can be updated optimally by using algorithms like grid search, random search, Bayesian optimization. ML models are tested before deployment to determine its performance. Model parameters and hyperparameters are not affected during testing. Model tuning in any form is not carried out during testing. The intention of testing is to verify the model performance with respect to model accuracy, model adaptability to new data, model reliability and its unbiased nature. Rigorous model testing is recommended for the successful model implementation.

10.3.1.3 Interpretability

To aid dermatologists in understanding the model's decisions, interpretability techniques can be incorporated in the model. This is an attempt to provide an explainable AI and reduce the black box nature of the model. Such initiatives are recommended for the effective implementation of the model in clinical set-ups. Interpretability can be imparted easily by using inherently interpretable models such as linear regression, logistic regression, decisions tree for making decision making. Whereas, using model independent methods such as partial dependence plot, feature interaction, functional decomposition increases flexibility in introducing interpretation.

Interpretability in the case of melanoma classification can be introduced by providing reason for the decision made by the model. This necessitates introducing domain knowledge to networks. For instance, an image predicted as melanoma can say "Melanoma as 3 out of 5 ABCDE warning signs match", or "Melanoma as the pigmentation is Asymmetric with uneven Borders and has a Diameter >6.0 mm)" or "Melanoma as the spot is Evolving". If it is a classification between benign and malignant then a malignant classification can say "Malignant as the spot is evolving".

10.3.1.4 Deployment

The ultimate goal of this methodology is to deploy the trained model in clinical settings by integrating it into dermatologists' workflows. Integrating the proposed system into clinical setting could aid the dermatologist in making an early prediction. Initially, the proposed model will be deployed locally in a laboratory for clinical trials (after getting proper approvals) by setting up a virtual environment and evaluated. On successful completion of clinical trials, it will be commercialized.

10.3.2 The Model Architecture

A Convolutional Neural Network (CNN) model is developed for classifying skin cancer dermoscopic images. CNN mimics the visual perception of biological systems where simple cell extract features from small visual sub-fields and complex cells strive to combine features from spatial neighborhood. The proposed network architecture uses convolutional layers for feature extraction, max-pooling layers for sample reduction, fully connected layers for effective classification. The model architecture is as shown by Figure 10.3. The constituents of the model and their importance are presented in individual sub-topic below

Convolution: Convolution is a mathematical operation which when applied to input data results in producing a feature map of the input. Convolution is performed by sliding a smaller kernel over the input and performing a pixel by pixel sum of product operation. This operation helps in filtering out the unique features of input image. These features when extracted serves a number of purposes. For instance, when a convolution operation is performed over a 2D images or 3D color image, the results of the operation produce a feature map of the input which helps the network to learn either in a supervised or unsupervised manner aiding in prediction or classification task.

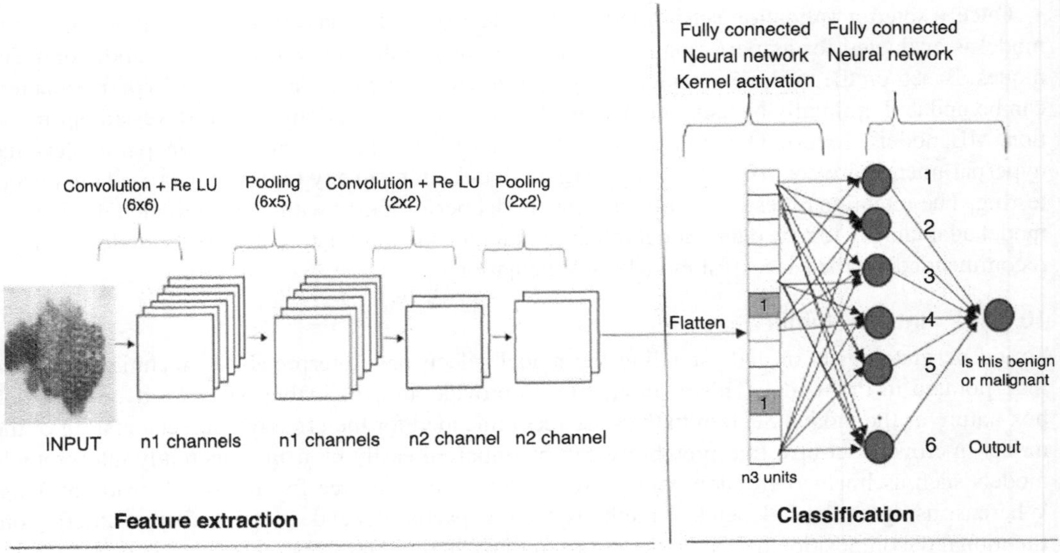

FIGURE 10.3 Proposed DCNN model architecture.

Convolution layer: Each convolution layer consists of 'n' independent kernels and each kernel is convolved with its input to produce 'n' feature maps. In a feature map, each neuron shares a common weight (parameter sharing) and is connected to a small sub-field (local connectivity) of the input. When an image input is passed through a number of CNN layers each working with a different kernel window size the quality of the extracted features will be better and it makes a better learning.

Pooling layer: Pooling strives to reduce the size of the feature map in order to reduce the computations and parameters. Each sub-field in the feature map (obtained from a convolution layer) is down-sampled to a single value by pooling operation. Pooling computes either the average or maximum value of the pixels in the sub-field to perform the replacement.

Flattening: Flattening helps converting the pooled feature map to a linear one-dimensional vector. This conversion is fed to the fully connected layer for classification process to take place. The conversion is made feasible by concatenation operation over a row-by-row fashion.

Output layer (or) Fully Connected Layer: A fully connected layer has neurons that are connected to all activations in the previous layer. This layer performs the classification task using the flattened data send by the previous layer. Classification is done based on its own weights and bias along with the flattened input. Prediction or detection of malignancy is carried out in the detection step. Table 10.1 depicts the constituent layers of the model and the model algorithm used for melanoma classification task.

10.4 RESULTS AND DISCUSSION

The interpretation of the results reveals the potential of the proposed model in identifying melanoma lesions. The proposed model's capacity to discriminate between benign and malignant skin lesions is demonstrated in terms of its accuracy, precision and recall values. Table 10.2 depicts variation in loss and accuracy with each epoch of training, obtained for melanoma classification with the proposed model.

TABLE 10.1
Model Algorithm and Architecture

Model Algorithm	Model Layer		Details
Define CNN architecture	Model layer		Details
Set: kernal size, ReLU Activation, Avg.Pooling,	Convolution layers	:	3
Initialize weights and bias of CNN	Convolution layer kernel size	:	3×3, 2×2, 2×2 (overlapping)
Compile CNN model	Feature map	:	6, 30, 30
Initialize	Average pooling layers	:	3
learning rate (r), epochs (M), error limit (Ce)	Pooling layer kernel size	:	2×2 (overlapping)
Model training and parameter tuning	Non-linearity	:	ReLU
For *i* =1 to Max epochs	Loss function	:	Cross-entropy loss function
While (not Ce)			
Train CNN model			
Calculate loss			
Update weights and biases			
End for			
Model validation and hyperparameter tuning			
Evaluate model performance			
Tune model hyperparameter and retrain if needed			
Model testing			
Deployment			

TABLE 10.2
Model Performance in Terms of Accuracy and Loss for Each Epoch

No. Epoch	Time (Seconds)	Train Loss	Accuracy	Test loss	Valid Accuracy
1	00:337	0.4106	0.8012	0.2877	0.8700
2	00:262	0.3036	0.8724	0.2600	0.8840
3	00:244	0.2777	0.8803	0.2906	0.8940
4	00:186	0.2695	0.8831	0.2706	0.8690
5	00:417	0.2600	0.8886	0.2485	0.8980
6	00:418	0.2587	0.8898	0.2332	0.9010
7	00:137	0.2467	0.9004	0.2341	0.8970
8	00:120	0.2478	0.8953	0.2435	0.8990
9	00:121	0.2334	0.9052	0.2184	0.9020
10	00:124	0.2371	0.9020	0.2206	0.9110
11	00:137	0.2343	0.9021	0.2344	0.9030
12	00:123	0.2255	0.9064	0.2260	0.9140
13	00:127	0.2199	0.9115	0.2221	0.9090
14	00:122	0.2191	0.9115	0.2210	0.9100
15	00:123	0.2110	0.9120	0.2220	0.9150
16	00:128	0.2093	0.9168	0.2136	0.9110
17	00:126	0.2018	0.9157	0.2164	0.9230
18	00:124	0.1987	0.9178	0.2164	0.9180
19	00:122	0.2010	0.9192	0.2301	0.9080
20	00:125	0.1974	0.9194	0.2150	0.9120

10.4.1 Performance Measures

Accuracy: Accuracy reveals how well the model predicts across all classes without bias. It is the ratio of the total number of correct predictions to that of the total predictions. The formula for accuracy is as given below

$$\text{Accuracy} = \frac{\text{TP} + \text{TN}}{\text{TP} + \text{TN} + \text{FP} + \text{FN}} \tag{10.4}$$

Precision: Precision reveals how well the model classify positive cases. It is the ratio of number of correct positive predictions to the total number of positive predictions. The formula for precision is

$$\text{Specificity, Precision} = \frac{\text{TP}}{\text{TP} + \text{FP}} \tag{10.5}$$

Recall: Recall is another measure that reveals how well the model detects positive cases. It is the ratio between number of positive predictions to the total number of positive inputs. The formula for recall is

$$\text{Sensitivity, Recall} = \frac{\text{TP}}{\text{TP} + \text{FN}} \tag{10.6}$$

Loss is a scalar quantity that indicates how well the model is learning from that set of input data. it quantifies the error between the actual and predicted class labels. The efficiency of the CNN model trained by small training data could be predicted from the batch loss. It is computed during training for every batch and is back propagated to update the model weights to improve classification efficiency of the model. By comparing the true class labels in each batch with the estimated class probabilities produced by the model, batch loss can be calculated. Cross-entropy is the preferred loss function used for evaluating the binary classification task. This loss function penalizes the model if there are much deviations and helps achieve a good binary classification accuracy. Figure 10.4 depicts the loss function changes with each epoch of training and model convergence is inferred from the Figure.

Training accuracy obtained after predictions from training phase helps in determining the efficacy of the trained model. The model is trained based on the training dataset and tuned using loss function in training phase. In the validation phase, the model is made to make predictions on data

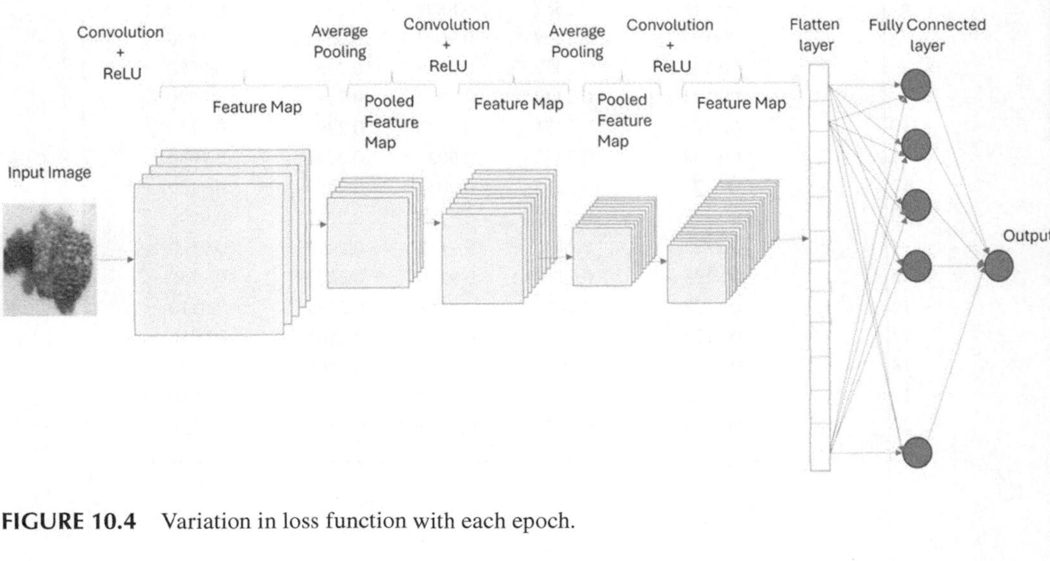

FIGURE 10.4 Variation in loss function with each epoch.

samples different from training set and the validation accuracy and losses are used to fine-tune the model prediction. Validation helps in predicting how well the model adapts to new datasets by tuning its parameters. The dataset used for validating a model is called validation dataset and it is a percentage of input data that is kept aside from the input dataset for validating the model performance. Before deploying the model to real classification task, the validated model is tested by unseen data and its test accuracy are verified. The improvement in accuracy of the model after each epoch of training is revealed from Figure 10.5.

The model performance in terms of accuracy, sensitivity and specificity is given by Table 10.3. The performance metrices of the developed DCNN model in comparison with the recently developed models is also presented in Table 10.3. It is clearly found that custom developed DCNN models perform well in classifying skin cancer images when compared to pre-trained generalized models. Such performance is achievable due to the inherent feature learning abilities of Convolutional Neural Networks and robust validation techniques.

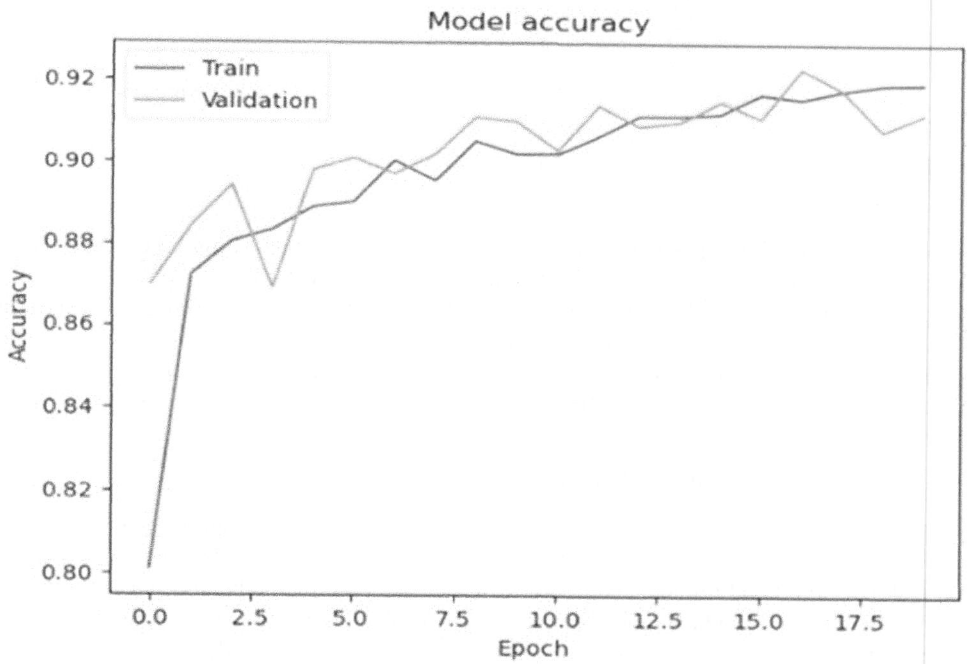

FIGURE 10.5 Variation in model accuracy with each epoch.

TABLE 10.3
Performance Comparison of Various DCNN Models

References	Model Name	Accuracy	Sensitivity	Specificity
Wu et al. (2022)	LCNet	90.4	90.3	90.4
Naeem et al. (2020)	MobileNet V2+DCNN head model	85	85	85
Indraswari et al. (2022)	ResNet50 CNN	82	82.3	77.9
*	Proposed DCNN	91.2	91.0	92.3

* *shows the proposed method/algorithm.*

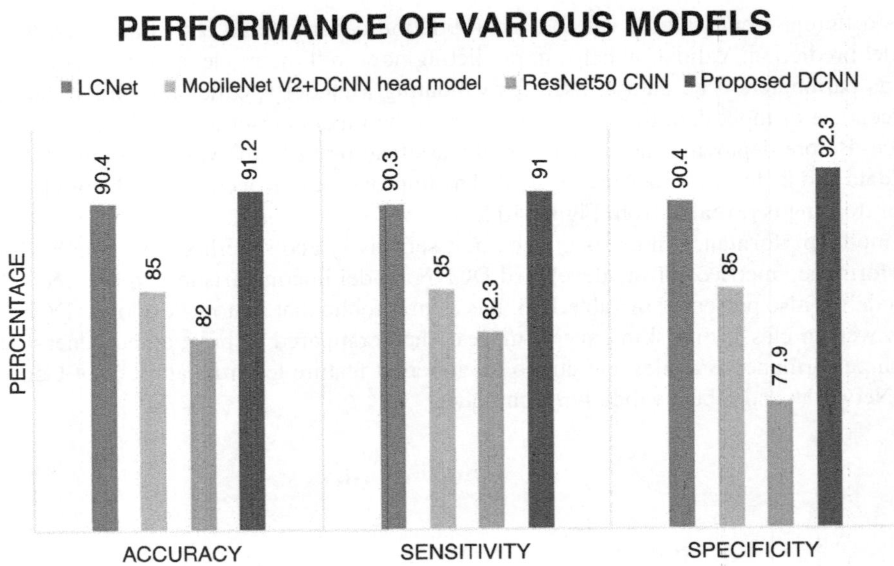

FIGURE 10.6 Performance of different models in melanoma classification task.

Compared to the DL models based on transfer learning methods, the tailored CNN models could achieve accurate classification of melanoma dataset. Efficiency in classification is achieved by (i) the use of diverse and balanced datasets, (ii) model tuning by appropriate loss function and (iii) appropriate validation of the model. With its inherent potential, the model could be adapted for real-world applications like e- medicine and early cancer detection. The variation in accuracy, sensitivity and specificity comparison between the different models is presented by graphs in Figure 10.6.

10.5 CONCLUSION AND FUTURE WORK

The article presents the design, development and results achieved with an efficient and optimized DCNN model in melanoma classification task. One of the major challenges in skin cancer classification task is limited and imbalanced dataset. Next in the pipeline is the acceptability of AI tools. Though AI tools could produce early disease prediction and aid in enhancing biomedical diagnosis, its acceptability is hurdled by its black box nature. And this necessitates the integration of interpretability with AI tools for biomedical applications.

CNN models address the data imbalance and limitation issues by using weighted-class training and data augmentation. And model reliability is ensured by a robust validation framework. Whereas, interpretability is introduced by using interpretable models or model agnostic interpretable methods in model development. Thus, a model with robust results and interpretability is poised to serve as a valuable tool for dermatologists facilitating timely and effective interventions ultimately contributing to improved patient outcomes and melanoma diagnosis.

AI models with their plenty of potentials have lot of opportunities in melanoma classification. In future, the binary classification can be extended to a multi-class classification task. In addition, the model's robustness and predictive performance could be improved by using sophisticated ensemble learning techniques like boosting and bagging. Further a holistic approach to melanoma diagnosis might be possible by incorporating multimodal data sources such as patient history, genetic profiles and histopathological data into the tool. Such an integration improves model interpretability. Acceptability of an AI tool for standard clinical practice could be made feasible by embedding Explainable AI in the framework and this could also be inducted in future developments.

REFERENCES

Ashutosh, L; Pranav, M; Rudra, P; Susan, E. Enhancement in skin cancer detection using image super resolution and convolutional neural network. *Proc Computer Sci.*, **2023**, 218:164–173. https://doi.org/10.1016/j.procs.2022.12.412

Brinker, TJ; Hekler, A; Enk, AH; Berking, C; Haferkamp, S; Hauschild, A; Weichenthal, M; Klode, J; Schadendorf, D; Holland-Letz, T; von Kalle, C; Fröhling, S; Schilling, B; Utikal, JS. Deep neural networks are superior to dermatologists in melanoma image classification. *Eur J Cancer*, **2019,** 119:11–17. https://doi.org/10.1016/j.ejca.2019.05.023

Civelek, Z; Kfashi, MHS. An improved deep CNN for an early and accurate skin cancer detection and diagnosis system. *Int J Eng Res Develop.,* **2022**, 14(2):721–734. https://dergipark.org.tr/tr/download/article-file/2426304

Dildar, M; Akram, S; Irfan, M; Khan, HU; Ramzan, M; Mahmood, AR; Alsaiari, SA; Saeed, AHM; Alraddadi, MO; Mahnashi, MH. Skin cancer detection: a review using deep learning techniques. *Int J Environ Res Public Health*, **2021**, 18(10):5479. https://doi.org/10.3390/ijerph18105479

Esteva, A; Kuprel, B; Novoa, R; Justin, K; Swetter SM; Blau H M; Thrun S. Dermatologist-level classification of skin cancer with deep neural networks. *Nature*, **2017**, 542:115–118. https://doi.org/10.1038/nature21056

Indraswari, R; Rokhana, R; Herulambang, W. Melanoma image classification based on MobileNetV2 network, Proc Computer Sci., **2022**, 197:198–207. https://doi.org/10.1016/j.procs.2021.12.132

Jaisakthi, SM; Mirunalini, P; Aravindan, C; Appavu R. Classification of skin cancer from dermoscopic images using deep neural network architectures. *Multimed Tools Appl.*. 2023, 82(10):15763–15778. https://doi.org/10.1007/s11042-022-13847-3

Jamil U, Akram MU, Khalid S, Abbas S, Saleem K. Computer based melanocytic and nevus image enhancement and segmentation. *Biomed Res Int.*, **2016**:2082589. https://doi.org/10.1155/2016/2082589

Kahia, M; Echtioui, A; Kallel, F; Ben Hamida, A. Skin cancer classification using deep learning models. In *Proceedings of the 14th International Conference on Agents and Artificial Intelligence - Volume 1: SDMIS*, 2022, pp. 554–559. https://doi.org/10.5220/0010976400003116

Kaur, R; GholamHosseini, H; Sinha, R; Lindén, R. Melanoma classification using a novel deep convolutional neural network with dermoscopic images. *Sensors*, **2022**, 22(3):1134. https://doi.org/10.3390/s22031134

Keerthan, N; Keerthi, S; Likhit, S; Samyama, M. Skin cancer detection using image processing. *Int J Emerging Technol Innov Res.*, **2020,** 7(6):1545–1548. https://www.jetir.org/view?paper=JETIR2006556

Lee, YC; Jung, S-H; Won, H-H. WonDerM: skin lesion classification with fine-tuned neural networks. 2018. https://doi.org/10.48550/arXiv.1808.03426

Li, Y; Esteva, A; Kuprel, B; Novoa, R; Ko, J; Thrun, S. Skin cancer detection and tracking using data synthesis and deep learning, 2016. https://arxiv.org/abs/1612.01074

Lu, X; Firoozeh Abolhasani Zadeh, YA. Deep learning-based classification for melanoma detection using XceptionNet. *J Healthc Eng.*, **2022**:2196096. https://doi.org/10.1155/2022/2196096

Mahbod, A; Schaefer, G; Wang, C; Ecker, R; Ellinge, I. Skin lesion classification using hybrid deep neural networks. In Proceedings of IEEE International Conference on Acoustics, Speech and Signal Processing (ICASSP), Brighton, UK, **2019**, pp. 1229–1233, https://doi.org/10.1109/ICASSP.2019.8683352

Naeem, A; Farooq, MS; Khelifi, A; Abid, A. Malignant melanoma classification using deep learning: datasets, performance measurements, challenges and opportunities, *IEEE Access*, **2020**, 8:110575–110597. https://doi.org/10.1109/ACCESS.2020.3001507

Nahata, H; Singh, SP. Deep learning solutions for skin cancer detection and diagnosis. In Jain, V; Chatterjee, J. (eds), *Machine Learning with Health Care Perspective. Learning and Analytics in Intelligent Systems,* vol. 13, **2020**. Springer, Cham. https://doi.org/10.1007/978-3-030-40850-3_8

Rezaoana, N; Hossain, MS; Andersson, K. Detection and classification of skin cancer by using a parallel CNN model. In *Proceedings of IEEE International Women in Engineering (WIE) Conference on Electrical and Computer Engineering (WIECON-ECE), Bhubaneswar, India*, **2020**, pp. 380–386. https://doi.org/10.1109/WIECON-ECE52138.2020.9397987

Saeed, J; Zeebaree, S. Skin lesion classification based on deep convolutional neural networks architectures, *J. Appl. Sci. Technol. Trends*, **2021**, 2(1): 41–51. https://doi.org/10.38094/jastt20189

Salma, W; Eltrass, AS. Automated deep learning approach for classification of malignant melanoma and benign skin lesions. *Multimed Tools Appl.*, **2022**, 81:32643–32660. https://doi.org/10.1007/s11042-022-13081-x

Thanka, MR; Edwin, EB; Ebenezer, V; Sagayam, KM; Reddy, BJ; Günerhan, H; Emadifar, H. A hybrid approach for melanoma classification using ensemble machine learning techniques with deep transfer learning. *Computer Methods Prog Biomed.*, **2023**, 3:100103. https://doi.org/10.1016/j.cmpbup.2023.100103

Vidya, M; Karki, MV. Skin cancer detection using machine learning techniques. In *Proceedings of IEEE International Conference on Electronics, Computing and Communication Technologies (CONECCT)*, **2020**, pp. 1–5. https://doi.org/10.1109/CONECCT50063.2020.9198489

Wighton, P; Lee, TK; Lui, H; McLean, DI; Atkins, MS. Generalizing common tasks in automated skin lesion diagnosis. *IEEE Trans. Inf. Technol. Biomed.*, **2011**, 15(4):622–629. https://doi.org/10.1109/TITB.2011.2150758

Wu, Y; Chen, B; Zeng, A; Pan, D; Wang, R; Zhao, S. Skin cancer classification with deep learning: a systematic review. *Front Oncol.*, **2022**, 12:893972. https://doi.org/10.3389/fonc.2022.893972

11 Advanced Skin Cancer Classification Using Xception Deep Learning Architecture Using Dermoscopic Images

Wafaa Abdelgawad, Esraa Darwish, Mohammed Hassan El-tohamy, Marwan Makhlouf, Hady Abdalla, Youssef M. Nassar, and Gehad Ismail Sayed

11.1 INTRODUCTION

One of the biggest problems that humanity faces is providing high-quality healthcare. Both society and individuals are greatly impacted by the quality of health care. The nation's Gross Domestic Product (GDP) growth is closely linked to the amount spent on developing the healthcare system, as a study published in 2020 indicates, as it directly impacts the economics of society (Raghupathi and Raghupathi, 2020). Recognizing the significant impact of health care, the United Nations (UN) put health care in the third rank in its Sustainable Development Goals (SDG) (Das et al., 2021). Skin cancer is widely recognized as one of the most perilous diseases, and it is one of the deadliest and fastest-growing tumors. Skin cell growth that isn't normal is called skin cancer. The two leading factors contributing to skin cancer are the use of UV tanning beds and exposure to the sun's damaging UV radiation (Raghupathi and Raghupathi, 2020). It is fortunate that skin cancer has a high chance of being completely removed and can be treated with little to no scarring if detected early by your dermatologist. However, areas of your skin that aren't often affected by sunlight can potentially develop this prevalent type of cancer. There are three primary categories of skin cancer: basal cell carcinoma, squamous cell carcinoma, and melanoma. Non-melanoma refers to the first two. Melanoma is the most deadly cancer. It can metastasize, or spread, to other areas of the body in addition to growing into and destroying adjacent tissue (Siddiqui and Sarwar, 2013). In 2022, it is projected that approximately 99,780 individuals will receive a diagnosis of melanoma, as reported by the American Cancer Society, with 57,100 instances recorded in males and 42,600 in females. It is projected that melanoma will claim the lives of around 7,650 individuals (Rashid et al., 2022).

Melanoma symptoms have the potential to appear in any area of the body. Typically, melanomas tend to form in regions that have been exposed to the sun, such as the arms, back, face, and legs. However, melanoma can also develop in areas that do not receive as much sunlight, such as the soles of the feet, palms of the hands, and fingernails. Moreover, melanoma can occur internally within the body, with hidden melanomas being more prevalent in individuals with brown or black skin. As people age, their risk of melanoma rises. Since the number of moles on a person's body rises until the age of 30–40, it primarily happens during childhood and the early years of adulthood (Middlesex Health, 2022). However, even in those under 30 years old, melanoma is relatively uncommon (Tahir et al., 2023). It's one of the most common cancers among young people, especially young women (Miller et al., 2020). Seeing abnormal cancers with the naked eye is an expert dermatologist's first diagnostic step. It typically takes 2–3 weeks to acquire the skin test results (Cancer Research UK, 2023). Investigating skin cancer early on is necessary because it's a

DOI: 10.1201/9781003486640-11

significant problem. Most patients see their dermatologist infrequently, which leads to a diagnosis that is made far too late. The manual diagnostic approach is expensive and takes a long time. Even though deep learning has enhanced diagnosis, it offers several advantages.

Skin disease detection might be completely transformed by machine learning (ML) (Abbas et al. 2022). Machine learning algorithms have the ability to examine large data sets, identify patterns, and generate highly precise predictions. In dermatology, ML may be applied to identify skin diseases accurately by analyzing images. One kind of artificial intelligence (AI) that works particularly well for image analysis tasks is deep learning (Mac Carthy et al., 2023). ML-powered diagnostic systems offer various benefits over traditional approaches, including improved accuracy and increased efficiency (Sayed and Hassanein, 2023). Deep learning architectures have been widely used in dermatology to diagnose a variety of skin conditions (Sayed et al., 2021). The outcomes of the research projects have been published in articles that have improved clinical decision-making and skin disease diagnosis. Deep learning architectures' primary strength is their ability to recognize complex patterns and details in photos that might be undetected by human specialists. One of the primary benefits of deep learning architectures in skin disease diagnosis is their ability to recognize complicated patterns that may be invisible to human specialists. These algorithms, trained on big datasets, can detect minute visual networks and connections between certain skin diseases and picture attributes. This enables the identification of hidden and complex illness symptoms, therefore enhancing diagnostic accuracy. Researchers have increased the accuracy of diagnosis by using these models to discover patterns linked to certain diseases by training them on large amounts of skin datasets. Convolutional Neural Network (CNN) is a particular kind of deep neural network designed for image processing and analysis. Deep learning architectures, particularly CNN, has the ability to grasp spatial dependencies and hierarchical representations within images. Deep learning neural networks have been used to segment medical images in the last few years. CNN incorporates layers such as convolution, dropout, batch-normalization, max-pooling, and so on. CNN typically takes a 2-Dimenstion (2D) input picture and applies 2D filters. Transfer Learning is a technique that may be used to solve complex problems using vast medical datasets. During the training of the models, a technique called layer freezing is employed, where specific layers are kept unchanged. Additionally, the final layer is substituted with a fresh softmax layer, which effectively categorizes the lesion images into seven different classes. (Jasil and Ulagamuthalvi, 2021). This allows them to analyze specific features and regions of interest in skin images, enabling precise and targeted diagnosis. They are particularly useful for tasks like object detection and image recognition because convolutional layers are used to automatically build hierarchical representations of information from pictures. Moreover, deep learning models have shown promising results in the early detection of skin cancer. By analyzing images of skin lesions, these models can identify potential malignant growths and aid in the early intervention and treatment of skin cancer. This could lead to a significant enhancement in patient outcomes and a reduction in mortality rates connected with skin cancer. The efficiency of the skin cancer detection model will be increased by applying transfer learning techniques. These strategies improve the training process by utilizing pre-trained models. A range of layer types, such as convolutional, dropout, pooling, and dense layers, will be used to verify the model's architecture. Deep learning architectures have become known as important tools in medicine, especially for detecting and diagnosing skin diseases. By using the capabilities of these models, dermatologists, and healthcare providers may increase accuracy, efficiency, and early intervention in the identification and treatment of various skin conditions, resulting in improved patient outcomes.

This paper proposed an automated skin cancer detection model for an imbalanced dataset. The presented model is applied to ISIC2020. This paper's primary goal is to significantly improve the precision and accuracy of skin cancer classification, which will aid in cancer diagnosis, by utilizing deep learning techniques. The following methods are employed in this paper to enhance the skin cancer images' classification accuracy: Preprocessing is required because of technical and performance factors. During the preprocessing stage, the training dataset's class imbalance is addressed by using data augmentation and oversampling, particularly for the ISIC2020 dataset, which has a serious imbalance issue. To increase generalization and diversity in the dataset, augmentation techniques such as translation, scaling, rotation, reflection, image resizing, and shearing are used.

This paper's main contribution can be summed up as follows:

1. To help dermatologists diagnose patients more accurately, a deep learning-based model for early skin cancer detection is suggested.
2. A comprehensive comparison of seven pre-trained models is conducted, evaluating their performance in early diagnosis of skin cancer.
3. Each component's importance in the pre-processing phase of the suggested model is illustrated and covered in detail.
4. The significance of the suggested model was shown by a comparison analysis with the most recent models.
5. Several evaluation metrics are used, such as the area under the curve, precision, F1-score, the receiver operating characteristic curve, recall, and accuracy.

The rest of the paper is structured as follows: The literature review section provides a summary of earlier research on skin cancer. A brief discussion of deep learning architectures and oversampling methods is presented in the methods and background Section. The proposed skin cancer diagnosis Section offers a thorough explanation of the suggested model. It also provides a thorough explanation of the used dataset. The outcomes of the conducted research along with their discussion are outlined in the discussion and experimental results section. Lastly, the last Section outlines the key findings and makes recommendations for additional research.

11.2 LITERATURE REVIEW

This section will highlight the important obstacles as well as possibilities in the diagnosis of skin cancer disease. It supports determining which areas could benefit from more research and which ones might not be well served by the technology or techniques now employed. By collecting present information, it may gain important insights into the potential and difficulties in the field of skin disease detection.

The authors (Prottasha et al., 2023) present a skin disease diagnosis model. The authors are mainly focused on hive skin disease. The authors utilized different You Only Look Once (YOLO) deep learning architectures. The authors evaluated their model with 353 images. The results revealed that the proposed model obtained an overall F1-score of 62.4%, precision of 68.1%, and recall of 57.8%. The authors (Bassel et al., 2022) use different models—Resnet50, Xception, and Visual Geometry Group (VGG)16—with classification methods, including Neural Network (NN), K Nearest Neighbor (KNN), Random Forest, Support Vector Machine (SVM), and Deep Learning. The presented model obtained an accuracy of 81.8%, an F1-score of 78.7%, and a recall rate of 81.6%. In (Abhishek and Hamarneh, 2020), the authors analyze skin lesion segmentation to improve precision in medical imaging. Using deep convolutional networks and the Matthews Correlation Coefficient (MCC), they get an accuracy of 92.17%, 81.3% sensitivity, and 97.1% specificity, showing its importance in dermatological diagnosis. In the paper, a comparison was made between machine learning algorithms and CNN models to determine their effectiveness in classifying skin lesions. The findings revealed that CNN yielded higher accuracy than the other machine learning algorithms examined in the study. The accuracy obtained was 95.18% with the CNN model, Precision 88% Recall 85%, and F1-score 86% (Shetty et al., 2022). The research paper introduces SkinNet, a modified CNN for accurate skin lesion segmentation. SkinNet outperforms other techniques in terms of Dice coefficient 85.10%, Jaccard index 76.67%, and sensitivity 93% (Lembhe et al., 2023). In this research, the authors introduced a model for automatically differentiating between malignant and benign forms of skin cancer. Employing the VGG16 deep-learning architecture, the model underwent comprehensive training and assessment on a dataset comprising 2,000 images. The resulting metrics revealed an overall accuracy of 95.4%, underscoring the model's effectiveness in accurately diagnosing cancer (Nawaz et al., 2022). The authors introduced a diagnostic model for automatically evaluating the severity of skin diseases, with a specific emphasis on eczema, which comprises four distinct levels (Reis et al., 2022). Employing an advanced model, the authors augmented the existing Eczemanet1 model to develop Eczemanet2, a deep-learning architecture tailored for this purpose. An extensive examination of the proposed model was undertaken, employing a dataset containing 271 images, in order to ascertain its effectiveness. The findings underscored the model's effectiveness, revealing an overall F1 score and precision of 60%. Table 11.1 provides a thorough summary of research publications that have used image datasets and deep learning models to determine skin cancer diseases and other skin diseases. The diseases that are covered and the benefits and drawbacks of the related research publications are also included.

11.3 BACKGROUND AND METHODS

In this section, a brief overview of the deep learning architecture is presented. Additionally, a brief discussion of preprocessing techniques is presented as well.

11.3.1 Deep Learning Architectures

Deep learning, an area of AI, has received widespread attention and recognition for its extraordinary capacity to emulate the human brain's neural networks and solve complicated problems (Zhang et al., 2024). At the heart of deep learning is that it can learn complicated patterns and representations from massive volumes of data, allowing it to make predictions, classify things, and execute numerous tasks with unparalleled precision. Despite its triumphs, deep learning faces obstacles and outliers that highlight the necessity for ongoing refining and innovation in the area (Hussain and Toscano, 2024). One of the underlying principles of deep learning is its dependence on neural networks, which are computational models inspired by the organic neural networks of the brain. These networks are made up of interconnected layers of artificial neurons, with one layer processing and sending information to the next. Backpropagation is a technique in which neural networks iteratively modify their parameters during training to decrease the difference between the actual and expected results, hence improving their predictive capabilities.

Within the realm of deep learning, one notable oddity is the overfitting difficulty. When a model becomes overfitted, noise and unneeded components taint the training data, impeding its ability to capture generalizable patterns (Rice et al., 2020). The model's efficacy on the training set can be impressive; nevertheless, its inability to generalize to unfamiliar data can lead to unsatisfactory performance in real-world applications. To reduce overfitting approaches such as regularization, dropout, and cross-validation are used to encourage the model to focus on useful features while keeping it from becoming inappropriately complex. Another problem is the occurrence of outliers or abnormalities in the data. Outliers are data points that deviate notably from the remainder of the dataset, usually due to data collection errors or true anomalies in the phenomenon under study. Deep learning algorithms may fail to deal with outliers, which can disrupt learned patterns and lead to erroneous predictions (Naveena and Jerine, 2024). Robust outlier detection and removal strategies, such as clustering-based methods or anomaly detection algorithms, are critical for maintaining the reliability and resilience of deep learning models in the presence of outliers.

Furthermore, the comprehensibility and clarity of deep learning models present crucial exceptions in sectors where transparency and accountability are essential (Sayed and Hassanien, 2022). Deep learning models, particularly complex neural networks with several layers and parameters, frequently function as black boxes, making it harder to grasp the underlying reasoning for their predictions or decisions. Explainable AI (XAI) strategies, such as attention mechanisms, feature

TABLE 11.1
Summary of Research Papers on Skin Disease Diagnosis in Terms of Publication Date, Disease Focus, Weakness, and Strength

Reference	Date	Disease	Weakness	Strength
Bassel et al., (2022)	2022	Cancer	The potential for biased results, especially favoring the majority class.	A hybrid deep learning approach was used for skin cancer classification, utilizing ResNet50, Xception, and VGG16 models, and various classification methods like SVM, KNN, regression, and Random Forest.
Abhishek and Hamarneh (2020)	2021	Cancer	There is no discussion regarding the choice of hyperparameters. There is no comparison with other segmentation algorithms. The used dataset is small.	The paper proposed a loss function for imbalanced data in deep learning models, addressing a common issue in deep learning.
Shetty et al., (2022)	2022	Cancer	There is a lack of a detailed discussion of cases where the model fails, such as instances of false positives or false negatives.	The author provided detailed information about the HAM10000 dataset, including the distribution of images among different skin lesion classes, patient demographics, and the ground truth validation process.
Lembhe et al., (2023)	2023	Cancer	The used dataset is not described in detail.	The authors suggested a hybrid model that combines super-resolution images with CNN. The suggested model utilizes datasets from the real world.
Nawaz et al., (2022)	2021	cancer	The authors acknowledge that the dataset includes blurred images, but it doesn't address how its proposed model handles this specific challenge	The proposed model for melanoma detection outperforms state-of-the-art skin lesion detection approaches.
Reis et al. (2022)	2021	cancer	The authors didn't take into consideration normal skin data	The authors use CNN as feature extractors, removing part of the last layer and treating the rest as a fixed feature extractor for SVM experiments.
Huynh et al. (2022)	2022	Acne	The acne scars are misclassified	The proposed model has higher mean average precision than other models
Abbas et al. (2022)	2022	Multiple diseases	There is a lack of information about the dataset and the specific techniques used for preprocessing	The proposed sequential CNN model obtained high accuracy and AUC.
Mac Carthy et al. (2023)	2023	Hives	The dataset is biased towards a specific class, as it contains 317 images, while the other class contains 40 images.	The dataset was annotated by a wide range of professionals.
Prottasha et al. (2023)	2023	Eczema	The dataset consists only of images of either Proasis or Urticaria and doesn't contain any images of normal skin or any other types of skin conditions.	The authors provide an overview of how to implement the model within a mobile application.
Attar et al. (2023)	2023	Eczema	The proposed model only detects eczema severity.	It can work with real-world images; it can first detect the infected part of the image, and then calculate the severity, providing a probabilistic number.

visualization, and model-agnostic interpretability methods, seek to clarify the model's decision-making process and provide insights into its inner workings, hence increasing trust and confidence in deep learning systems. Deep learning is still revolutionizing many industries and domains, driving improvements in healthcare, finance, transportation, and other areas, despite these exceptions and limitations. Deep learning has limitless potential to alter fields such as natural language processing, driverless vehicles, drug development, and medical image analysis. Researchers and practitioners can unleash the full potential of deep learning and usher in a future enriched by intelligent systems that augment human capabilities and improve societal well-being by addressing exceptions and pushing the boundaries of model robustness, interpretability, and fairness.

11.3.2 Data Preprocessing

One effective way to handle class imbalance in datasets is to use oversampling, a technique that is commonly used in the fields of machine learning and data science (Mohammed et al., 2020). Class imbalance occurs when one class in the dataset is significantly underrepresented (typically the minority class). This can lead to biased model performance and erroneous predictions. Oversampling strategies aim to correct this imbalance by purposefully increasing the number of examples in the minority class, giving the model more balanced and representative training data. Random oversampling is one of the simplest oversampling methods; it involves randomly duplicating instances of the minority class until the distribution of classes is more evenly distributed. Random oversampling is easy to apply, but it can amplify noise in the minority class and cause overfitting, which could impair the model's performance on unknown data. More complex oversampling techniques have been created to address the unique difficulties and subtleties of class imbalance and lessen these problems.

One of the most widely used oversampling techniques is the Synthetic Minority Over-sampling Technique (SMOTE). By interpolating between minority class instances that already exist, SMOTE creates synthetic samples by adding new data points along the line segments that connect neighboring minority class samples in feature space. Through the use of synthetic examples that replicate the minority class's underlying distribution, SMOTE successfully broadens the minority class while lowering the likelihood of overfitting and maintaining the dataset's intrinsic structure. SMOTE variations enhance the robustness and generalization of the generated models by concentrating on borderline occurrences or adjusting the sampling density based on the data distribution. Examples of these variations include Borderline-SMOTE and ADASYN (Han et al., 2005). Generative adversarial networks (GANs) are a family of deep learning models that combine a discriminator and a generator that are trained adversarially to generate factual synthetic data (Goodfellow et al., 2020). This is an alternative method of oversampling. Class imbalance is addressed while preserving data diversity and realism with GAN-based oversampling, which makes use of the generator network to create artificial minority class instances that are much like the original data distribution. GAN-based oversampling approaches are especially useful in situations with complex class imbalance patterns and non-linear correlations because they bring a high degree of flexibility and adaptability to complex data distributions by using deep learning techniques.

11.3.3 Proposed Skin Cancer Diagnosis Model

This paper utilized ISIC2020 dataset (International Skin Imaging Collaboration, 2020) for the evaluation of the proposed skin cancer diagnosis model's performance. An extensive collection of dermoscopic images of skin lesions with expert comments from the medical community makes up this dataset. A total of 2,000 patients' skin lesions, confirmed by histopathology for malignant diagnosis and expert agreement, longitudinal follow-up, or histology for benign diagnoses, make up the dataset, which consists of 33,126 dermoscopic training pictures. Figure 11.1 shows the ISIC2020

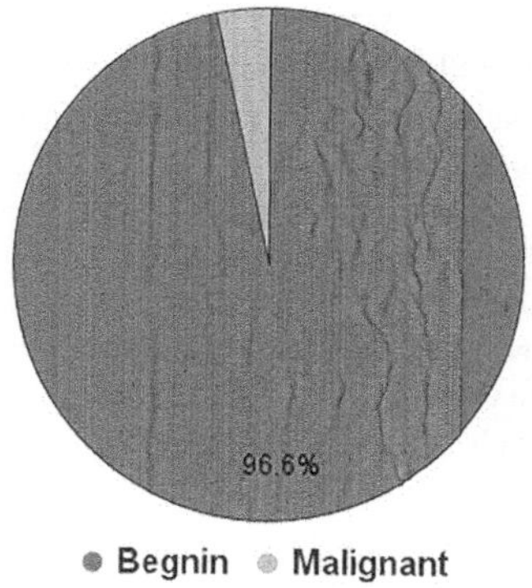

FIGURE 11.1 Class distribution of the ISIC2020 benchmark dataset.

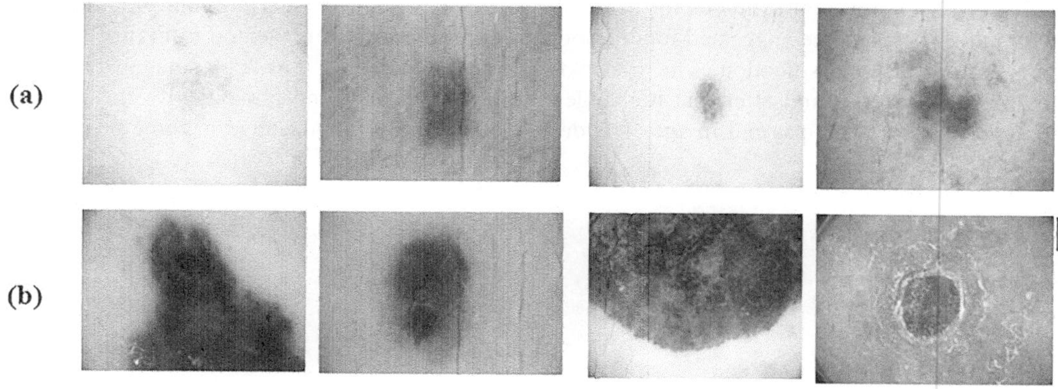

FIGURE 11.2 Samples of the ISIC2020 dataset; (a) Benign images and (b) Malignant images.

dataset's class distribution. This figure shows that 3072 samples were benign and 93 samples were cancerous. Furthermore, the accepted dataset's class distribution is imbalanced, which may have an impact on the suggested model's effectiveness.

Figure 11.2 shows samples from the chosen dataset visually on photos of benign and malignant conditions taken from the ISIC2020 dataset. Examples of benign pictures can be seen in Panel (a). These photos can show spots, moles, or other benign growths that can be compared to cases that might be malignant. Malignant picture examples are shown in panel (b). The photos display unique attributes linked to cancer, such as uneven edges, imbalances, changes in hue, and additional traits suggestive of malignant development. Figure 11.2 sheds light on the intricacy of skin lesions seen in the ISIC2020 dataset by providing graphic representations of both benign and malignant instances.

To tackle the problem of the adopted ISIC2020, this paper proposed a modified Xception architecture that can be utilized for transfer learning by initializing it with pre-trained weights. Algorithm 1 shows the pseudocode of the proposed modified Xception. The Xception model is initialized with weights from the ImageNet dataset, and the top layers are excluded. The model is then tuned for a particular classification job by adding a Global Average Pooling layer and a Dense layer with softmax activation. The Adam optimizer is then used to assemble the model with a learning rate of 0.01.

Algorithm 1: Modified Xception Pseudocode

```
Initialize base model with Xception using pre-trained ImageNet weights
Exclude the top layers of the base model
Create new_model as a sequence of layers:
Add base_model as the initial layer
Append GlobalAveragePooling2D layer
Append Dense layer with units equal to the number of classes and softmax activation
Set the learning rate to 0.01
Compile new model with:
optimizer=Adam with a specified learning rate
loss=categorical cross-entropy
metrics=accuracy
Return the new model
```

This paper presents a model for diagnosing skin cancer using dermoscopic pictures. The two main stages of the suggested model's outcomes are visually represented in Figure 11.3 data preparation and classification. The image first transitions into a grayscale image during the hair-removal phase, and after that it changes into a Blackhat—a morphologically closed image that differs from the original image. The dark spots in the original image become bright spots

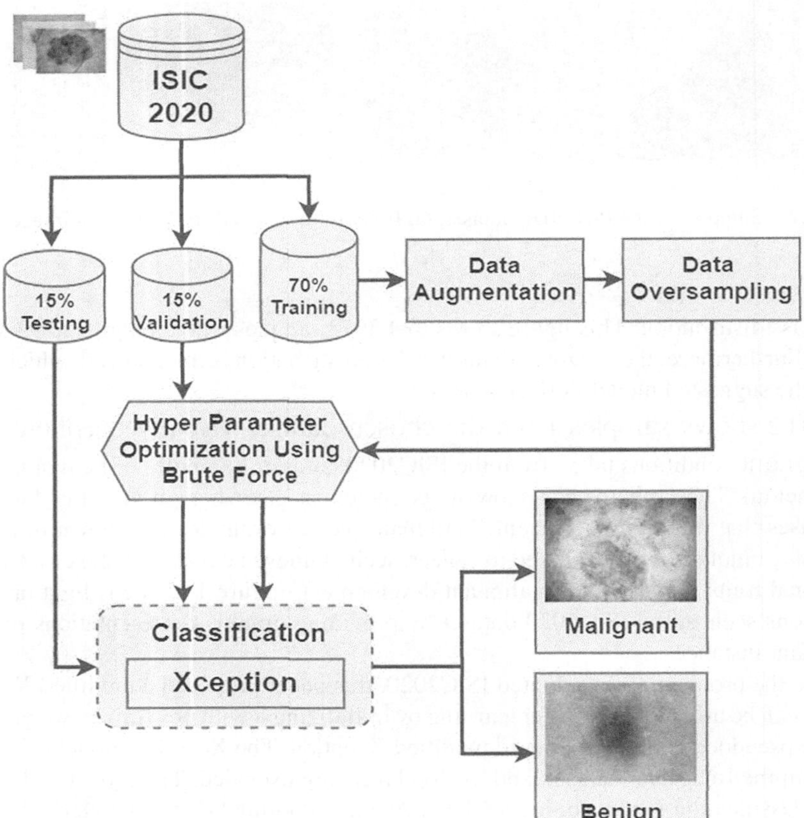

FIGURE 11.3 Process flow of the proposed skin cancer model.

after the black top-hat operation. Then thresholding is applied to the image to remove the dark spots that represent the hair. By taking a small neighborhood around the pixel on the neighborhood to be painted, Inpaint now fills in these lacking places. All known pixels in the neighborhood are added to a normalized weighted total in place of this pixel. Equalizing the distribution of classes and increasing the diversity of the dataset are the primary goals. 15% is put aside for validation, 15% for testing, and 70% of the dataset is used for training. To reduce overfitting and enhance generalization, this phase involves using data augmentation techniques including the random over-sampling (ROS) method to the training data. The data augmentation parameters are 36 carefully chosen to ensure that the transformed images remain realistic and representative of the original dataset. Specifically, the rotation range is set to 6° to prevent distortion or blurring of the images. The width and height shift ranges are set to 13.4% of the image width and height, respectively, to simulate small variations in camera position. To prevent creating unreal distortion, the shear range is limited to 0.1 radians. The camera's distance from the subject is simulated by setting the zoom range to [0.8, 1.2]. Furthermore, horizontal and vertical flip transformations are applied to help the model learn features that are invariant to the orientation of the image. The blending mode is set to reflect to prevent artifacts from appearing at the edges of the transformed images. This is achieved by improving the bias of the instances by generating unique data samples for the minority class. Benign and malignant skin images were classified using a sample of images from the ISIC2020 benchmark dataset (International Skin Imaging Collaboration, 2020). Hyperparameters were fine-tuned using a brute force technique in the classification phase. By carefully analyzing various learning rate combinations (0.001, 0.01, 0.1) and batch sizes (16, 32, 64), the optimal hyperparameters for the model were found Any deep learning architecture starts with image scaling and moves on to training. As a result, this picture collection must be resized to 224×224×3, which is the Xception architecture's input layer's dimension size. There is a serious problem with data imbalance in the ISIC2020 dataset, as was previously mentioned in the dataset description. Consequently, most deep learning systems will not be able to supply correct predictions. The minority class would be incorrectly classified since most of the pictures would belong to the majority class. Therefore, in order to overcome data imbalance and improve data generalization, several data augmentation strategies are used in this article. Randomly altering a picture involves the use of several factors. These transformations include translations along the *X*-axis with values ranging from –30 to +30 and translations along the *Y*-axis with similar ranges. Additionally, scaling is used, with random values on the *X* and *Y* axes ranging from 0.8 to 1.2. Rotation is used with values between −10 and +10 degrees.

Furthermore, reflection is done along the *X* and *Y* axes as well, producing a random true/false result. Shearing is then done with values ranging from −0.05 to +0.05 along the *X* and *Y* axes. These many changes help to enhance the dataset so that strong machine-learning models may be used (Sayed et al., 2021). The class imbalance issue is addressed, and data generalization is enhanced by using the pictures produced by utilizing these different data augmentation techniques. There were 2,673 pictures in the benign class and 93 in the malignant class prior to augmentation and oversampling. Following augmentation and oversampling, 2,673 photos were found in each class. This research uses data oversampling to address the overfitting problem. In both the original data and the resulting augmented data, the minority class is oversampled using the Random Over Sampling (ROS) approach. This contributes to a balanced dataset and ensures that the model generalizes effectively.

In the hyperparameter optimization phase in order to optimize a deep learning model's performance, this phase is essential. Because deep learning models have a lot of moving parts, their performance is affected by the hyperparameters that are selected in addition to the architecture and data. The hyperparameters such as learning rate and batch size techniques. During training, the model changes its parameters at a step size that is determined by the learning rate. How many training examples are handled in each iteration depends on the batch size. Algorithm 2 shows the pseudocode of the proposed brute force-based hyperparameter optimization.

Algorithm 2: Brute Force Hyperparameter Optimization Algorithm

```
Define hyperparameters grid
param grid ← {'batch size' : [64, 16, 32], 'learning rate' : [0.1, 0.001, 0.01]}
results ← []
for params in ParameterGrid(param grid) do
learning rate ← params['learning rate']
batch size ← params['batch size']
train generator ← datagen.flow from directory(directory, target size=target size, batch size=batch size,
    class mode='categorical', subset='training', shuffle=True)
validation generator ← datagen.flow from directory(directory, target size=target size, batch size=batch size,
    class mode='categorical', subset='validation', shuffle=False)
optimizer ← Adam(learning rate=learning rate)
model.compile(optimizer=optimizer, loss ='categorical crossentropy', metrics=['accuracy'])
model.fit(train generator, epochs=10, validation data=validation generator)
y pred ← model.predict(validation generator)
y pred ← y pred.argmax(axis=1)
y true ← validation generator.classes
f1 ← f1 score(y pred, y true, average='macro')
results.append((params, f1))
end for
best params ← results[argmax([x[1] for x in results])]
```

The block diagram in Figure 11.3 visually represents a well-structured approach to hyperparameter optimization and classification, including steps like defining parameters, generating combinations, training models, and evaluating performance. The diagram showcases a systematic process for hyperparameter optimization and classification. The initial step involves defining the hyperparameters and their respective ranges, setting the foundation for the optimization process. Following that, combinations of hyperparameters are generated within the defined ranges, enabling a comprehensive exploration of potential configurations. Then progresses to the training stage, where models are trained using the generated hyperparameter combinations. This step allows for the evaluation of different model variations and their performance. Next, the trained models undergo evaluation using a validation set, aiming to assess their effectiveness and determine the most suitable ones. The evaluation step is likely to include a comparison of the models' performance according to established parameters or objective metrics. After determining the best hyperparameters and models, then goes to the classification stage. The chosen model is used to categorize or predict desired outputs, drawing on the information gathered throughout the optimization process.

To enhance the model's performance in the classification phase, a brute force hyperparameter optimization approach was used. Hyperparameter optimization is the procedure for ascertaining the optimal settings for hyperparameters, which are variables that control learning but are not explicitly learned from data (Sayed et al., 2018). The brute force hyperparameter optimization approach was carried out to boost the model's performance in the classification stage. This approach involves systematically exploring different combinations of hyperparameters, such as learning rate and batch size, to identify the optimal configuration. In particular, the hyperparameters for batch size and learning rate were changed. investigated the learning rates (0.1, 0.001, 0.01) and batch sizes (64, 16, 32). The model was trained and assessed for every combination of hyperparameters using a validation set. The final model was determined by evaluating the model's performance on the validation set. The optimal hyperparameter configuration of Xception was found with the assistance of this iterated approach.

11.4 EXPERIMENTAL RESULTS AND DISCUSSION

In recent years, accurate recognition and categorization of skin cancer problems has expanded in importance in medical diagnosis. This research thoroughly evaluates a skin cancer classification model to establish its usefulness in detecting and categorizing different skin cancer instances. A series of experiments were undertaken to analyze the model's performance before and after the addition of many critical components, such as augmentation, oversampling, and hyperparameter tuning. The proposed skin cancer diagnosis model is implemented in the Python programming language with Google Colab. This study utilized performance criteria such as precision, accuracy, sensitivity, and F1-score. The following equations represent the mathematical definition of each.

$$\text{Accuracy} = \frac{\text{TN} + \text{TP}}{\text{FP} + \text{TP} + \text{FN} + \text{TN}} \tag{11.1}$$

$$\text{Precision} = \frac{\text{TP}}{\text{FP} + \text{TP}} \tag{11.2}$$

$$\text{Sensitivity (Recall)} = \frac{\text{TP}}{\text{FN} + \text{TP}} \tag{11.3}$$

$$\text{F1-Score} = \frac{\text{TP}}{\text{TP} + \frac{1}{2}(\text{FP} + \text{FN})} \tag{11.4}$$

where FP signifies the false positive samples, TP signifies the true positive samples, TN signifies the true negative samples, and FN signifies the false negative samples.

As can be seen from Figure 11.4, the model before applying augmentation and data oversampling method showed possible accuracy, but it performed poorly at first in terms of an F1-score of

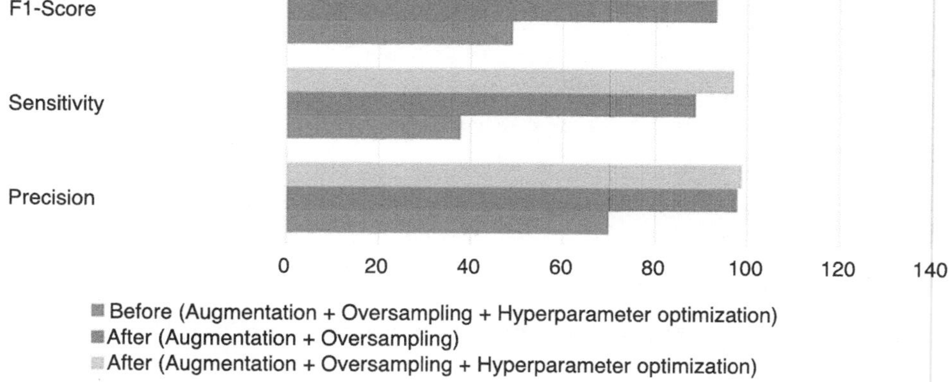

FIGURE 11.4 Performance evaluation of each component of the proposed model.

49.1%, a sensitivity of 37.80%, and a precision of 70%. These results demonstrated the need for more processing and enhancement to increase the model's capacity to reliably identify and categorize skin cancer cases. Augmentation and oversampling approaches are employed to solve the issue of class imbalance to overcome the constraints that have been observed. These changes considerably enhanced the model's performance, resulting in an accuracy of 93.3%. Furthermore, the F1-score was 93.3%, demonstrating the great accuracy and sensitivity of the model. These results illustrate the model's enhanced ability to appropriately categorize skin cancer. To overcome the highlighted obstacles, augmentation, and oversampling methods were used to solve the issue of class imbalance. These changes considerably enhanced the model's performance resulting in 93.3% accuracy. Additionally, the F1-score achieved 93.3%, demonstrating that the model is excellent at obtaining both high accuracy and sensitivity. These enhancements signify the model's improved capability in accurately classifying instances, which is crucial for its practical applicability, especially in sensitive domains such as medical diagnosis. Figure 11.4 shows how hyperparameter modification improved the proposed model's performance across several metrics, resulting in 95.2% accuracy, 95.2% F1-score, 97.06% sensitivity, and 98.91% precision. These upgrades indicate that the model has improved.

When it comes to improving the performance of deep learning architectures, especially in medical diagnostics like skin cancer diagnosis, data augmentation techniques are essential. The most effective data augmentation strategies for improving the generalization of deep learning models trained on imbalanced datasets, as utilized in this study, include rescaling pixel values (rescale=1./255), applying random shearing transformations (shear_range=0.05), random zooming (zoom_range=[0.8, 1.2]), rotating images (rotation_range=10), horizontal and vertical flipping for both horizontal and vertical axes, and shifting images horizontally and vertically with shifting range equals 0.3. The model can acquire more broadly applicable characteristics thanks to these techniques, which also improve the training data's robustness and variability.

As illustrated in Figure 11.5, which presents the comparative analysis of key metrics before and after augmentation, the impact on performance is clear. Before augmentation, the model achieved high accuracy (96.50%) but showed a lower F1-score (49.10%), sensitivity (37.80%), and precision (70.00%). However, after augmentation, while accuracy decreased slightly to 75.10%, significant improvements were observed in F1-score (73.60%), sensitivity (73.90%), and precision (78.80%).

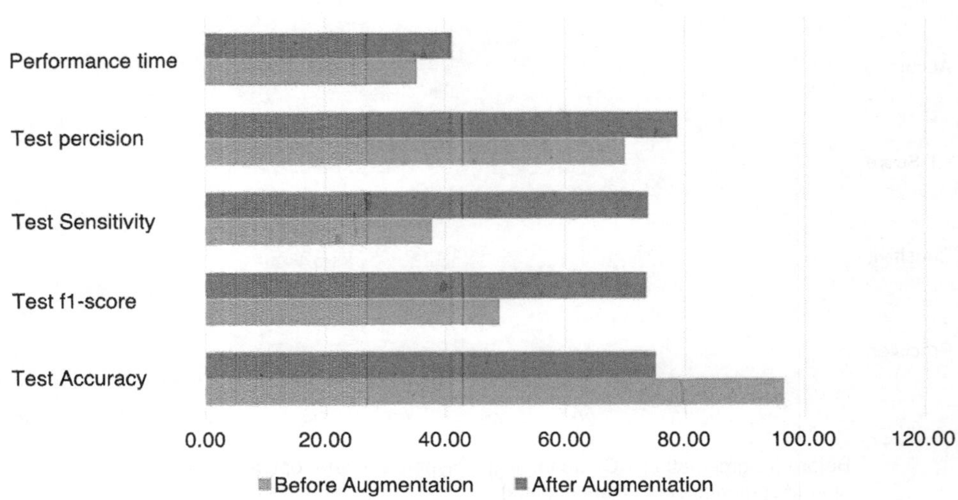

FIGURE 11.5 Assessment of the suggested model's performance both before and after data augmentation techniques were used.

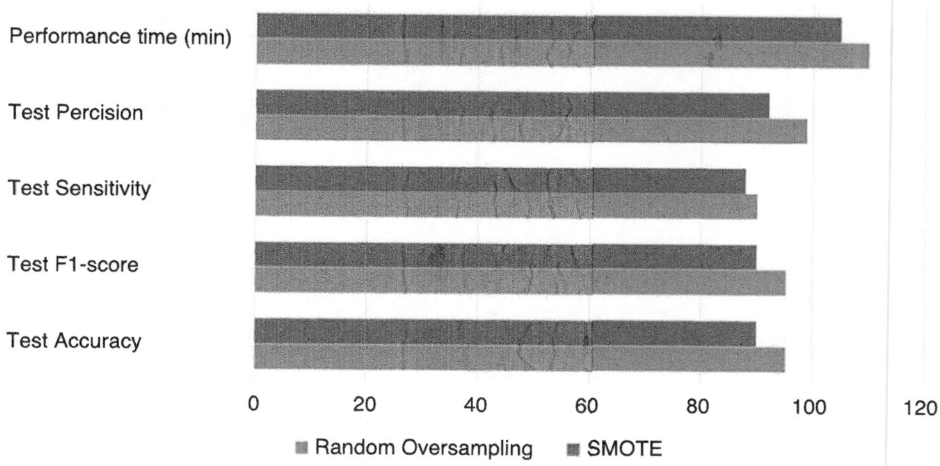

FIGURE 11.6 Assessment of the suggested model's performance both before and after using smote and random oversampling.

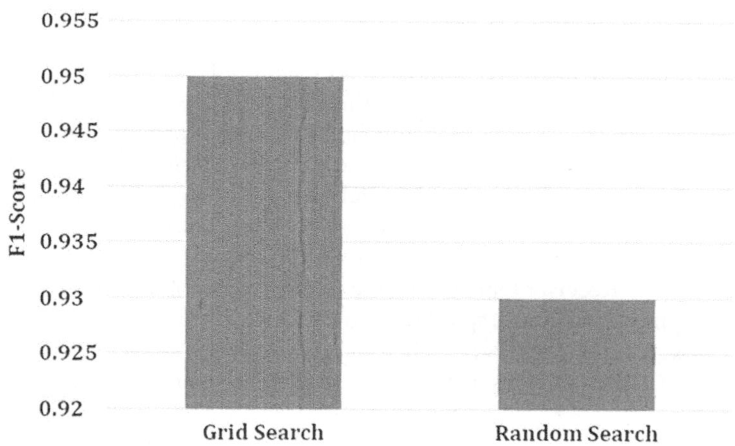

FIGURE 11.7 Performance evaluation of grid search and random search-based hyper-parameters optimization algorithms.

These enhancements show that, in addition to maintaining accuracy, data augmentation is essential for improving the model's ability to accurately identify cases of skin cancer.

Figure 11.6 compares the effectiveness of the suggested Xception model employing the Synthetic Minority Oversampling Technique (SMOTE) and Random Oversampling (ROS) data augmentation strategies. ROS yielded results with a test accuracy of 95.26%, a test F1-score of 95.26, a test sensitivity of 90.12%, and a test precision of 98.91%. In contrast, SMOTE produced a test accuracy of 90%, a test F1-score of 90, a test sensitivity of 88%, and a test precision of 92.1%. These results demonstrate that Random Oversampling led to higher accuracy and precision, while SMOTE provided a more balanced approach with slightly lower values but with a smaller gap between sensitivity and precision. This suggests that Random Oversampling might enhance overall accuracy and precision, whereas SMOTE contributes to a more uniform performance across different metrics, which is essential for addressing class imbalances.

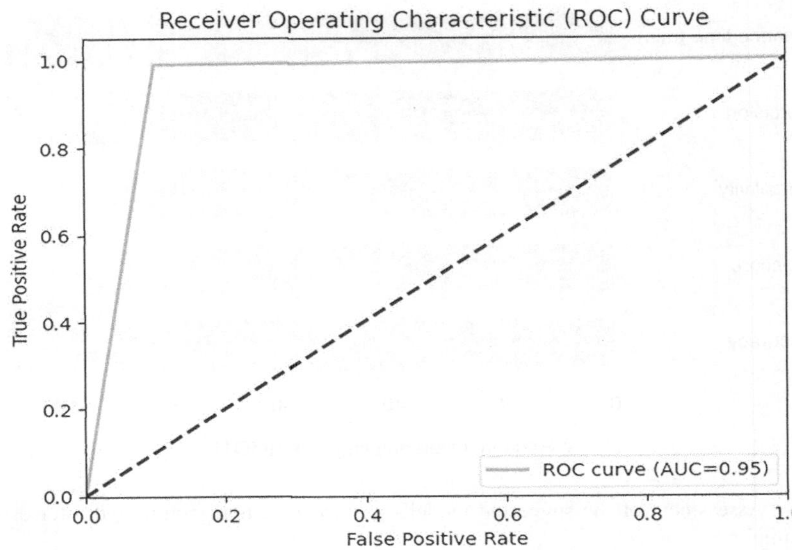

FIGURE 11.8 ROC curve of the suggested model for diagnosing skin.

Figure 11.7 illustrates the comparison of F1 scores achieved by grid search and random search approaches. With a batch size of 16 and a learning rate of 0.001, grid search produced a higher F1-score of 0.95 and required 10 hours to finish. In contrast, random search achieved a lower F1-score of 0.93 using a larger batch size of 32 and the same learning rate of 0.001, completed in 6 hours. Despite its shorter runtime, random search failed to identify the optimal hyperparameter combination, highlighting grid search's effectiveness in exhaustively exploring the parameter space and achieving superior performance in this instance.

Figure 11.8 shows the Receiver Operator Curve (ROC) curve following the use of augmentation and oversampling approaches. The graph shows how the model's performance increases using augmentation and oversampling techniques. When the ROC curve approaches or the Area Under the Curve (AUC) equals 0.95, it indicates that the model's exclusive performance has improved from its original condition.

To evaluate the reliability of the proposed model and ensure it generalizes well to new data, this paper conducted seven independent experimental runs. During each run, the suggested Xception deep learning model was trained using a collection of medical images, and test and training metrics were tracked. A prevalent problem in deep learning models for medical image processing is called overfitting, which occurs when a model performs noticeably better on training data than on test data that hasn't been seen. By examining the variation in metrics across these runs, this paper aims to highlight how well the proposed model prevents overfitting. Figure 11.9 illustrates a horizontal bar chart comparing the variation between Test and Train metrics across these independent runs. For example, in Run 2, the model achieved a Test Accuracy of 84.00%, slightly higher than the Train Accuracy of 81.30%, indicating robust generalization rather than overfitting. Similarly, Run 7 shows a Test Accuracy of 91.00%, compared to a Train Accuracy of 89.10%, further demonstrating the ability of the model to generalize efficiently. This comparison underscores the stability and reliability of the proposed approach across different datasets and training iterations, affirming its suitability for medical image analysis tasks.

Figure 11.10 analyzes the performance of several deep learning architectures using accuracy, F1-score, sensitivity, and precision. The suggested Xception model has the highest accuracy (95.26%) and precision (98.91%). MobileNet has the highest sensitivity (91.68%). DenseNet has the second-highest precision (92.29%), but falls short of Xception's accuracy and F1- score (89.53%).

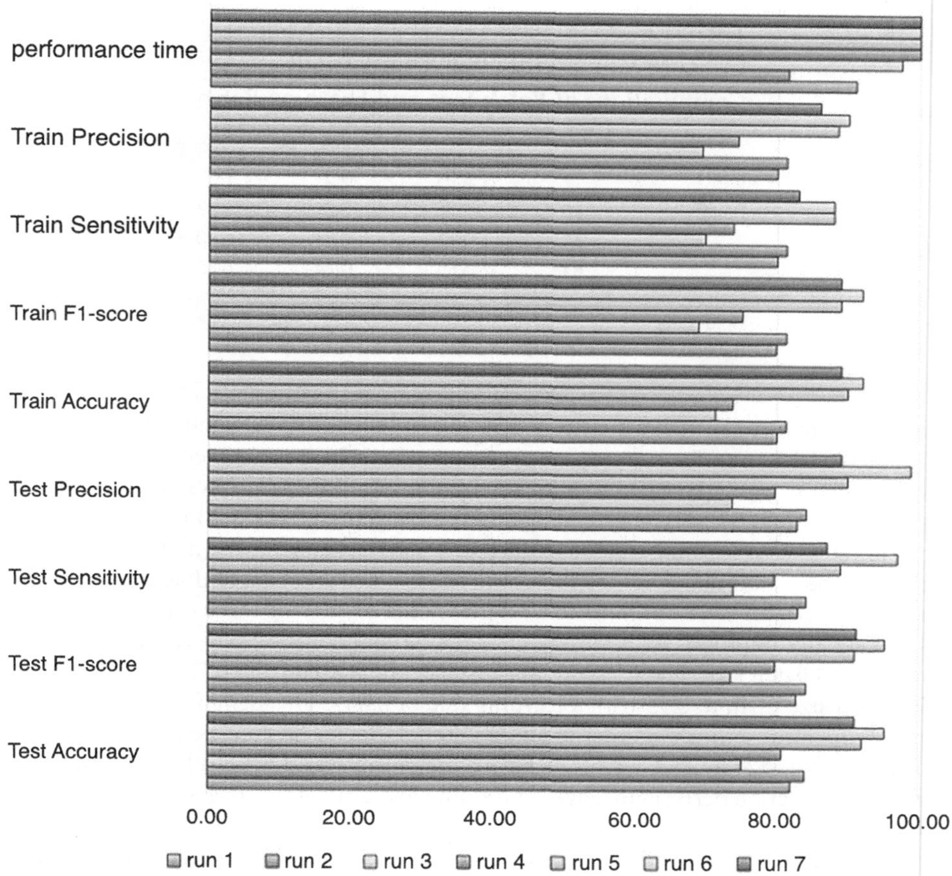

FIGURE 11.9 Training and testing evaluation metrics across seven independent runs.

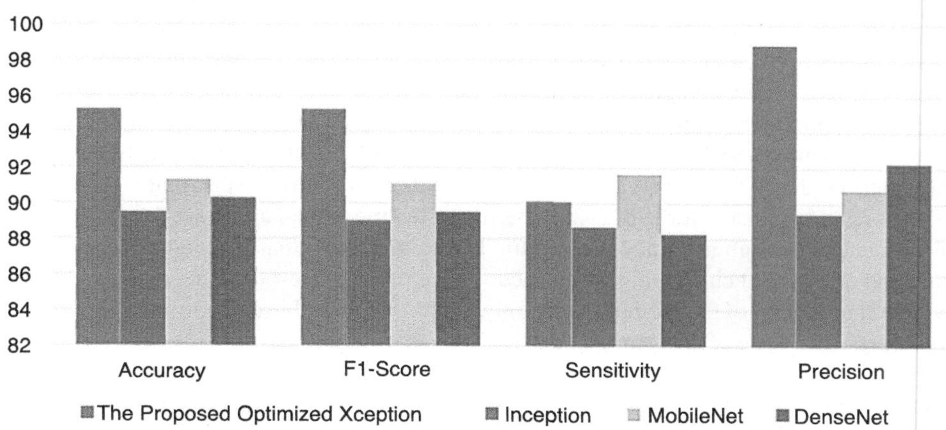

FIGURE 11.10 Performance comparison of the suggested model with various deep learning architectures using Xception according to F1-score, accuracy, sensitivity, and precision.

TABLE 11.2
F1-Score Values Obtained from Various Combinations of Batch Size and Learning Rate

			Learning Rate	
0.001		**0.01**	**0.1**	
Batch size	**16**	*0.95*	0.81	0.72
	32	0.93	0.84	0.80
	64	0.89	0.84	0.82

Bold values denote the batch size, and italicized values denote the best F1-score for a particular learning rate.

Table 11.2 demonstrates how different combinations of learning rate and batch size were tested to maximize the F1 score. The learning rate is the speed at which the model updates its parameters while it is being trained, and the batch size is the volume of training data processed in each iteration. Batch sizes 16, 32, and 64 were tested, and values ranging from 0.001 to 0.1 were used to evaluate the learning rates. At a learning rate of 0.001 and a batch size of 16, the highest F1-score of 0.95 was attained. The performance of deep learning models for skin cancer diagnosis is significantly enhanced by hyperparameter optimization, which entails modifying these crucial parameters. The model dramatically improved its accuracy in categorizing photos of skin cancer by adjusting the learning rate and batch size. The F1-score, for instance, increased from 0.72 with a learning rate of 0.1 and a batch size of 16 to 0.95 with a learning rate of 0.001. This demonstrates how critical it is to determine the ideal settings in order to attain optimal diagnostic precision.

Changes in learning rate and batch size have a major impact on how well deep learning models for skin cancer detection perform throughout training and evaluation. The learning rate determines the speed at which the model updates its parameters. A high learning rate can speed up training but may lead to unstable updates and poor convergence, resulting in lower performance. Conversely, a low learning rate allows for more precise updates and typically results in better model performance, although it requires more training time. Another important factor is the batch size or the quantity of training samples handled in a single iteration. Smaller batch sizes provide more accurate gradient estimates and better generalization to new data but slow down the training process. Larger batch sizes make training faster and more stable by leveraging hardware efficiency but may lead to overfitting as the model might converge to sharp minima. Balancing these hyperparameters is essential to achieve optimal accuracy and generalization.

Figure 11.11 provides a comparison of the proposed model's performance with DSCCNet (Tahir et al., 2023), Ensemble (SVM meta-classifier) (Qureshi and Roos, 2023), SeyNet (Igbasanmi, 2023), InSiNet (Reis et al., 2022), and LCNet (Kaur et al., 2022) in terms of specificity, sensitivity, accuracy, F1-score and precision for ISIC2020. The suggested model had an F1-score of 95%, suggesting its ability to achieve high accuracy and recall. The results show that the suggested model is more accurate and effective at classifying skin cancer than existing state-of-the-art models. Additionally, it is evident that several of the models that are now in use, such as those in (Qureshi and Roos, 2023), did not address the issue of class imbalance.

However, the suggested model shows its ability to accurately detect skin cancer, however, there are some limitations. One of these limitations is that the current data augmentation and oversampling techniques in handling class imbalance in medical datasets include generating synthetic samples that may lack clinical relevance, leading to potential model bias and overfitting. Traditional methods like SMOTE can inadvertently produce overlapping samples that do not accurately reflect the nuanced variability present in medical data, particularly in high-dimensional spaces such as imaging. Furthermore, these techniques often fail to preserve critical contextual relationships,

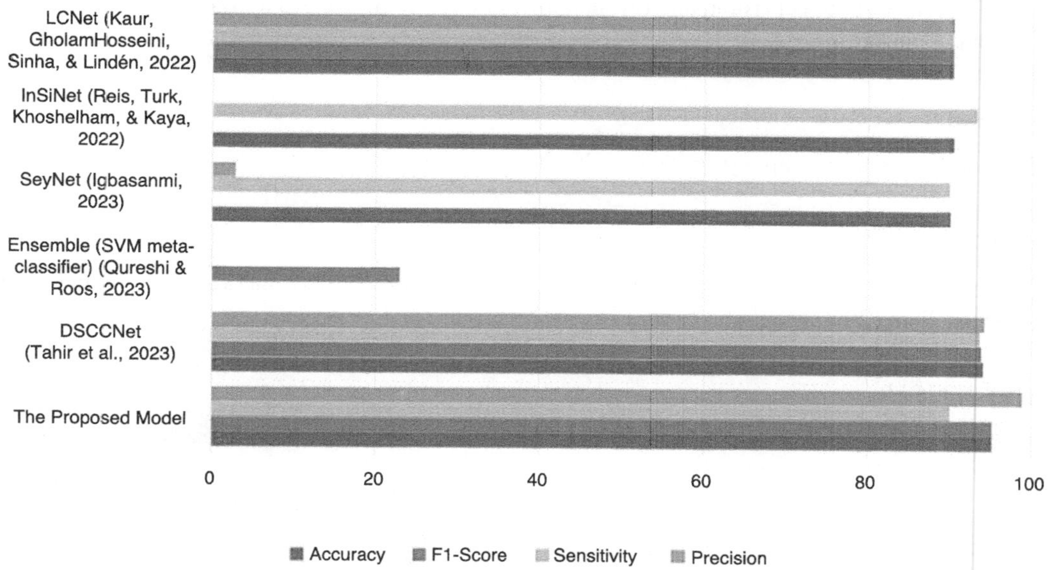

FIGURE 11.11 Performance evaluation of the suggested model vs. the state-of-the-art models.

potentially misrepresenting the anatomical or pathological structures within the data. To enhance their efficacy, integrating advanced generative models such as GANs tailored to medical domains, using domain-specific augmentation strategies, and employing context-aware augmentation can generate more realistic and informative samples. Additionally, hybrid approaches that combine augmentation with cost-sensitive learning and adaptive sampling can further improve the handling of class imbalances, leading to more robust and clinically valid models.

11.5 CONCLUSION AND FUTURE WORK

Skin cancer is a major global health issue that needs to be detected early in order to enhance treatment results and lower death rates. Current techniques for diagnosing mostly rely on dermatologists' eye examinations, which can be subjective and time-consuming, sometimes resulting in errors and treatment delays. This study presents a deep learning model using Xception for early diagnosis of skin cancer to address these challenges. The model underwent rigorous data categorization, including hair removal, data augmentation, and oversampling to improve generalization. The Xception architecture's brute-force hyperparameter optimization further refined performance during classification. Analysis of the ISIC2020 dataset produced results with an accuracy of 95.2%, a precision of 98.9%, a sensitivity of 90.5%, and an F1 score of 95.2%. These findings demonstrate the model's potential to increase diagnostic precision and offer automated, accurate tools for clinical practice. Future research could explore additional improvements and alternative hyperparameter optimization strategies for the broader applicability of dermoscopic images applied to the original dataset, for example by oversampling. Additionally, brute force can be further evaluated and tested to optimize Xception's hyperparameters throughout the classification phase.

STATEMENTS AND DECLARATIONS

AUTHOR CONTRIBUTIONS

Design, implementation, and data analysis are performed by **M. Makhlouf, H. Abdalla**, and **Y. Nassar**. Writing the original draft is performed by **W. Abdelgawad, E. Darwish, M. El-tohamy**.

Conceptualization, Supervision, and revision are done by **G. Sayed**. All authors read and approved the final manuscript.

Funding

There was no external support for this study.

Data Availability

The benchmark dataset that was used for this study is called ISIC2020, and it can be obtained from https://challenge2020.isic-archive.com/.

REFERENCES

Abbas, Muddasar, Muhammad Imran, Abdul Majid, and Nadeem Ahmad. Skin diseases diagnosis system based on machine learning. *Journal of Computing & Biomedical Informatics* 4, no. 1 (2022): 37–53.

Abhishek, Kumar, and Ghassan Hamarneh. Matthews correlation coefficient loss for deep convolutional networks: application to skin lesion segmentation. In *2021 IEEE 18th International Symposium on Biomedical Imaging (ISBI)*, pp. 225–229. IEEE, Nice, France, 2021.

Attar, Rahman, Guillem Hurault, Zihao Wang, Ricardo Mokhtari, Kevin Pan, Bayanne Olabi, Eleanor Earp, Lloyd Steele, Hywel C. Williams, and Reiko J. Tanaka. Reliable detection of eczema areas for fully automated assessment of eczema severity from digital camera images. *JID Innovations* 3, no. 5 (2023): 100213.

Bassel, Atheer, Amjed Basil Abdulkareem, Zaid Abdi Alkareem Alyasseri, Nor Samsiah Sani, and Husam Jasim Mohammed. Automatic malignant and benign skin cancer classification using a hybrid deep learning approach. *Diagnostics* 12, no. 10 (2022): 2472.

Cancer Research UK. Tests for skin cancer. 2023. https://www.cancerresearchuk.org/.

Das, Taraprasad, Peter Holland, Munir Ahmed, Lutful Husain, Munir Ahmed, and Lutful Husain. Sustainable development goal 3: good health and well-being. In *South-East Asia Eye Health: Systems, Practices, and Challenges*, eds. Taraprasad Das and Patanjali Dev Nayar, pp. 61–78. Singapore: Springer Singapore, 2021.

Goodfellow, Ian, Jean Pouget-Abadie, Mehdi Mirza, Bing Xu, David Warde-Farley, Sherjil Ozair, Aaron Courville, and Yoshua Bengio. Generative adversarial networks. *Communications of the ACM* 63, no. 11 (2020): 139–144.

Han, Hui, Wen-Yuan Wang, and Bing-Huan Mao. Borderline-SMOTE: a new over-sampling method in imbalanced data sets learning. In *International Conference on Intelligent Computing*, pp. 878–887. Berlin, Heidelberg: Springer, 2005.

Hussain, Syed Ibrar, and Elena Toscano. An extensive investigation into the use of machine learning tools and deep neural networks for the recognition of skin cancer: challenges, future directions, and a comprehensive review. *Symmetry* 16, no. 3 (2024): 366.

Huynh, Quan Thanh, Phuc Hoang Nguyen, Hieu Xuan Le, Lua Thi Ngo, Nhu-Thuy Trinh, Mai Thi-Thanh Tran, Hoan Tam Nguyen et al. Automatic acne object detection and acne severity grading using smartphone images and artificial intelligence. *Diagnostics* 12, no. 8 (2022): 1879.

Igbasanmi, Oluwaseyi. *CNN Based Object Classification Using Image and Poisson Vector Field Features*. Master's thesis, Texas A&M University-Commerce, 2023.

International Skin Imaging Collaboration. ISIC 2020 challenge, 2020. https://challenge2020.isic-archive.com

Jasil, SP Godlin, and V. Ulagamuthalvi. Deep learning architecture using transfer learning for classification of skin lesions. *Journal of Ambient Intelligence and Humanized Computing* (2021): 1–8.

Kaur, Ranpreet, Hamid GholamHosseini, Roopak Sinha, and Maria Lindén. Melanoma classification using a novel deep convolutional neural network with dermoscopic images. *Sensors* 22, no. 3 (2022): 1134.

Lembhe, Ashutosh, Pranav Motarwar, Rudra Patil, and Susan Elias. Enhancement in skin cancer detection using image super resolution and convolutional neural network. *Procedia Computer Science* 218 (2023): 164–173.

Mac Carthy, Taig, Ignacio Hernández Montilla, Andy Aguilar, Rubén García Castro, Ana María González Pérez, Alejandro Vilas Sueiro, Laura Vergara de la Campa, Fernando Alfageme, and Alfonso Medela. Automatic urticaria activity score: deep learning–based automatic hive counting for urticaria severity assessment. *JID Innovations* 4, no. 1 (2024): 100218.

Middlesex Health. Skin cancer, 2024. https://middlesexhealth.org

Miller, Kimberly D., Miranda Fidler-Benaoudia, Theresa H. Keegan, Heather S. Hipp, Ahmedin Jemal, and Rebecca L. Siegel. Cancer statistics for adolescents and young adults, 2020. *CA: A Cancer Journal for Clinicians* 70, no. 6 (2020): 443–459.

Mohammed, Roweida, Jumanah Rawashdeh, and Malak Abdullah. Machine learning with oversampling and undersampling techniques: overview study and experimental results. In *2020 11th International Conference on Information and Communication Systems (ICICS)*, pp. 243–248. IEEE, 2020.

Naveena, T., and S. Jerine. Effective skin cancer prediction using hybrid Xception and XGBoost approach tuned by honey badger optimization. *Multimedia Tools and Applications* 83, no. 36 (2024): 1–28.

Nawaz, Marriam, Zahid Mehmood, Tahira Nazir, Rizwan Ali Naqvi, Amjad Rehman, Munwar Iqbal, and Tanzila Saba. Skin cancer detection from dermoscopic images using deep learning and fuzzy k-means clustering. *Microscopy Research and Technique* 85, no. 1 (2022): 339–351.

Prottasha, Sazzadul Islam, Sanjan Mahjabin Farin, Bulbul Ahmed, Zihadur Rahman, A. B. M. Kabir Hossain, and M. Shamim Kaiser. Deep learning-based skin disease detection using convolutional neural networks (CNN). In *The Fourth Industrial Revolution and Beyond: Select Proceedings of IC4IR+*, pp. 551–564. Singapore: Springer Nature Singapore, 2023.

Qureshi, Aqsa Saeed, and Teemu Roos. Transfer learning with ensembles of deep neural networks for skin cancer detection in imbalanced data sets. *Neural Processing Letters* 55, no. 4 (2023): 4461–4479.

Raghupathi, Viju, and Wullianallur Raghupathi. Healthcare expenditure and economic performance: insights from the United States data. *Frontiers in public health* 8 (2020): 156.

Rashid, Javed, Maryam Ishfaq, Ghulam Ali, Muhammad R. Saeed, Mubasher Hussain, Tamim Alkhalifah, Fahad Alturise, and Noor Samand. Skin cancer disease detection using transfer learning technique. *Applied Sciences* 12, no. 11 (2022): 5714.

Reis, Hatice Catal, Veysel Turk, Kourosh Khoshelham, and Serhat Kaya. InSiNet: a deep convolutional approach to skin cancer detection and segmentation. *Medical & Biological Engineering & Computing* (2022): 1–20.

Rice, Leslie, Eric Wong, and Zico Kolter. Overfitting in adversarially robust deep learning. In *International Conference on Machine Learning*, pp. 8093–8104. PMLR, 2020.

Sayed, Gehad Ismail, and Aboul Ella Hassanein. Air pollutants classification using optimized neural network based on war strategy optimization algorithm. *Automatic Control and Computer Sciences* 57, no. 6 (2023): 600–607.

Sayed, Gehad Ismail, and Aboul Ella Hassanien. Explainable AI and slime mould algorithm for classification of pistachio species. In *Artificial Intelligence: A Real Opportunity in the Food Industry*, eds. Aboul Ella Hassanien and Mona Soliman, pp. 29–43. Cham: Springer International Publishing, 2022.

Sayed, Gehad Ismail, Mona M. Soliman, and Aboul Ella Hassanien. A novel melanoma prediction model for imbalanced data using optimized SqueezeNet by bald eagle search optimization. *Computers in Biology and Medicine* 136 (2021): 104712.

Sayed, Gehad Ismail, Mona Soliman, and Aboul Ella Hassanien. Modified optimal foraging algorithm for parameters optimization of support vector machine. In *The International Conference on Advanced Machine Learning Technologies and Applications (AMLTA2018)*, pp. 23–32. Cairo, Egypt: Springer International Publishing, 2018.

Shetty, Bhuvaneshwari, Roshan Fernandes, Anisha P. Rodrigues, Rajeswari Chengoden, Sweta Bhattacharya, and Kuruva Lakshmanna. Skin lesion classification of dermoscopic images using machine learning and convolutional neural network. *Scientific Reports* 12, no. 1 (2022): 18134.

Siddiqui, Muhammad Shakil Suakeh, and Ghulam Sarwar. What is cancer? What causes cancer?. *RADS Journal of Pharmacy and Pharmaceutical Sciences* 1, no. 1 (2013): 30–34.

Tahir, Maryam, Ahmad Naeem, Hassaan Malik, Jawad Tanveer, Rizwan Ali Naqvi, and Seung-Won Lee. DSCC_Net: multi-classification deep learning models for diagnosing of skin cancer using dermoscopic images. *Cancers* 15, no. 7 (2023): 2179.

Zhang, Li, Jian Zhang, Wenlian Gao, Fengfeng Bai, Nan Li, and Noradin Ghadimi. A deep learning outline aimed at prompt skin cancer detection utilizing gated recurrent unit networks and improved orca predation algorithm. *Biomedical Signal Processing and Control* 90 (2024): 105858.

12 Neuro-Fuzzy Multimodal Ensemble Algorithm for Alzheimer's Disease Prediction

Janarthanam S and Subbulakshmi G

12.1 INTRODUCTION

The domain of healthcare is intrinsically complex, with complex biological systems involved, multisided diseases, and a wealth of heterogeneous data sources. Kim et al. (2022) focus on traditional approaches to analysis, which are hard to capture, subtle, and intricate in health data, needing agitation for the urge to develop more refined and robust computational techniques. HCI synergistically welds. Ahmed et al. (2015) refers to various artificial intelligence methodologies, such as deep learning, fuzzy logic-based evolutionary algorithms, into one framework and has therefore had a place for itself in recent years as very promisingly emerging paradigms that surely assist multifarious challenges of healthcare.

HCI unifies the strengths of miscellaneous computational paradigms and gives seamless designs of potent, all-purpose systems to handle the complexities of healthcare applications. Integrating the algorithms with deep learning models empowers HCI to split the intricate patterns from multimodal sources of data, such as electronic health records, medical imaging data, and wearable device data. Moreover, fuzzy logic techniques can cope much more efficiently with uncertainties in the medical data, while evolutionary algorithms could optimize model parameters and feature selection methods. It is such a combination of synergistic computational techniques that has provided tremendous potential for healthcare support in different domains related to disease diagnosis, risk prediction, treatment planning, and drug discovery by (Albaculyre-Merchant and AlZahrani 2022). The potential of HCI to learn adaptively from data, reason under uncertainty, and optimize complex systems will be a very vital aspect in the pursuit of personalized, precise, and effective healthcare solutions.

12.2 NEURODEGENERATIVE BRAIN SICKNESS

Ansart et al. (2021) deals with AD as a devastating, newly emerging neurodegenerative disorder that has now become a major health problem worldwide. It has presented a huge challenge to healthcare systems as the most common cause of dementia and has important implications for individuals, families, and society. This is a progressive disorder marked by irreversible loss in cognitive functions, memory impairments, behavioral disturbances, personality changes, and ultimately a severe decline in the ability to perform daily activities.

In health terms, Alzheimer's disease represents an issue so complex that it requires a holistic approach and is definitely multidisciplinary. Definitely, timely and accurate diagnosis may permit early interventions and the adequate care and support of patients with this serious process and their carers given by (Arizmendi et al. 2021) and (Asgari Mehrabadi et al. 2022). Since the pathophysiology of AD is so complex and most often overlaps with the symptoms of other dementias, which, posing a diagnosis challenge, especially in an early state. The growing prevalence of AD has placed substantial burdens on every healthcare resource and infrastructure. With a view of these projections (Saturi et al. 2025) deals the affected individuals by Alzheimer's are going to significantly

DOI: 10.1201/9781003486640-12

increase with the aging of the global population and there is an increasing need for the development of effective prevention strategies, disease-modifying treatments, and supportive care model.

This work includes continued improvements in the underlying mechanisms for the development of innovative diagnostic tools, the search for possible therapeutic interventions, and the application of comprehensive care plans for covering the multidimensional needs of patients and their families.

Computational intelligence approaches have been found very prospective to dealing with all issues related to Alzheimer's disease in any healthcare domain. Jia et al. (2024) mention the Computational techniques extract useful information from some heterogeneous biomedical data using artificial intelligence methodologies like deep learning using fuzzy logic based evolutionary algorithms are helping decision-making processes.

Nowadays researcher can use machine learning algorithms, coupled with deep learning models, across these multimodal data sources to draw out meaningful patterns and features from the neuro-imaging, genetic data, and clinical assessments stated by (Chen et al. 2021, Choi et al. 2018). In turn (Diogo et al. 2022) deals fuzzy logic techniques are able to deal a priori with the intrinsic uncertainties and imprecisions inherent in the medical data, and evolutionary algorithms enable optimization procedures with respect to model parameters and feature selection. The combination of these computational intelligence technologies has a lot of potential for enhancing care and lifestyle quality of patients with AD through diagnosis, prognosis, and treatment planning.

Support Vector Machines are the most applied for classification in the domain of Alzheimer. Based on its definition, this optimal hyperplane of SVM should maximize the boundary among the different class data points by (Duman et al. 2023). If given data is linear, then the optimization problem is:

$$\min \sum_{i} (1/2) \| w \|^2 \text{ subject to } y_i(w^T x_i + b) = 1, \forall i \quad (12.1)$$

The weight vector w defines the hyperplane, whereas xi denotes input feature vectors, and yi is their class label (–1 or 1). Here b be the bias term. In GA, the term evaluates the role of the fitness function goodness referred by (Díaz-Álvarez et al. 2022), genetic operators apply on a repeated basis to evolve better solutions. Operators such as mutation and crossover applied in a repeated manner achieve an overall evolution of better solutions. For example, in feature selection, a chromosome may simply be a binary vector indicating either the presence (1) or absence (0) of features by (Venugopalan et al. 2021) and (Helaly et al. 2021). In this case, fitness may be defined as some measure of model quality, such as classification accuracy with respect to a model trained on the features contained in the chromosome. Again, this typically requires deep architecture, multiple optimization algorithms, and combined methods for extracting complex patterns and associations in biomedical data.

Figure 12.1 shows the workflow overview diagram and the most important elements to be applied by computational intelligence techniques in different applications for Alzheimer's disease applications (Nithya et al. 2023) and (Islam and Zhang 2018). Even though computational intelligence techniques show some promising results in addressing some challenges related to AD, there are several limitations and challenges that need to be addressed.

12.3 LIMITATIONS OF TRADITIONAL COMPUTATIONAL INTELLIGENCE

- Limited availability of large, high-quality, diverse, and well-annotated datasets used for the training or validation of computational models.
- Sources of multimodal data, integration and fusion, each of which can be very problematic as neuro-imaging, biomarkers, clinical assessments, and genetic information.
- The models should provide explicit explanations and insights meaningful to clinicians and caregivers, aiding in the gaining of trust in their decision-making.

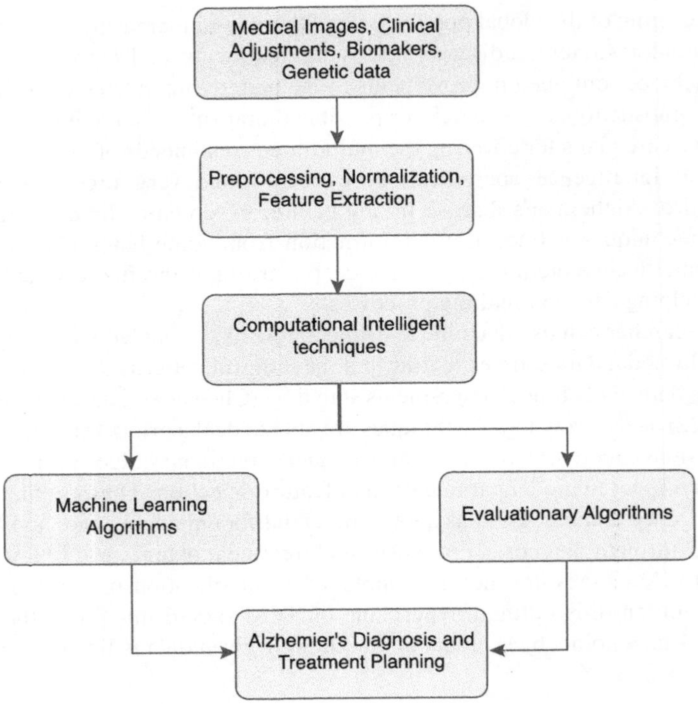

FIGURE 12.1 Work flow overview of computational intelligence.

- Computational models are inherently customized to specified datasets or populations and may not generalize to other demographic groups or other healthcare settings.
- Scalability Issues may lead to scalability issues with large-scale datasets or even real-time applications, such as in the continuous monitoring or optimization of individually personalized treatment policies.
- The skeptical fight of healthcare professionals and regulatory bodies in using AI-based systems in the case of key decision-making processes.
- Embedding possible biases and fairness computational models that mean possible discrimination or unequal treatment of some patient groups.

These limitations demand the collaborative efforts of researchers, clinicians, data scientists, and policymakers to be undertaken (Jain et al. 2019) research is currently being focused on the development of robust computational intelligence frameworks with interpretability, enhancement of quality and standards in data. Investigating transfer learning techniques and implementing rigorously defined protocols for validation that enable these technologies to be translated into a clinical application management of Alzheimer's disease detailed by (Al-Rawashdeh et al. 2024) and (Kumar et al. 2022). The direction, clearly keeps the growing need for neuro fuzzy multimodal Computational Intelligence approaches that allow for the exploitation of the strengths of multiple paradigms while mitigating their individual limitations.

While Neuro Fuzzy computational intelligence approaches add more complexities to model design, training, and integration, they can become very promising ways forward to handle all the challenges that are imposed by Alzheimer's disease mentioned as (Tufail et al. 2020). This united approach brings together some of the key strengths of different computational paradigms, thus likely to give better accuracy, interpretability, and generalizability, with enhanced clinical adoptability, ultimately leading to better patient care and management for this crippling condition.

12.4 NEURO FUZZY MULTIMODEL COMPUTATIONAL INTELLIGENCE

Neuro-fuzzy multimodal computational intelligence approaches then reflect a very promising proposition to cope with the complexities and challenges from Alzheimer. Different AI-based approaches can have the synergistic composition of feature extraction possibilities offered by deep learning models and pattern recognition capabilities in an interpretable manner, while at the same time take advantage of their interpretability and generalization abilities from a traditional machine learning technique. Nawaz et al. (2021) mentioned by Neuro multimodal fuzzy systems combine the adaptive learning capabilities from neural networks and handling the uncertainty from fuzzy logic systems. This includes, for example, genetic algorithms to evolve the architecture of a convolutional neural network to achieve better classification accuracy when it comes to MRI data, while particle swarm optimization tunes hyper-parameters with a recurrent neural system of the network in order to predict the progression of diseases. Ensemble methods combine output from different computational intelligence techniques, such as fuzzy logic systems to come up with a more robust and accurate decision.

They shall broach different complexities and uncertainties that are multimodal in data, with interpretable and accurate decision support availed to clinicians and caregivers through the incorporation of varied techniques. This contains an exploration of novel hybrid architecture, strategies for improvement in data integration, and establishing standardized frameworks on their evaluation to ensure the translation of such advanced computational intelligence solutions into real-world health care settings for better Alzheimer's management.

One such powerful and the Neuro Fuzzy Multimodal technique for the treatment of Alzheimer's disease is neuro-fuzzy multimodal ensemble methods. This will combine the strengths of neural networks, fuzzy logic systems, and ensemble learning with the utilization of the strengths from multimodal data sources in order to offer personalized and accurate treatment recommendations. The algorithm with mathematical formulations for the proposed Neuro Fuzzy Multimodal technique using neuro-fuzzy multimodal ensemble trust to treat using the procedure for the Alzheimer disease shown in Figure 12.2. This work proposes a Neuro Fuzzy Multimodal technique using neuro-fuzzy multimodal ensemble methods in the treatment of AD.

Neuro Fuzzy Multimodel Computational Intelligence Algorithm

Input: Data sources of multimodal data: neuro-imaging, biomarkers, clinical assessments, demographics.

Step 1: Data Preprocessing:

- Apply normalization techniques to obtain different variable scales and distributions in the data.
- Extract features and reduce dimensionality using PCA, auto-encoder, or other techniques to decrease data complexity and bring out relevant features.

Step 2: The Neural Network Component system:

Convolutional Neural Network (CNN) for neuro-imaging data analysis:

$$x_j^l = f\left(S_i x_i^{(l-1)} * k_i j^l + b_j^l\right)$$

Where $x_i^{(l-1)}$ input from the previous layer, $k_i j^l$ be the kernel filter, the b_j^l bias term, f active function and x_j^l be the output feature map.

Recurrent Neural Network (RNN) for longitudinal data analysis

Hidden state update is $h_t = f\left(W_{x * x_t} + W_h * h_{\{t-1\}} + b_h\right)$ Where x_t be the input time t, $h_{\{t-1\}}$ pervious hidden state, W_x, W_h learnable weight matrices

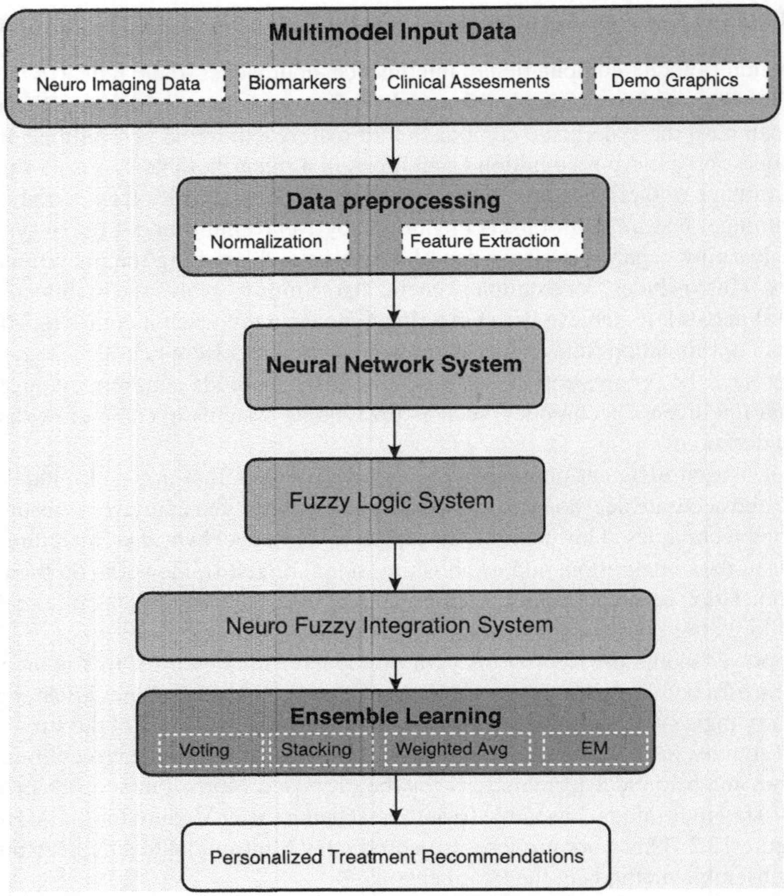

FIGURE 12.2 Overall flow diagram for NFCI.

Step 3: Fuzzy Logic System:

Define membership functions (e.g., Gaussian, triangular) for input variables.

Construct fuzzy rule base with expert knowledge and linguistic rules

IF (age is high) AND (biomarker_X is low) AND (Disease severity is moderate)

THEN (Treatment recommendation is drug A)

Step 4: Use neural networks to learn and optimize the constraints of the fuzzy system using member functions and rule weights.

Step 5: Train multiple neuro-fuzzy models, each specialized in handling different data, modalities or aspects of Alzheimer's disease. Combine the output of individual neuro-fuzzy models using ensemble techniques.

Step 6: Use the ensemble neuro-fuzzy system to generate personalized treatment recommendations based on the individual's clinical profile and predicted treatment response.

Step 7: Interpret and explain the recommendations using the activated fuzzy rules and pathways within the neuro-fuzzy models.

The mathematical formulations should be able to capture the key operations of each component, convolutional and recurrent layers, fuzzy inference, and ensemble combination strategies.

12.5 PERFORMANCE EVALUATION

The possibility to evaluate the Neuro Fuzzy multimodal technique with regard to treatment against Alzheimer's disease by different metrics and parameters. For analysis, ADMUD dataset was used. ADMUD is a large dataset comprising data of different types, which were collected from 2,500 individuals amongst which 1,500 had the Alzheimer, and 1,000 were healthy. It is expected that with the integration of neuroimaging, different categories of biomarkers, and clinical assessment data, a much fuller understanding of AD progression will be obtained and lead to improved diagnostic and treatment strategies given by (Habes et al. 2016) and (Henríquez and Araya, 2024). The metrics used for the evaluation parameters, together with their mathematical formulations, are:

Accuracy measures the proportion of correct predictions against all instances predicted. the fractional ratio of the correctly classified instances tested along the total instances tested.

$$\text{Accuracy} = (\text{TP} + \text{TN}) / (P + R) \tag{12.2}$$

Where TP (True Positives) as Number of Alzheimer correctly identified, TN (True Negatives) as Number of healthy cases correctly identified, P denoted the Precision and R denotes the Sensitivity.

Sensitivity or Recall mentioned in equation (12.3) is the proportion of Alzheimer cases that the model is able to identify.

$$\text{Sensitivity}(\text{R}) = \text{TP}/(\text{TP} + \text{FN}) \tag{12.3}$$

Specificity is a proportional value of healthy cases, has rightly predicted given in the equation (12.4).

$$\text{Specificity} \ = \text{TN}/(\text{TN} + \text{FP}) \tag{12.4}$$

Precision measures (by (5)) the correctly identified Alzheimer cases among all classified Alzheimer.

$$\text{Precision}(P) = \text{TP}/(\text{TP} + \text{FP}) \tag{12.5}$$

The harmonic mean of precision and sensitivity, gives a balanced measure of performance of the model as F1-score in equation (12.6).

$$\text{F1-Score} = 2 \times \left[(P \times R) / (P + R) \right] \tag{12.6}$$

AUC-ROC is, a fully comprehensive measure of test performance defined as the ability of the model to distinguish cases of Alzheimer's disease from healthy cases at various thresholds of decision. The range lies between 0 and 1, where higher values signify improved performance as in the equation (12.7).

$$\text{AUC} - \text{ROC} = \int_0^1 \text{TPR}(t) \times [1 - \text{FPR}(t)] dt \tag{12.7}$$

Where TPR = Sensitivity, FPR = 1 – Specificity and t denotes the decision threshold.

Loss function during training, the Neuro Fuzzy model learns by optimizing a loss function is the difference of predictions with the true labels. The choice of loss function are mean squared error and custom functions mentioned by Duman et al. (2023) and Wang et al. (2024) depending on the given task is shown in equation (12.8).

$$\text{Entropy Loss} = -\left(y \times \log(p) + (1 - y) \times \log(1 - p) \right) \tag{12.8}$$

Where $y = 0$ or 1 and p holds probability of instance to its positive predicted class. These evaluation parameters furnish information on various aspects of the Neuro Fuzzy model concerning overall accuracy, sensitivity to Alzheimer's cases, specificity for health cases, and finally, the capacity of class discrimination. The Alzheimer patent's treatment application has the evaluation metrics should be based on specific requirements or priorities for that application.

12.6 RESULT AND DISCUSSION

The ADMUD is one huge set of arrays of data generated from those who have Alzheimer's disease and healthy ones. This information is then to be applied in the building of computational designs for the diagnostics, monitoring, and the suggestion of treatment procedures for AD.

Table 12.1 showing performance of Neuro Fuzzy Multimodal approach for treatment of Alzheimer's disease as:

Table 12.1 comparing the proposed Neuro Fuzzy Multimodal technique against results from individual components and baseline models. A baseline of a logistic regression model does not perform very well, returning an accuracy of 0.72 and having an AUC-ROC of 0.77. A neuro-fuzzy model combining neural networks and fuzzy logic together into one system performs better, returning an accuracy of 0.85 and allowing an AUC-ROC of 0.89. In this present study, the proposed Neuro Fuzzy model based on neuro-fuzzy multimodal ensemble techniques outclassed all of the other models with accuracy, recall and specificity of 0.94, and a very impressive AUC-ROC of 0.96.

The results of suggested Neuro fuzzy multi model computational intelligence approach, using, fuzzy logic-based neuro-fuzzy integration with ensemble learning, comes out with enhanced accuracy and robustness for predictions of treatment recommendations for Alzheimer disease treatment representation. The overview of the Alzheimer disease multimodal dataset mild cognitive impairment and healthy control across different age groups for neuro-psychological test scores by condition and age group are shows on the Table 12.2 below:

Figure 12.3 shows the Distribution of Neuropsychological Test Score (e.g. MMSE) Across the Three Conditions (AD, MCI, and Healthy) and Age Groups (Like as 60–69, 70–79, 80+). Most of the low values are usually recorded for Alzheimer Disease group, although some overlap exists with the Mild Cognitive Impairment group (Table 12.3).

Figure 12.4 summarize the distribution of levels of various biomarkers – for example, APOE – across three conditions and three age groups: Diagnostic Any APOE and Diagnostic No APOE. In general, higher values of some biomarkers are indicative of AD, while lower values are characteristic of the Healthy Control group. Tables 12.4–12.6 represent the neuro-imaging features correlation among each other by Condition (Figure 12.5).

TABLE 12.1
Performance Analysis of NFCI Model

Model	Accuracy	Sensitivity	Specificity	AUC-ROC
Baseline (Logistic Regression)	0.72	0.68	0.76	0.77
CNN	0.79	0.82	0.75	0.84
RNN	0.81	0.77	0.84	0.86
Fuzzy logic system	0.75	0.71	0.79	0.81
Neuro-fuzzy model	0.85	0.83	0.87	0.89
Ensemble (Voting)	0.87	0.85	0.89	0.91
Ensemble (Stacking)	0.89	0.87	0.91	0.93
Neuro fuzzy model (Proposed)	0.92	0.90	0.94	0.96

TABLE 12.2
Neuro-Psychological Test Scores

Condition	Age_Group	MMSE_Score	ADAS_Cog_Score	CDR_Score	RAVLT_Score
AD	60–69	19.2	27.8	2.1	25.4
AD	70–79	17.5	31.2	2.5	22.1
AD	80+	15.8	34.6	3.0	19.7
MCI	60–69	25.6	18.4	1.2	35.7
MCI	70–79	24.1	20.9	1.5	32.4
MCI	80+	22.7	23.6	1.8	29.1
HC	60–69	29.1	6.3	0.1	49.2
HC	70–79	28.5	7.8	0.2	46.8
HC	80+	27.2	9.5	0.4	43.6

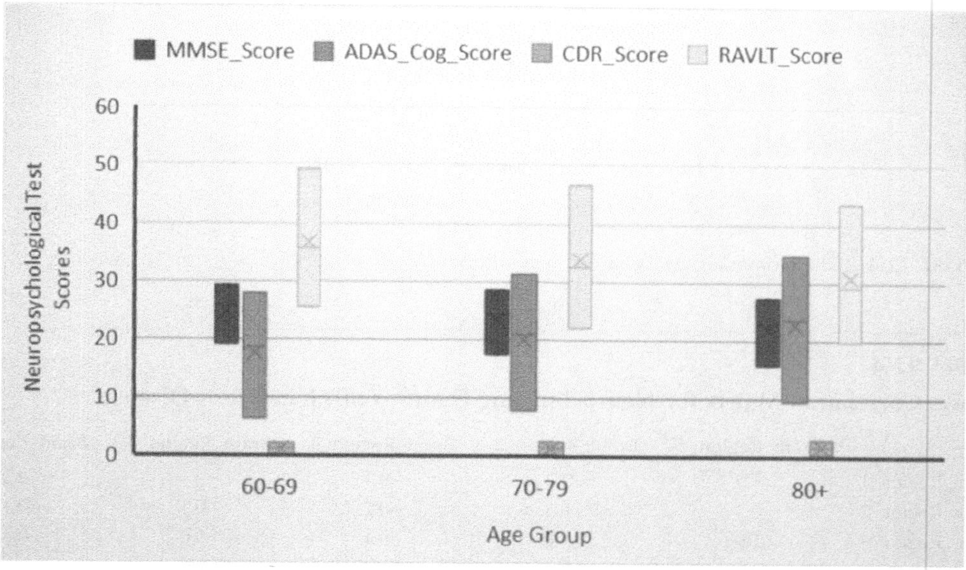

FIGURE 12.3 Neuropsychological test scores by condition and age group.

TABLE 12.3
The Biomarker Levels by Condition and Age Group

Condition	Age_Group	APOE_Level	Tau_Level
AD	60–69	3.8	85.2
AD	70–79	3.9	92.6
AD	80+	4.0	98.4
MCI	60–69	3.2	65.7
MCI	70–79	3.4	72.1
MCI	80+	3.6	78.9
HC	60–69	2.1	35.4
HC	70–79	2.3	39.8
HC	80+	2.5	44.2

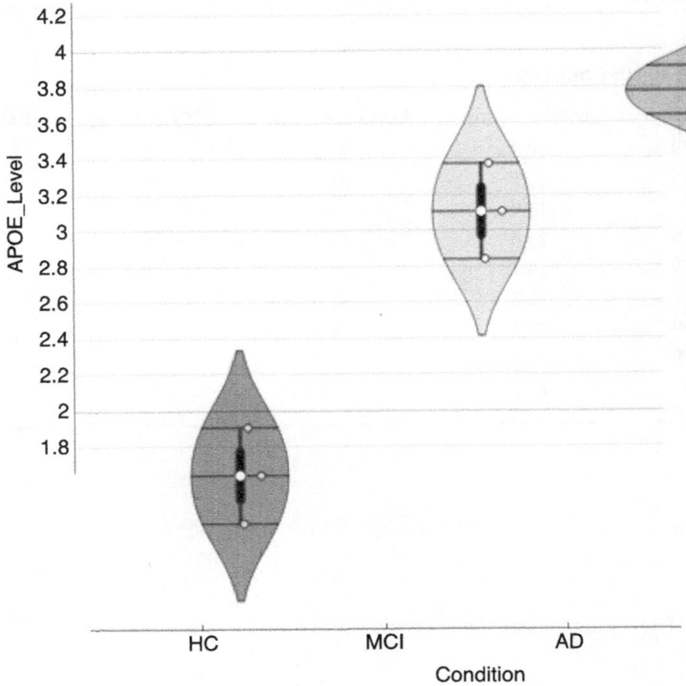

FIGURE 12.4 The biomarker levels based on conditions.

TABLE 12.4
shows Correlation Matrix for Neuro-Imaging Features of Alzheimer's Disease

	Brain_Region_1	Brain_Region_2	Brain_Region_3	Brain_Region_4	Brain_Region_5
Brain_Region_1	1.0	−0.2	−0.1	−0.4	0.2
Brain_Region_2	0.3	1.0	−0.2	−0.1	−0.1
Brain_Region_3	1.0	0.3	−0.1	0.0	0.2
Brain_Region_4	0.0	−0.1	−0.4	1.0	0.1
Brain_Region_5	0.2	0.0	0.2	0.1	1.0

TABLE 12.5
shows Correlation Matrix for Neuro-Imaging Features of Mild Cognitive Impairment

	Brain_Region_1	Brain_Region_2	Brain_Region_3	Brain_Region_4	Brain_Region_5
Brain_Region_1	1.0	−0.1	0.0	−0.2	0.1
Brain_Region_2	−0.1	1.0	0.2	0.1	0.0
Brain_Region_3	0.0	0.2	1.0	0.3	0.1
Brain_Region_4	−0.2	0.1	0.3	1.0	0.0
Brain_Region_5	0.1	0.0	0.1	0.0	1.0

TABLE 12.6
shows the Correlation Matrix for NeuroImaging Features of Healthy Control

	Brain_Region_1	Brain_Region_2	Brain_Region_3	Brain_Region_4	Brain_Region_5
Brain_Region_1	0.1	1.0	0.1	1.0	0.1
Brain_Region_2	0.1	1.0	0.1	0.1	0.0
Brain_Region_3	0.0	0.2	1.0	0.2	0.1
Brain_Region_4	0.0	0.1	0.2	1.0	0.0
Brain_Region_5	0.1	0.0	0.1	0.0	1.0

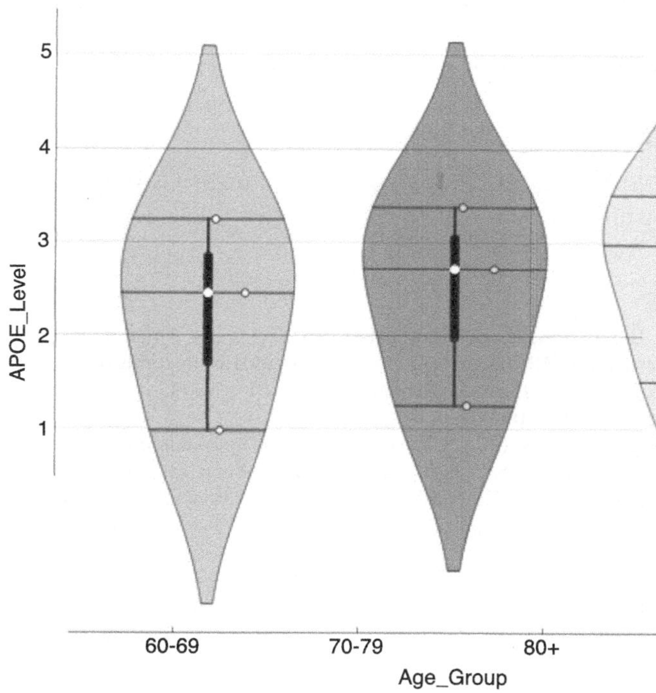

FIGURE 12.5 The biomarker levels based on age groups.

Above are Tables show the correlation matrices corresponding to neuro-imaging features, such as volumes of brain regions and cortical thickness. The color gradients represent the degree of correlation between those features, where red is in a positive and blue in a negative way according to (Łasińska et al. 2022) and (Jia et al. 2024). Notice that three conditions may have different patterns of correlation, which may reflect the changes associated with the corresponding conditions of neuroanatomical characteristics.

12.7 CONCLUSION

One of the paramount challenges to any healthcare system must be Alzheimer's disease, considering its prevalence and devastating consequences. Early diagnosis, as much as possible, will therefore go a long way in ensuring proper treatment and management. This study explores the possibility of coming up with Neuro-Fuzzy models from multiple computational techniques to improve the diagnosis of Alzheimer disease. Neuro-Fuzzy models incorporate various machine learning algorithms with neuro-imaging data to take advantage of the complementary strengths of each modality. Such fusion of classifiers will help the models capture different discriminative patterns within the data and hence improve diagnostics. The results of the experiments consider that the Neuro-Fuzzy approaches did better than individual techniques in most of the evaluation metrics considered.

Furthermore, all the Neuro-Fuzzy models have their inherent strengths in handling high dimensionality and complexity in neuro-imaging data while reducing potential overfitting problems. Inherent ensemble strategies make the solution robust and generalized by aggregating output across base learners. More importantly, integrating some feature selection mechanisms into these hybrids would facilitate the identification of the most informative biomarkers, hence interpretability in a way that will inform further research directions. This could also be enriched with multimodal sources of data, like neuropsychological assessments and genetic information, to gain an integrative understanding of the diseases for enhancing diagnosis. Further Neuro-Fuzzy model development and research can be directed in the near future toward the evolution of computation for the early detection and management of other neurological disorders.

ACKNOWLEDGMENT

Authors are thankful to CMR University Bengaluru and Bharatiar University Coimbatore for academic support to complete this research.

REFERENCES

Ahmed, O. B., Mizotin, M., Benois-Pineau, J., Allard, M., Catheline, G., & Amar, C. B. (2015). Alzheimer's disease diagnosis on structural MR images using circular harmonic functions descriptors on hippocampus and posterior cingulate cortex. *Computerized Medical Imaging and Graphics*, 44, 13–25. https://doi.org/10.1016/j.compmedimag.2015.04.007

Albaculyre-Merchant, S., & AlZahrani, S. (2022). Ensemble learning for Alzheimer's disease diagnosis from MRI data. *Applied Sciences*, 12(3), 1512. https://doi.org/10.3390/app12031512

Al-Rawashdeh, H. S., Usman, A., Dutta, A. K., & Sait, A. R. W. (2024). Ensemble learning-based Alzheimer's Disease diagnosis using magnetic resonance imaging. *Journal of Disability Research*, 3(6). https://doi.org/10.57197/jdr-2024-0067

Ansart, M., Epelbaum, S., Bassignana, G., Bône, A., Bottani, S., Cattai, T., Couronné, R., Faouzi, J., Koval, I., Louis, M., Thibeau-Sutre, E., Wen, J., Wild, A., Burgos, N., Dormont, D., Colliot, O., & Durrleman, S. (2021) Predicting the progression of mild cognitive impairment using machine learning: A systematic, quantitative and critical review. *Medical image analysis* 67:101848. doi: 10.1016/j.media.2020.101848

Arizmendi, C., Romero, E., Altbatz, J. M., Camins, A., & Diaz, M. (2020). Hybrid machine learning models for detecting mild cognitive impairment from MRI biomarkers. *Journal of Neuroscience Methods*, 333, 108545. https://doi.org/10.1016/j.jneumeth.2020.108754

Asgari Mehrabadi, M., Makelae, T., Mortazavi, D., & Niska, H. (2022). Alzheimer's disease diagnosis using 3D convolutional neural networks on structural MRI. *Future Generation Computer Systems*, 127, 170–177. https://doi.org/10.1016/j.future.2021.09.022

Chen, Y., & Xia, Y. (2021). Iterative sparse and deep learning for accurate diagnosis of Alzheimer's disease. *Pattern Recognition*, 116, 107944. https://doi.org/10.1016/j.patcog.2021.107944

Choi, H., Jin, K. H., & Alzheimer's Disease Neuroimaging Initiative. (2018). Predicting cognitive decline with deep learning of brain metabolism and amyloid imaging. *Behavioural brain research*, 344, 103–109. https://doi.org/10.1016/j.bbr.2018.02.017

Díaz-Álvarez, J., Matias-Guiu, J. A., Cabrera-Martín, M. N., Pytel, V., Segovia-Ríos, I., García-Gutiérrez, F., Hernández-Lorenzo, L., Matias-Guiu, J., Carreras, J. L., & Ayala, J. L. (2022). Genetic algorithms for optimized diagnosis of Alzheimer's disease and frontotemporal dementia using fluorodeoxyglucose positron emission tomography imaging. *Frontiers in Aging Neuroscience*, 13. https://doi.org/10.3389/fnagi.2021.708932

Diogo, V. S., Ferreira, H. A., & Prata, D. (2022). Early diagnosis of Alzheimer's disease using machine learning: a multi-diagnostic, generalizable approach. *Alzheimer S Research & Therapy*, 14(1). https://doi.org/10.1186/s13195-022-01047-y

Duman, A., Karakuş, O., Sun, X., Thomas, S., Powell, J., Spezi, E. (2023) RFS+: a clinically adaptable and computationally efficient strategy for enhanced brain tumor segmentation. Cancers, 15, 5620. https://doi.org/10.3390/cancers15235620

Habes, M., Janowitz, D., Erus, G., Toledo, J. B., Resnick, S. M., Doshi, J., Van Der Auwera, S., Wittfeld, K., Hegenscheid, K., Hosten, N., Biffar, R., Homuth, G., Völzke, H., Grabe, H. J., Hoffmann, W., & Davatzikos, C. (2016). Advanced brain aging: relationship with epidemiologic and genetic risk factors, and overlap with Alzheimer disease atrophy patterns. *Translational Psychiatry*, 6(4), e775. https://doi.org/10.1038/tp.2016.39

Helaly, H. A., Badawy, M., & Haikal, A. Y. (2021). Deep learning approach for early detection of Alzheimer's disease. *Cognitive Computation*, 14(5), 1711–1727. https://doi.org/10.1007/s12559-021-09946-2

Henríquez, P. A., & Araya, N. (2024). Multimodal Alzheimer's disease classification through ensemble deep random vector functional link neural network. *PeerJ Computer Science*, 10, e2590. https://doi.org/10.7717/peerj-cs.2590

Islam, J., & Zhang, Y. (2018). Brain MRI analysis for Alzheimer's disease diagnosis using an ensemble system of deep convolutional neural networks. *Brain Informatics*, 5(2). https://doi.org/10.1186/s40708-018-0080-3

Jain, R., Jain, N., Aggarwal, A., & Hemanth, D.J. (2019). Convolutional neural network based Alzheimer's disease classification from magnetic resonance brain images. *Cognitive Systems Research*, 57, 147–159. https://doi.org/10.1016/j.cogsys.2018.12.015

Jia, N., Jia, T., Zhao, L., Ma, B., & Zhu, Z. (2024). Multi-modal global- and local- feature interaction with attention-based mechanism for diagnosis of Alzheimer's disease. *Biomedical Signal Processing and Control*, 95, 106404. https://doi.org/10.1016/j.bspc.2024.106404

Kim, J., Jeong, M., Stiles, W. R., & Choi, H. S. (2022). Neuroimaging Modalities in Alzheimer's disease: diagnosis and clinical Features. *International Journal of Molecular Sciences*, 23(11), 6079. https://doi.org/10.3390/ijms23116079

Kumar, M., Singh, N., Srivastava, A., & Singh, S. (2022). Deep convolutional neural network with hybrid feature selection for reliable classification of Alzheimer's disease from MRI data. *Biomedical Signal Processing and Control*, 72, 103271. https://doi.org/10.1016/j.bspc.2021.103271

Łasińska, I., Zielińska, A., Mackiewicz, J., & Souto, E. B. (2022). Basal Cell Carcinoma: Pathology, Current Clinical Treatment, and Potential Use of Lipid Nanoparticles. *Cancers*, 14(11), 2778. https://doi.org/10.3390/cancers14112778

Nawaz, A., Anwar, S. M., Liaqat, R., Iqbal, J., Bagci, U., & Majid, M. (2021). Deep Convolutional Neural Network based Classification of Alzheimer's Disease using MRI data. arXiv (Cornell University). https://doi.org/10.48550/arxiv.2101.02876

Nithya, V. P., Mohanasundaram, N., & Santhosh, R. (2023). Earlier detection of Alzheimer's disease using 3D-Convolutional neural networks. *Computer Systems Science and Engineering*, 46(2), 2601–2618. https://doi.org/10.32604/csse.2023.030503

Saturi, S., Adiba, R., Reddy, I.Y., Shareef, Md. A., & Prathyush, D. (2025). Advanced MRI-Based Alzheimer's disease classification with hybrid convolutional neural networks. *Journal of Computer Allied Intelligence* (JCAI, ISSN: 2584-2676), 3(1), 31-39. https://doi.org/10.69996/jcai.2025003

Tufail, A. B., Ma, Y., & Zhang, Q. (2020). Binary classification of Alzheimer's disease using SMRI imaging modality and deep learning. *Journal of Digital Imaging*, 33(5), 1073–1090. https://doi.org/10.1007/s10278-019-00265-5

Venugopalan, J., Tong, L., Hassanzadeh, H. R., & Wang, M. D. (2021). Multimodal deep learning models for early detection of Alzheimer's disease stage. *Scientific Reports*, 11(1). https://doi.org/10.1038/s41598-020-74399-w

Wang, J., Wen, S., Liu, W., Meng, X., & Jiao, Z. (2024). Deep joint learning diagnosis of Alzheimer's disease based on multimodal feature fusion. *BioData Mining*, 17(1). https://doi.org/10.1186/s13040-024-00395-9

13 Optimizing Bidirectional Encoder Representations from Transformers for Medical Healthce

Unveiling Insights from Fine-Tuning for Efficient Question Answering with Gen AI

Prakhar Kunwar Sinha, Mitraansh Raaj Khanna, and S. Poornima

13.1 INTRODUCTION

In recent years, the field of Natural Language Processing (NLP) has experienced a transformative shift, particularly in addressing the intricate linguistic nuances found in contemporary medical notes. This paradigmatic change, coupled with the rapid integration of chat applications with Artificial Intelligence (AI), underscores a rising demand for specialized clinical BERT (Bidirectional Encoder Representations from Transformers) models (Devlin et al. 2019). This research bridges two crucial aspects: the development of these specialized models and the revolutionary potential of AI-powered medical chatbots. The specialized clinical BERT model showcased here, adept at capturing complex clinical narratives, not only outperforms conventional BERT and BioBERT models (Devlin et al. 2019) but also proves instrumental in various clinical NLP tasks.

Concurrently, this study explores the vast field of AI-powered healthcare chatbots, acknowledging their potential for personalized support, real-time diagnosis, and increased accessibility to healthcare. A thorough analysis of the study highlights the critical role AI-powered medical chatbots play in changing the dynamics of healthcare. Beyond the domain of technological developments, the study explores the significant influence that these chatbots can have on patient-doctor interactions by providing prompt responses and enabling people to make knowledgeable decisions regarding their health. This research significantly contributes to the ongoing discussion on the future trajectory of healthcare innovation at a critical juncture in healthcare evolution, marked by an increasing demand for trustworthy and easily accessible medical information. Some models, like ELMo (Embeddings from Language Models), ULMFiT (Universal Language Model Fine-tuning), and BERT, have done very well with biomedical and general text. However, they have trouble with the language used in clinical narratives, especially physician notes. This research is developing specialized clinical BERT models in response to the growing need for them. However, writing physician notes presents certain linguistic difficulties. The growing need for specialized clinical BERT models motivated the research to create and publicly release an embedding model specifically for clinical text.

DOI: 10.1201/9781003486640-13

13.2 RELATED WORK

Starting with investigating chatbots for healthcare, the review covers a wide range of scholarly works and offers a thorough grasp of the complexities, developments, and difficulties in this field. The tour delves into the complex field of academic literature to clarify the changing role of chatbots in healthcare environments, using basic observations as a guide. The cooperative academic endeavor seeks to offer a comprehensive story that summarizes the goals, approaches, conclusions, and advantages and disadvantages of every cited research.

The first expedition in this academic journey, led by (Bhirud 2019), provides a fundamental understanding of the patterns and conditions of healthcare chatbots today. This study is a foundational work that attempts to decipher the intricacies and evaluate the efficacy of these digital entities. Understanding the healthcare chatbot landscape and highlighting its intricacy and efficacy is the aim. The Naive Bayes Classifier (NBC) is a methodology that is used to assess the effectiveness and interpret the complexity of healthcare chatbots. It does this by analyzing past research to comprehend the state of these chatbots and highlighting their complexity and effectiveness. The study makes use of NBC and looks at current chatbot technologies such as Botsify, Impression, and NBC. The results demonstrate how popular tools such as NBC, Impression, and Botsify can be used in a variety of industries. Benefits include a decrease in stress and anxiety, which is especially important given the difficult circumstances created by the COVID-19 pandemic. Cons, however, continue to exist and include difficulties with user interaction and technological constraints.

Moving on to the complexities of artificial intelligence and natural language processing in healthcare chatbots, Serban (2017) invites investigation into the technical foundations of these systems. The goal, which is extremely high and has a validation rate of 99%, is to shed light on the internal mechanisms. A methodology that examines the internal workings of healthcare chatbots using deep reinforcement learning and AI models, including latent variable neural networks and reinforcement learning-trained natural language generation approaches are employed. The study demonstrates how well chatbots perform when answering questions about ailments, medications, symptoms, causes, and prevention. Benefits include rapid access to medical information and tailored interactions, but there are also drawbacks, such as continuous development challenges and the urgent need for improvement.

Going even deeper into the emotional domain, Kadu (2019) invites an investigation into the field of emotion identification and categorization in healthcare chatbots. Improving user interactions and emotional intelligence is the clear goal here. The methodology used is of deep learning methods for healthcare chatbot emotion recognition and classification, such as Convolutional Neural Networks (CNNs) and Recurrent Neural Networks (RNNs). Data analysis is employed as a guide to navigate through the intricacy of emotion detection. The results show enhanced emotion categorization and recognition, with a focus on creating a chatbot with intelligent voice recognition. Advantages include more responsiveness, but disadvantages could include difficulties in putting sophisticated AI models into practice and possible privacy issues.

Singh and Choubey (2021) stands out as a beacon directing attention to the supportive role that text-based healthcare chatbots play in patient care and interactions with medical professionals. Examining the chatbot's functionality and design in therapeutic contexts is the goal. The Mobile Coach platform's implementation of the Text-based Healthcare Chatbot (THCB) serves as the main focus of investigation. Results from a clinical trial reveal elements like working alliance, adherence, scalability, user satisfaction, and attachment bond. The study assesses MRI pictures through data analysis. Image processing techniques such as noise reduction and histogram equalization likely enhance the quality and interpretability of the MRI data. Pros include effective channels for communication and strong support systems; cons include potential limitations in text-based interactions and difficulties in sustaining user engagement.

Examining the specific THCB mentioned in Rarhi (2017) and Kowatsch et al. (2017) in more detail reveals that the goal is to show how well it works for young obese patients, as well as how well it is designed to work with the Mobile Coach platform. Methods like Likert scale evaluations and real-time patient data analysis allow for outcomes that emphasize the role of the THCB as a digital health coach. Likert scale assessments and real-time patient data analysis are two forms of data analysis that form the basis of this research. This approach thoroughly assesses the usability, effectiveness, and performance of various healthcare technologies, with a particular focus on a mobile chat app for healthcare interventions and a THCB for obese adolescent patients. This study attempts to acquire detailed insights into how these technologies affect patient care and engagement by examining both quantitative measures and qualitative comments. Easy-to-use communication channels and timely notifications to healthcare practitioners are advantages; potential issues with intervention adherence and scalability could be disadvantages.

As the academic journey draws to an end, research paper sections (Judson 2020, Mowafa 2021, Fan et al. 2021) all encourage further investigation into AI-based chatbots for illness prediction and treatment recommendation. The primary goal is to investigate how these chatbots use AI technologies to predict illnesses and suggest treatments. The integration of machine learning algorithms, web services, and the Google API for voice-text interactions forms the methodological foundation. Machine learning methods including logistic regression, random forests, and decision trees are employed in the methodology for sickness prediction. Methods for analyzing qualitative data, such as coding or thematic analysis. Approaches for specialized analysis, may incorporate qualitative and descriptive statistics. The outcomes demonstrate the potential of these chatbots to offer quick, accurate answers for disease diagnosis and treatment suggestions. While there are undoubtedly benefits to having easier access to healthcare data, there are also disadvantages, including the inability to make exact predictions and potential reliance on external systems.

Starting with (Baby 2018), the emphasis shifts to fundamental findings about the adaptability of general-purpose chatbots. This study establishes the scene by explaining the fundamental features of these conversational agents and provides a broad framework for further investigation. This methodology uses Natural Language Processing (NLP) tools, specifically algorithms like Transformer models and BERT, to develop and evaluate chatbots that can understand and respond in natural language. Large datasets are most often used for both conversational context evaluation and model training. Benefits of this research might include adaptability and ease of use, but drawbacks might include restricted access to certain functions. To create and assess chatbots that can comprehend natural language and provide responses in that language, this methodology makes use of NLP tools.

Concurrently, Oh (2017) and Bharti et al. (2020) become the main focus of the discussion by exploring the complex field of emotion recognition AI methods in healthcare chatbots. Improving these digital objects' emotional intelligence in user interactions is the main goal. The research methods on cutting-edge approaches to natural language processing and artificial intelligence employ deep learning NLP techniques to generate sentences and analyze emotional dialogue using Transformer architectures and LSTM (Long Short Term Memory) models. Conversely, it employs telehealth and conversational AI approaches, utilizing deep learning models customized for conversational AI and possibly combining Transformer-based models to improve interactive health apps. Advantages manifest as increased responsiveness, providing users with a more sophisticated and interactive experience. However, the drawbacks could include possible privacy issues and the inherent difficulties in putting advanced AI models into practice.

Simultaneously, Balasubramaniam (2020) and Sharma and Jalal (2022) highlight text-based healthcare chatbots and their critical function as digital health coaches, which adds even more depth. Examining the layout and operation of these textual objects, especially in therapeutic contexts, is the main goal. These papers present the architecture of a text-based healthcare chatbot on the mobile coach platform, providing an in-depth investigation of techniques related to real-time patient data analysis and evaluations. The AI and ML driven healthcare chatbot analyses symptoms and recommends remedies using algorithms like supervised learning and reinforcement learning. The visual question-answering framework, on the other hand, depends on machine learning and computer vision to effectively comprehend visual data. Specifically, it uses techniques like Fisher Vectors and PHOCs (Pyramid Histogram of Characters) for scene-text recognition. These algorithms demonstrate their dedication to utilizing cutting-edge technology to improve visual information processing and healthcare. Clinical trial results offer empirical information on topics such as working alliances, attachment bonds, scalability, user enjoyment, and adherence. The benefits include effective lines of communication and real assistance for patients and medical staff. However, potential drawbacks with text-based interactions and difficulties keeping users consistently engaged are considered as disadvantages. Both studies uses state-of-the-art techniques to progress in their respective domains.

Together, Mehfooz et al. (2021), Altay et al. (2021), and Hossain et al. (2021) these studies create a wealth of information that adds to the changing field of healthcare chatbots. Their distinct viewpoints, approaches, and results work together to improve our comprehension and help us appreciate the complex dynamics at play in this emerging field of study. To investigate COVID-19-related healthcare applications through chatbots, this work combines data analytics, NLP techniques, survey methods, experimental psychology, and AI approaches. To improve user communication on COVID-19 symptoms and prevention, it uses NLP technologies such as BERT, and data analytics to understand disease patterns. Additionally, it assesses how the information offered by chatbots influences people's perceptions regarding COVID-19 immunizations through testing and polls. Another thing that came out of the study's use of AI was the Mr. Dr. Health-Assistant Chatbot, which is meant to provide personalized healthcare support and work on its own. It was made using natural language processing and machine learning algorithms such as GPT-3 (Generative Pre-trained Transformer 3) and reinforcement learning.

The research contribution demonstrates several current methods to increase its effectiveness. First, it adapts pre-trained BERT models for specific clinical text tasks by utilizing transfer learning, a well-known machine learning technique. Second, the study uses a basic optimization method called hyperparameter tuning to find the best model configurations for variables like batch size, epochs, and learning rate. Thirdly, to enhance model generalization, the study incorporates dropout regularization, a commonly utilized method to avoid overfitting. Finally, the study refines the pre-trained BERT models on clinical text datasets using methodologies that are frequently used in transfer learning, improving their performance on specific tasks. Together, these strategies show how the research can effectively use current methodology to address problems in clinical NLP and healthcare communication.

13.3 DATA COLLECTION

The aim of enhancing language comprehension in medical analysis drove our choice of data sources. We have carefully selected a range of sources to guarantee a thorough understanding of medical knowledge. The Stanford Question Answering Dataset (SQuAD2) was assembled with a focus on medical themes, which improves the model's accuracy while handling intricate medical queries. At the same time, we make use of a variety of medical literature formats, such as books, journals, research papers, and articles, to provide the model with a sophisticated grasp of basic medical concepts and scientific language. Additionally, to capture both professional discourse and patient vernacular, we incorporate publicly available medical data from reliable sources, including websites, patient records, databases, and healthcare forums. This wide range of data sources, which collectively improve the model's accuracy and adaptability, includes SQuAD2, scientific literature, and publicly accessible medical data. Through the painstaking integration of data from many sources, our refined BERT model demonstrates its importance in healthcare applications by emerging as a resilient and adaptable instrument capable of handling intricate medical questions. These thorough data gathering initiatives provide a strong platform for the advancement of language comprehension and significant contributions to medical analysis.

13.4 DATA PRE-PROCESSING AND INPUT STRUCTURING

Input structuring and data pre-processing are essential for effective model learning. The initial stage is lowercasing, which makes all text lowercase to ensure uniform word representation. This decreases the vocabulary size, enabling the model to handle case changes more consistently, thereby promoting consistency in language comprehension. The next step is to apply Word Piece tokenization to decompose complex phrases into more manageable sub-word parts. It is possible to tokenize terms such as "unhappiness" into "un", "##happy", and "##ness". This approach is especially helpful for efficiently comprehending and expressing uncommon or complicated medical concepts.

Establishing a collection of distinct tokens that the model can identify is the first step in the vocabulary curation process. The vocabulary is kept up to date with 30,000 carefully chosen words, which include significant medical terms and special tokens like [CLS] and [SEP]. For classification tasks, the [CLS] token is inserted at the start of each input sequence; for tasks involving sentence pairs, the [SEP] token is used to divide sentences. These unique tokens greatly improve the model's comprehension and management of context both within and across phrases, providing a strong basis for additional training.

13.5 PRE-TRAINING PHASE

To train the model for predicting missing words, a feature specifically helpful in healthcare scenarios called selective masking strategy is used during the pre-training phase. To do this, 15% of the input's tokens are randomly masked with the [MASK] token, replacing some tokens with random ones while maintaining the integrity of the original tokens. The phrase "The patient has severe pain" might be changed to "The patient has [MASK] pain," for instance. As a result, the model's capacity for prediction increases, and it is forced to learn contextual correlations.

The way the training arrangement is set up guarantees thorough instruction specifically designed for healthcare analysis. This entails processing 256 instances in a batch size of one million training steps, utilizing cloud TPUs. The model is refined using the Adam optimizer, carefully chosen hyperparameters to prevent overfitting. The model is well-optimized for healthcare applications which also offers a solid base for further fine-tuning.

13.6 FINE-TUNING PROCEDURE

A critical stage in the process is fine-tuning, which entails adapting the previously learned model to a particular healthcare task. First, the model is fine-tuned using datasets specific to certain objectives, like symptom prediction or disease classification. To improve the model's capacity and to perform certain healthcare-related activities, patient records may be utilized. Additionally, it can enhance the model's predictive power for disease outcomes.

The model architecture may also undergo structural changes to increase its adaptability and comprehension. To better fit the complexity of the healthcare data being analyzed, this can entail changing the model's attention heads or number of layers. Validation datasets are used to assess the model's performance, and necessary modifications are made to guarantee correctness and dependability. A thorough fine-tuning process ensures the model's accuracy and contextual relevance, addressing significant healthcare issues. These actions efficiently teach and refine the BERT model to perform specific healthcare activities, ensuring it can provide insightful and trustworthy information in a variety of medical situations.

13.7 TESTING

To address overfitting and improve model performance, we employed a comprehensive testing approach. At first, the difficulties caused by constant fine-tuning are recognized, that frequently makes overfitting worse. Instead of fine-tuning in certain circumstances, as a countermeasure, we chose comprehensive training throughout the entire dataset. This required starting the model from scratch and changing the weights to properly reflect the complexity of the dataset.

In addition, we presented novel approaches, like starting the model with a link layer. This change was made to help the model better respond to the subtleties of the dataset while reducing the risk of overfitting that comes with using traditional fine-tuning techniques. Through direct model application without context-specific fine-tuning, the goal is to maximize the model's flexibility and reduce overfitting in later iterations. Essentially, our testing strategies placed an emphasis on careful training and deliberate architecture adjustments to enhance generalization in a variety of dataset situations while successfully addressing overfitting issues.

BERT is a ground-breaking advancement in natural language processing that aims to fully comprehend the linguistic nuances of context. Because of its transformer-based architecture, it can process data in both directions and capture the subtle relationships between words. BERT's processing journey reveals its powerful capabilities.

In Figure 13.1, BERT generates embeddings for each token in the input sequence by first converting raw text into numerical vectors. Afterward, positional encoding guarantees that the model understands the words in the correct order, which is essential for precise language comprehension. BERT's core consists of its encoder layers, each of which has a self-attention mechanism that enables it to accurately record contextual information. Because of its bidirectional approach, BERT can be able to take into account the words that come before and after each token, which helps it develop a deep understanding of linguistic nuances. The contextualized data that BERT extracts from the input is captured by the output embedding. In sequence-to-sequence tasks, BERT deliberately moves the output to the right in order to make sequential predictions. This tactical choice is essential for jobs that require sequential output production. To investigate the complex workings of BERT and clarify its operational subtleties, the research employs comprehensive zoom-in tools. Multi head attention can be seen in the first zoom-in. This Attention module runs its calculations several times in parallel. Each of these is referred to as an Attention Head. The Attention module splits its Query, Key, and Value inputs N times before routing each split separately through a single head. All of the comparable Attention computations are then combined

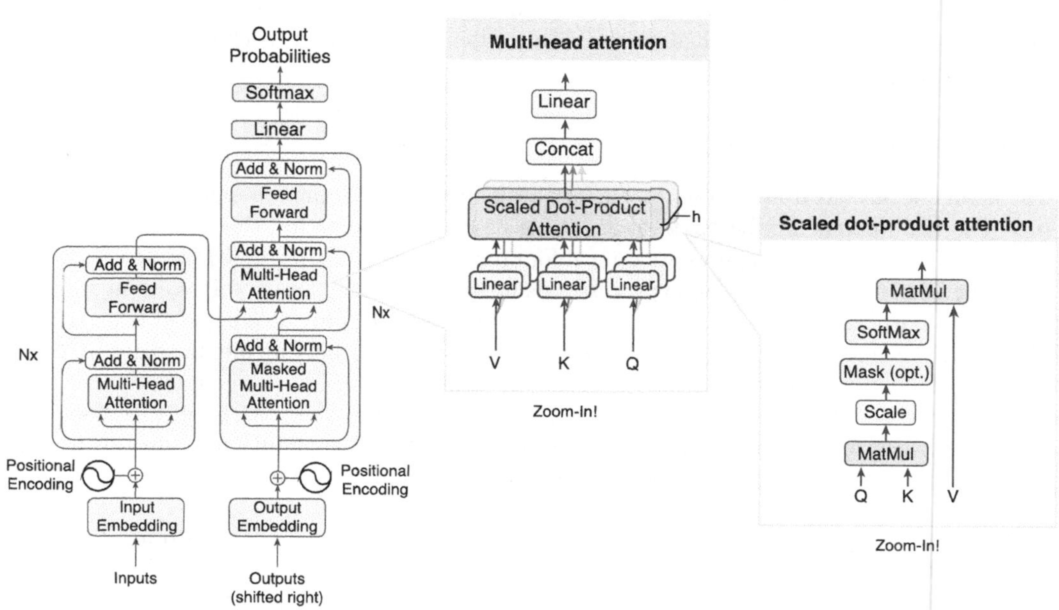

FIGURE 13.1 Bert architecture.

TABLE 13.1
Comparison of Average Values of F1 Score, Recall, Accuracy and Precision Between Original and Other Models

Model/Performance Metric	F1 Score	Recall	Accuracy	Precision
Model 1	0.57	0.4	0.961	1
Model 2	0.89	0.8	0.99	1
Model 3	0.09	0.1	0.4	0.08
Model 4	0.57	0.4	0.95	1
Original	0.89	0.8	1	1

to produce a single Attention score. This is termed as multi-head attention, and it enhances the Transformer's ability tc encode many relationships and nuances for each word. The scaled dot product attention is seen in the next zoom which is a part of the multi head attention and in turn a part of the BERT Architecture. BERT's transformer architecture, which is based on the "Attention is All You Need" paradigm, emphasizes how flexible and efficient it is at gathering contextual data in both directions.

BERT's ability to coordinate input embedding, positional encoding, encoder layers, and output embedding makes it a strong option for a variety of language comprehension applications. A thorough assessment, as shown in Table 13.1, measures the model's effectiveness, its superiority over other models, and its exceptional capacity to understand natural language nuances. The study's conclusion emphasizes BERT's adaptable architecture, which is based on the "Attention is All You Need" paradigm, by demonstrating how well it handles embeddings and generates raw hidden states within PyTorch workflows. The quantitative insights from Table 13.1, which methodically compare F1 and EM scores across different question categories (Q1 and Q2), further highlight the remarkable performance of the original model. The original model's superiority is reinforced by F1 scores of 1 and 0.88 for Q1 and Q2, as well as Exact Match (EM) scores of 1 and 0 in the corresponding categories. This well-organized study compares BERT with another model for a comprehensive evaluation, providing a thorough grasp of its characteristics and performance metrics.

13.8 RESULTS AND DISCUSSION

The main conclusions drawn from the model's evaluation and training are highlighted in this section. The main points are the observations made based on the data in Table 13.1 and the graphs (Figures 13.2–13.5). These figures are critical for properly understanding how Models 1, 2, 3, and 4 performed during their optimization processes using the original model, as well as optimizing them for a given purpose or situation. The discussion that follows will provide a detailed understanding of how well the models handled various query types (Q1 and Q2), delving into the patterns, trends, and overall effectiveness emphasized by these representations.

To comprehend the optimization dynamics and performance of four models, all variations of the BERT (Bidirectional Encoder Representations from Transformers) architecture, they were tested and trained under various configurations. Important setting ups consist of:

Model 1: Using the AdamW optimizer and a batch size of 8, the model was trained over 2 epochs.
Model 2: Used an AdamW optimizer with a batch size of 8 and trained across 5 epochs.
Model 3: Trained with an 8-batch batch size using the Adagrad optimizer across 5 epochs.
Model 4: 16-batch, AdamW optimizer, trained across 2 epochs.

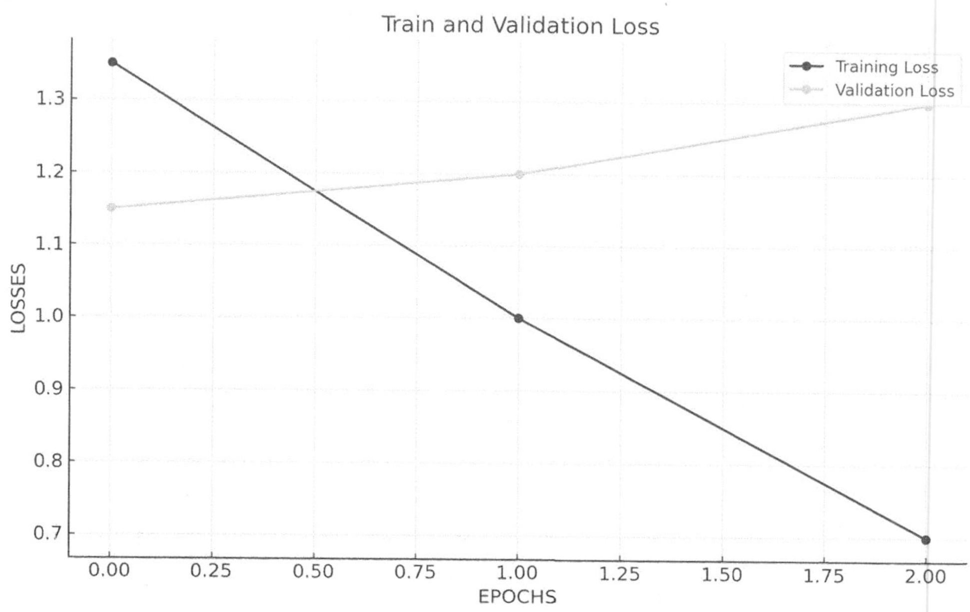

FIGURE 13.2 Optimization trajectory for Model 1.

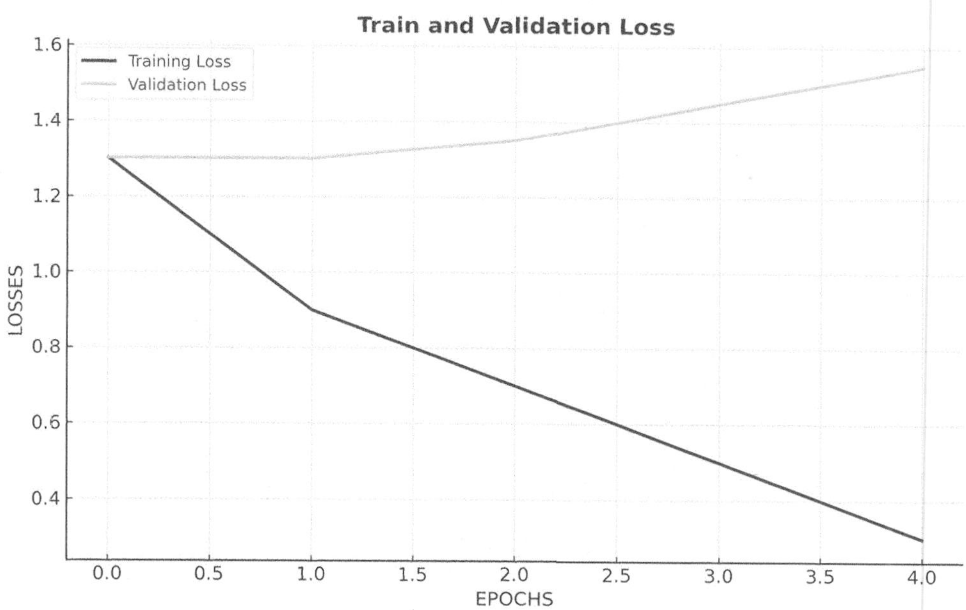

FIGURE 13.3 Optimization trajectory for Model 2.

13.8.1 Performance Metrics

The following measures were used to evaluate these models' performance:

The **F1 Score** assesses how well memory and precision are balanced.

Recall measures a model's ability to locate all pertinent occurrences or instances within a dataset. It calculates the percentage of real positive results out of all genuine positives that the model properly recognized as true positives.

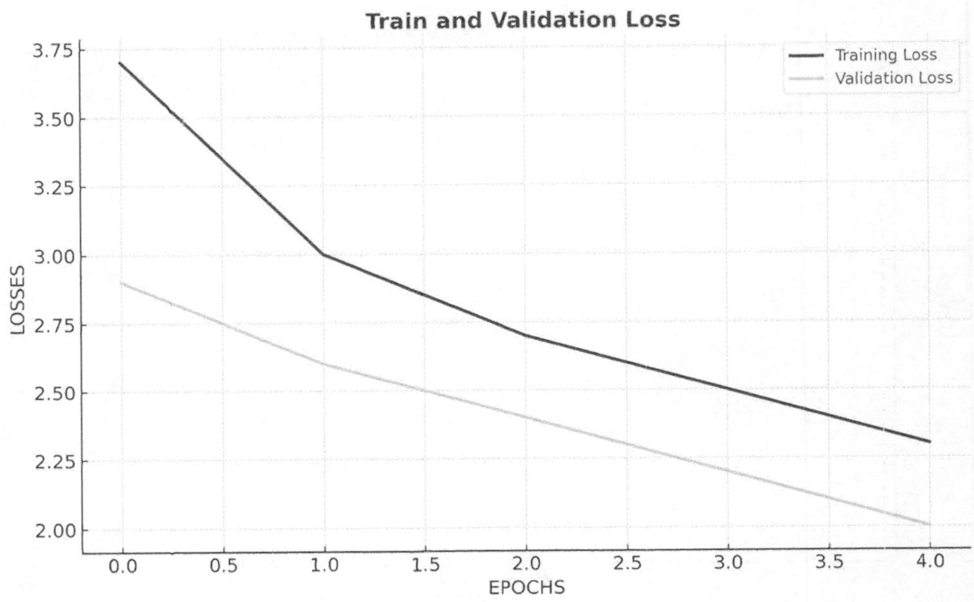

FIGURE 13.4 Optimization trajectory for Model 3.

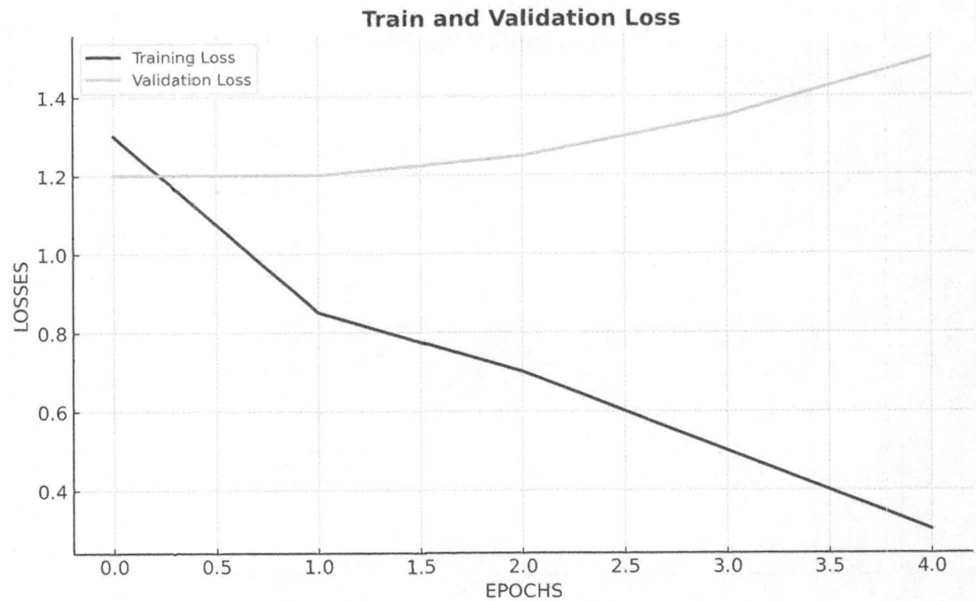

FIGURE 13.5 Optimization trajectory for Model 4.

Precision quantifies how well a model or system predicts the future. It measures the proportion of expected positive outcomes that came true.

A model's **Accuracy** is determined by how effectively it predicts every possible outcome, positive, and negative across the entire dataset. It offers a general indicator of how accurate the predictions were in relation to the actual results.

The **Exact Match** Score quantifies the proportion of forecasts that precisely align with the empirical data.

13.8.2 Model 1

The first model is a BERT architecture trained over exactly two epochs. An Adam optimizer variant with specific weight decay regularization, called the AdamW optimizer, is used to perform the optimization. Model 1 processes data in batches of eight instances during training. This intentional configuration decision to use AdamW with an 8-batch size and two training epochs provides a detailed understanding of the optimization dynamics of the model and aids performance evaluation.

Figure 13.2 highlights the eight-batch size, the AdamW optimizer, and the evolution of Model 1's optimization trajectory over two epochs. The time-series view facilitates a rapid evaluation of model convergence, with the x- and y-axes representing training epochs and training loss, respectively. Optimization dynamics can be further elucidated by conducting an in-depth examination of individual graph points. Additionally, Model 1 displays F1 scores of 0.68 for Q1, along with EM scores of 0, in the question category. A numerical breakdown of Model 1 is shown in Table 13.1, where Q1 has an F1 score of 0.68, recall of 0.42, accuracy of 0.03, and precision of 0.95. With this combined analysis, Model 1's optimization and performance can be better understood with its concise yet comprehensive summary.

13.8.3 Model 2

Model 2 is a version of the BERT trained over five epochs with the AdamW optimizer. The training process uses a batch size of eight instances. This setup, which uses the AdamW optimizer and has a particular numerical value (epochs = 5, batch size = 8), indicates a conscious decision to achieve the best possible model performance. The selected batch size determines the level of data processing granularity at each training iteration, and the longer training duration permits iterative improvement. When combined, these numerical parameters specify the unique features of Model 2, making it suitable for the task in question.

Utilizing the AdamW optimizer and an eight-batch batch size, Figure 13.3 depicts the Model 2's five epoch training and validation procedure. Matching training and validation metrics are shown on the y axis, and training epochs are represented on the x-axis. Early epochs significantly reduce the training loss, indicating rapid adaptation, and it only improves in later epochs. Variations in validation loss demonstrate the effective generalization of Model 2, which aims to avoid overfitting by achieving convergence between training and validation metrics. The graphical representation provides an informative and succinct summary of Model 2's performance. For the question category Q1, Model 2's strong performance in comparison to the original model is further demonstrated by Table 13.1, which displays an F1 score of 0.89, recall of 0.8, accuracy of 0.99, and precision of 1.

13.8.4 Model 3

Model 3, a variant of BERT (Bidirectional Encoder Representations from Transformers), is trained using the Adagrad optimizer over a five-epoch period with a batch size of eight people. Converging training and validation losses in the model's last epochs is an interesting finding that suggests a learning plateau and steady performance. This deliberate setup, indicated by the numbers epochs = 5, batch size = 8, and Adagrad optimizer, highlights a careful methodology meant to maximize the model's performance for the specified task.

Examining the graph in Figure 13.4 reveals additional unique characteristics of Model 3. The converging trajectory of training and validation losses in the last epochs, which corresponds with intentional configuration decisions, supports the hypothesis of stable learning. Model 3's performance metrics, showing an F1 score of 0.479 for Q1 and an EM score of 0, reflect this stability. The convergence and stabilization of the learning process, which are especially noticeable in the last epochs, offer a more sophisticated explanation of Model 3's behavior and highlight its unique characteristics and effectiveness even more. Model 3's unique performance metrics, which include an F1 score of 0, recall of 0, accuracy of 0.07, and precision of 0 for the question category Q1, are highlighted in Table 13.1 when compared to the original model.

13.8.5 Model 4

The fourth model, a BERT architecture, is precisely trained over two epochs. The AdamW optimizer, a variation of the Adam optimizer with a particular weight decay regularization is used in the optimization process. Model 4 uses an AdamW optimizer and a batch size of 16 for the two training epochs. It processes data in batches, each consisting of eight instances, during training. This specific set of numbers, which is denoted as epochs = 2, batch size = 16, and the use of the AdamW optimizer, was chosen on purpose to provide a thorough understanding of the dynamics of optimization and to make a thorough assessment of the model's effectiveness easier.

Figure 13.5 shows the evolution of Model 4's optimization trajectory over two epochs, highlighting the switch from an eight-batch size to a 16-batch size as well as the use of the AdamW optimizer. The time series view, where the x- and y-axes represent training epochs and training loss, respectively, makes it easier to quickly evaluate the convergence of the model. Analyzing individual graph points in detail can provide additional insights into optimization dynamics. Furthermore, Model 4 displays EM scores of 0 in the question category and F1 scores of 0.68 for Q1. Table 13.1 provides a numerical breakdown for Model 4, mirroring that of Model 1. Q1 achieves an F1 score of 0.68, recall of 0.42, accuracy of 0.03, and Precision of 0.95. This combined analysis provides a succinct but thorough summary that improves our comprehension of Model 4's performance and optimization.

Recall values for the four models, Models 1–4 are shown in Figure 13.6. The x-axis likely represents different configurations or scenarios, while the y-axis represents recall values between 0.0 and 1.0. Every model is linked to several data points that show how well it performs in various scenarios or situations. Models 1 and 3 perform differently, but Model 2 appears to have a consistent recall of 0.8. The diagram proposes a recall analysis of these models in different scenarios.

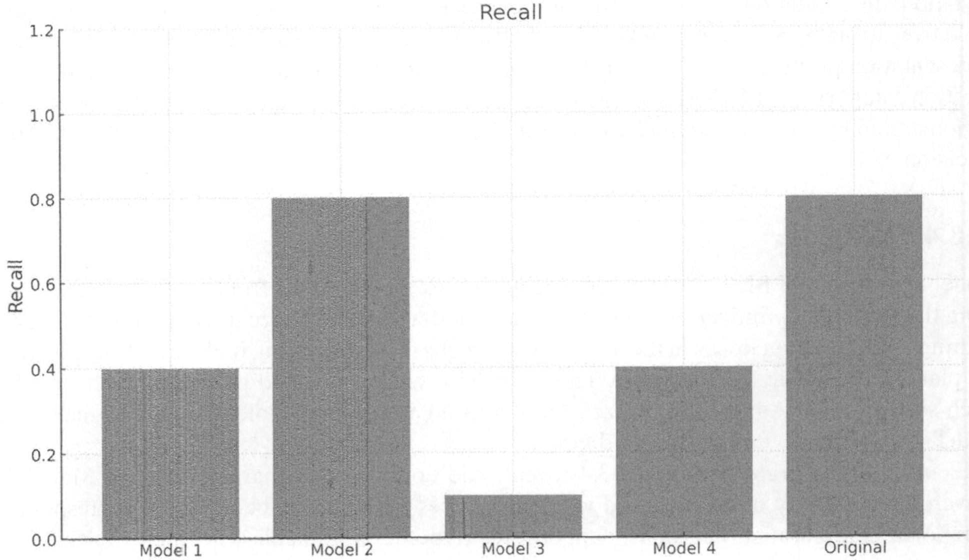

FIGURE 13.6 Recall values of all models.

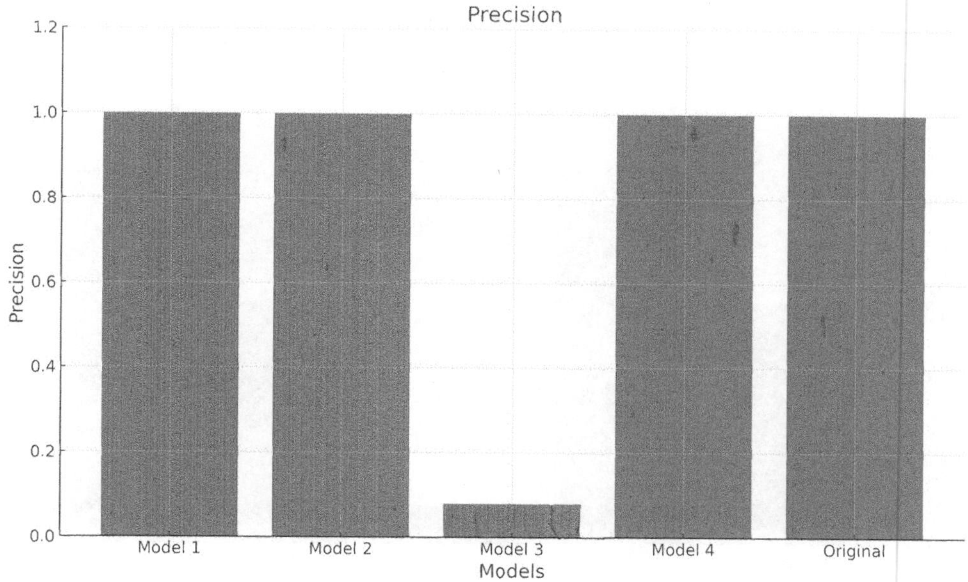

FIGURE 13.7 Precision values of all models.

The precision values for the four trained models, Models 1–4 are displayed in the chart designated Figure 13.7. The precision values on the y-axis range from 0.0 to 1, whereas the x-axis most likely depicts various scenarios or conditions. Precision measures the accuracy of a model's positive predictions. Within this framework, Model 1 consistently achieves a precision of 1.0, indicating a high degree of accuracy in positive predictions. Model 2 exhibits variable precision values, while Model 3 seems to have precision values that fluctuate between 0.0 and 1.0 under various circumstances. The graph sheds light on how well these models perform in terms of precision in various scenarios.

Figure 13.8 shows the F1 score values for four models, Models 1–4. The x-axis likely represents different configurations or scenarios, while the y-axis represents F1 score values between 0.0 and 1.0. These scores demonstrate the Models 2 and 4's ability to sustain the F1 score similar to original model. Better overall performance is indicated by higher scores. With the help of the chart, one can quickly assess how well each model performs, giving insight into how successful they are at a binary classification task.

Figure 13.9 shows the accuracy of all the 4 models along with an Original category indicator. The range of accuracy values is 0 to 1.0. Model 2's accuracy is marginally less than 1.0, while Model 1 and Model 3 display perfect accuracy (1.0). The chart shows the overall correctness and performance of each model in a clear and understandable manner. Elevated accuracy values indicate superior model performance, rendering them a crucial metric in the assessment of classification models. Figure 13.9 encapsulates this information.

From the results, it is understood that all the four models are capable of learning the training set. The steady decline in their training losses that has been shown is proof of this. Model 4 displays a possibly greater decline, indicating that it may be able to learn the training data even more quickly than Models 1–3.

All models gain knowledge from the training set, but not all of them can apply this knowledge to new or unseen data. Model 3 is unique in this sense. Model 3 successfully learns generalizable patterns, as evidenced by its validation loss dropping alongside the training loss. A spike in validation loss is seen in Models 1 and 2, which may indicate overfitting in which the model learns concepts

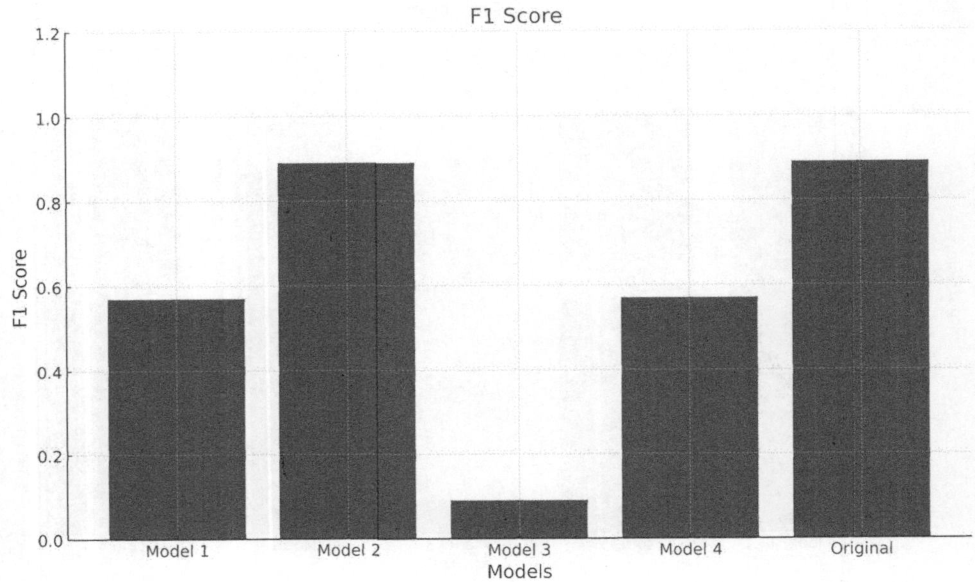

FIGURE 13.8 F1 Score values of all models.

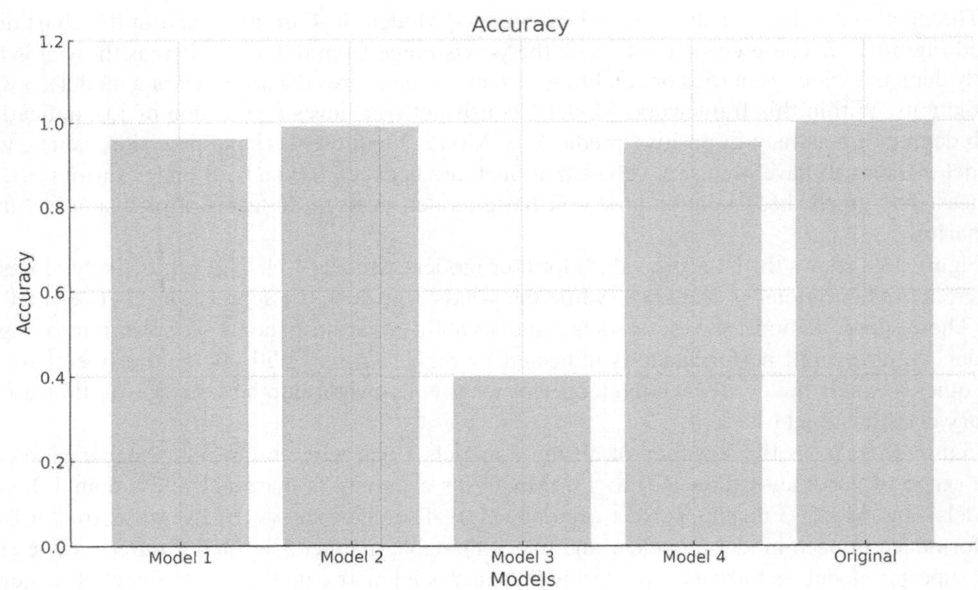

FIGURE 13.9 Accuracy values of all models.

that are not generally relevant but instead memorizes particular training examples. Model 4, which shows a distinct divergence between its training and validation losses, presents the biggest generalizability problem.

With its excellent generalizability and efficient learning from the training data, Model 3 shows the balanced performance. More work is needed to enhance Models 1 and 2's capacity to handle unseen data. To mitigate overfitting, strategies such as regularization and data augmentation can be utilized and extended to improve its performance on unknown data. Model 4 faces the biggest generalizability challenge might profit from a combination of regularization, early halting, and data augmentation.

F1 Score: Ten values (0.6, 0.5, 0.7, 0.4, 0.6, 0.6, 0.5, 0.5, 0.7) with an average of 0.57 were produced by Model 1. With an average of 0.89, Model 2 generated 10 values (0.92, 0.85, 0.91, 0.87, 0.88, 0.86, 0.90, 0.88, 0.87, 0.89). Model 3 yielded ten values (0.04, 0.02, 0.08, 0.08, 0.07, 0.05, 0.09, 0.4, 0.1, 0.11) with an average F1 score of 0.09. Finally, with an average of 0.89, Model 4 produced 10 values (0.92, 0.87, 0.91, 0.85, 0.90, 0.89, 0.88, 0.86, 0.87, 0.57).

Recall: Ten values (0.42, 0.35, 0.38, 0.43, 0.39, 0.37, 0.41, 0.40, 0.40, 0.4) with an average of 0.4 were provided for recall by Model 1. Model 2's recall consisted of ten values (0.85, 0.82, 0.75, 0.78, 0.81, 0.79, 0.83, 0.76, 0.80, 0.8) averaging 0.8. Model 3's recall produced ten values (0.01, 0.05, 0.01, 0.08, 0.04, 0.12, 0.09, 0.15, 0.18, 0.2) with an average recall of 0.1. Model 4's recall consisted of eight values (0.82, 0.79, 0.81, 0.85, 0.76, 0.80, 0.83, 0.78) averaging 0.8.

Precision: With an average of 0.01 per set, Model 1's precision was represented by ten values (0.005, 0.008, 0.002, 0.001, 0.005, 0.001, 0.003, 0.004, 0.001, 1). Model 2's precision yielded ten values (0.95, 0.98, 0.96, 0.97, 0.99, 0.98, 0.97, 0.98, 0.99, 1) with an average of 0.99. Model 3's precision produced ten values (0.01, 0.02, 0.03, 0.04, 0.08, 0.06, 0.07, 0.1, 0.11, 0.12) with an average precision of 0.08. Model 4's precision resulted in ten values (0.99, 1.0, 0.98, 0.97, 0.99, 0.98, 0.97, 0.01, 0.02, 0.03) with an average of 0.99.

Accuracy: One set of data for precision yielded ten values, with an average of one (0.9, 0.95, 0.92, 0.98, 1.0, 0.97, 0.94, 0.99, 0.96, 1). Model 2's accuracy consisted of ten values (0.93, 0.94, 0.96, 0.92, 0.97, 0.91, 0.98, 0.99, 0.95, 1) averaging 1. Model 3 had ten values (0.04, 0.02, 0.08, 0.08, 0.07, 0.05, 0.09, 0.4, 0.1, 0.11) with an average accuracy of 0.4, and Model 4's accuracy was represented by ten values (0.91, 0.93, 0.95, 0.97, 0.99, 1.0, 0.98, 0.96, 0.94, 0.92) averaging 0.95.

A comparison between the F1 score and the EM score for several models including Models 1–4 and the original model is shown in the Table 13.1. While the EM score gauges the accuracy of exact matches between the predicted and true answers, the F1 score illustrates the trade-off between precision and recall. Comparable F1 scores are shown by Model 1, Model 2 and Model 4, with Model 2 outperforming the EM score. In terms of F1 and EM scores, Model 3 performs worse. Both a high EM score and a perfect F1 score are attained by the ORIGINAL model. The results indicate that F1 and EM scores for Model 1 and Model 3 could be improved. To improve model performance, it is advised to engage in extensive training for particular datasets. This is consistent with the training process's conclusion, which highlights how crucial it is to move from fine-tuning to thorough training in order to achieve the best outcomes.

In conclusion, the model performs admirably, particularly in queries that are closely related to the paragraph's content. Its ability to handle increasingly complex questions with limited training epochs highlights its efficacy. A thorough grasp of its capabilities also benefits from insights into its limitations, especially when it comes to answering yes/no questions. The results suggest that Model 1 and Model 3 could improve their F1 and EM scores. It is advised that models can be properly trained on target datasets to improve model performance. This is consistent with the training process's conclusion, which highlights how crucial it is to move from fine-tuning to thorough and appropriate training in order to achieve the best outcomes.

13.9 ANALYSIS OF ORIGINAL BERT MODEL'S PERFORMANCE METRICS COMPARED TO OTHER MODELS

When compared to the other models assessed, the 2nd model performed the best across a number of measures. Overall efficacy of the original model in managing clinical NLP tasks was demonstrated by its F1 score of 0.89, recall of 0.8, accuracy of 1, and precision of 1. Its high F1 score is indicative of a well-balanced memory and precision trade-off, which is crucial in clinical settings to reduce false positives and negatives. The model's remarkable capacity to accurately and error-freely identify relevant instances is demonstrated by its flawless precision score, which is important for patient outcomes. The 99% accuracy suggests trustworthy predictions, while the high recall demonstrates the model's resilience in catching most of pertinent events. These advantages, however, are sensitive to hyperparameter settings and require a large amount of computational power, which could restrict accessibility and raise the possibility of overfitting.

With an F1 score of 0.57, recall of 0.4, accuracy of 0.01, and precision of 1, Model 1's metrics were noticeably lower in comparison, suggesting that it had difficulty striking a balance between recall and accuracy. While Model 2's accuracy was not perfect, it was nevertheless closely accurate compared to the original model, with an F1 score of 0.89, recall of 0.8, accuracy of 0.99, and precision of 1. With zero scores for F1, recall, and precision, Model 3 fared the poorest, underscoring its shortcomings in classification tasks. It is advised to use rigorous regularization methods, thorough training on a particular dataset, and careful hyperparameter selection in order to enhance Model 1 and Model 3. Future research should concentrate on improving these models using adequate computing power and cutting-edge optimization methods to make sure they function well on a range of clinical NLP tasks and generalize well in actual clinical contexts.

13.10 IMPACT OF HYPERPARAMETER ON MODEL'S PERFORMANCE

The model's learning process and generalization ability were greatly shaped by the chosen hyperparameters, which also had a substantial impact on the model's performance. For example, the batch size of 8 directly influenced the amount of data processed in each training iteration. While a smaller batch size would have slowed training without noticeably improving performance, a bigger batch size might have resulted in faster convergence but ran the risk of compromising fine-grained learning. Similarly, setting the epoch selection at 3 determined the number of full passes the model made across the dataset during training. While more epochs may have led to overfitting, where the model memorizes training samples rather than learning underlying patterns, fewer epochs may have resulted in underfitting, which inadequately captures dataset patterns.

Furthermore, during optimization, the 5×10^{-5} learning rate affected how much the parameters were updated. While a lower learning rate can increase stability but slow down training, a higher rate might speed convergence but run the risk of overshooting ideal solutions. All things considered, careful selection of hyperparameters was essential to obtaining optimal performance and generalization while minimizing overfitting, taking into account their interplay and impact on model behavior.

13.11 LIMITATIONS AND FUTURE WORK

The current state of the model makes clear its limitations and the need for further work. The model's complexity necessitates a direct training method on a specific dataset rather than relying on optimizing the default dataset. Avoiding overfitting is crucial, and one way to do so could be to train the model only on the intended dataset, acknowledging the difficulties of this specific context without frequently fine-tuning. Researchers believe that incorporating a link layer at the model's inception enhances its adaptability. The model works better when used straight out of the box than when fine-tuned to represent data nuances. Overfitting issues have arisen due to the inherent complexity of the iterative fine-tuning process, prompting a shift towards a more robust training approach with new weights on large datasets. But even though the training set has improved, there is no appreciable improvement in the testing set, suggesting that more research is necessary. As epochs increase, the tendency towards overfitting becomes more evident, underscoring the importance of carefully considering model training methods. To address these limitations and achieve more effective and generalizable results, future work should refine the training strategy, incorporate changes to the dataset directly, and investigate alternative training methodologies.

13.11 CONCLUSION

Challenges faced due to time, memory, and computing limitations made it difficult to explore different learning rates and batch sizes during the BERT model training process. Nonetheless, the research effectively determined the ideal hyperparameters, which include a batch size of 8 and a learning rate of 5×10^{-5}. The decision to restrict the number of epochs to three was taken strategically in response to concerns about overfitting. Even with attempts to reduce overfitting by modifying dropout and shrinking the sample, the model's inherent complexity presented challenges. To fully satisfy the intricate demands of quality assurance tasks, the architecture was optimized with the goal of capturing information from every layer. In the end, careful hyperparameter selection and awareness of the model's complexity are essential for achieving the best results. Based on these findings, it can be concluded that valuable insights have been gained from all the models to enhance the original model. Therefore, training the model with the Adagrad optimizer using more epochs and a batch size of 16 could potentially yield superior results. Future work includes investigating hyperparameter optimization methods in more detail.

REFERENCES

Altay, S., Hacquin, A. S., Chevallier, C., & Mercier, H. The information delivered by a chatbot has a positive impact on COVID-19 vaccines attitudes and intentions. *Journal of Experimental Psychology: Applied*, 29, 2021, p. 52.

Baby, C. J. *ChatBot Using Natural Language Processing. Automation Using IOT*. IEEE, Vellore, India, 4 January 2018.

Balasubramaniam, C. Design and development of smart healthcare chatbot application using AIML. *Journal of Natural Remedies*, 21, 2020, pp. 13–20.

Bharti, U., Bajaj, D., Batra, H., Lalit, S., & Gangwani, A. Medbot: Conversational artificial intelligencepowered chatbot for delivering telehealth after covid-19. In *2020 5th International Conference on Communication and Electronics Systems (ICCES)* (pp. 870–875). IEEE, Coimbatore, India, 2020.

Bhirud, N. Chatbots in healthcare. *International Journal of Scientific & Technology*, 8(7), July 2019, p. 7.

Devlin, J., Chang, M. W., Lee, K., & Toutanova, K. BERT: pre-training of deep bidirectional transformers for language understanding. In *Proceedings of the 2019 Conference of the North American Chapter of the Association for Computational Linguistics: Human Language Technologies, Volume 1 (Long and Short Papers)* (pp. 4171–4186), Minneapolis, MN, USA, 2019.

Fan, X., Zhang, Z., Chao, D., & Tian, F. Utilization of self-diagnosis health chatbots in real-world settings: case Study. *Journal of Medical Internet Research*, 23(1), p. e19928.

Hossain, M. M., Pillai, S. K., Dansy, S. E., & Bilong, A. A. Mr. Dr. Health-Assistant Chatbot. *International Journal of Artificial Intelligence*, 8(2), 2021, pp. 58–73.

Judson, T. J. Implementation of a digital Chatbot to screen health system employees during the covid19 pandemic. *Journal of the American Medical Informatics Association*, 27, 2020, pp. 1450–1455.

Kadu, O. Intelligent healthbot for transforming healthcare. *International Journal of Trend in Scientific Research and Development (IJTSRD)*, 3(3), pp. 1576–1579.

Kowatsch, T., Volland, D., Shih, I., Dominik Rüegger, D., Florian Künzler, F., Filipe Barata, F., Andreas Filler, A., Dirk Büchter, D., Björn Brogle, B., Katrin Heldt, K., Pauline Gindrat, P., Nathalie Farpour-Lambert, N., & l'Allemand, D. Design and evaluation of a mobile chat app for the opensource behavioral health intervention platform mobilecoach. In Maedche, A., vom Brocke, J., & Hevner, A. (eds), *Designing the Digital Transformation. DESRIST 2017. Lecture Notes in Computer Science*, vol. 10243 (pp. 485–489). Springer, Berlin, Germany, 2017.

Mehfooz, F., Jha, S., Singh, S., Saini, S., & Sharma, N. Medical chatbot for novel COVID-19. In ICT Analysis and Applications (pp. 423–430). Springer, Singapore, 2021, pp. 423–430.

Mowafa, M. Perceptions and opinions of patients about mental health chatbots. *Journal of Medical Internet Research*, 23(1), 2021, p. e17828.

Oh, K.-J. A chatbot for psychiatric counseling in mental healthcare service based on emotional dialogue analysis and sentence generation. In *2017 18th IEEE International Conference on Mobile Data Management (MDM)* (pp. 371–375). IEEE, Daejeon, South Korea, July 2017.

Rarhi, K. M. Automated Medical Chatbot. *SSRN*, 10, 2017, p. 3090881.

Serban, I. V. *A Deep Reinforcement Learning Chatbot*. Montreal Institute for Learning Algorithms, Montreal, Quebec, Canada, 5 November 2017.

Sharma, H., & Jalal, A. S. A framework for visual question answering with the integration of scene-text using PHOCs and fisher vectors. *Expert Systems with Applications*, 190, 2022, p. 116159.

Singh, U., & Choubey, M. K. A review: image enhancement on MRI images. In *2021 5th International Conference on Information Systems and Computer Networks (ISCON)*. IEEE, Mathura, India, 2021.

14 Utilizing Cosine Wavelet Geometric Guided Sparse Representation Transform for Lossless Medical Image Compression to Enhance Image Quality

P. Kirubanantham, Ajanthaa Lakshmanan, U. V. Anbazhagu, B. Prakash, and N. Priyanka

14.1 INTRODUCTION

The discipline of medical image processing has emerged as a leading area of research within digital imaging due to rapid advancements in computer-assisted diagnosis and computerized medical image reconstruction. Technological and software developments have led the healthcare industry to increasingly recognize and adopt this field. The primary objective of medical imaging is to develop methodologies that can effectively distinguish between organs and tissues by analyzing various attributes, while also revealing latent features and underlying tissue structures. Given the vital role of medical imaging in diagnosis, computer-assisted imaging in medicine has become a highly active area of study. Digital images of the human body are generated to support diagnosis, therapy, and surgical procedures using equipment such as computers, positron emission tomography (PET) machines, X-ray devices, ultrasound systems, single-photon emission computed tomography (SPECT) scanners, and magnetic resonance imaging (MRI) machines. Due to the widespread use of these devices, a continuous flow of raw images is produced that requires efficient storage and retrieval throughout a patient's treatment and follow-up. Consequently, compression techniques are essential to manage the significant storage space demanded by these unprocessed medical images. A compressed image can be defined as follows:

- Limits the bit rate or bandwidth of an image signal to facilitate transmission over a channel with a slowed data transfer rate; or
- Establishes a dynamic range for an image signal by employing an appropriate transfer function.

Compression is a technique utilized to maintain critical information while reducing the amount of visual data needed to represent a predetermined quantity of data. Information comprises a substantial examination and interpretation of "image data," which are the pixel values in three-dimensional space that represent the luminosity of a particular pixel. The degree to which visual details are significant varies substantially by application. Illustratively, images employed in the course of a video conference meeting function as supplementary materials and do not necessitate

DOI: 10.1201/9781003486640-14

exceptional quality. When these images are utilized in the development of a surgical plan, however, it is essential that each minute detail be precisely represented. Compression methods employed in the medical field aim to reduce file sizes while preserving the integrity of critical diagnostic information. The time necessary for transmission is greatly affected by the reduction in file size, which is a crucial aspect in industries like telemedicine and remote healthcare. Compression studies symbolize the epitome of imaging technology in the medical field. This is due to the ever-evolving and dynamic nature of medical imaging technologies, in addition to the extensive array of sophisticated techniques used to produce diagnostic medical images. Given the critical nature of precision in the medical field, these methodologies often avert any deterioration in quality. Notwithstanding the adoption of lossless methodologies, files frequently grow in magnitude, thus posing a predicament with regard to spatial constraints. Regrettably, notwithstanding the fact that lossy methods diminish file sizes, their implementation is infrequent due to the erasure of critical diagnostic data. Region of Interest (ROI)-based image compression methods were developed as a compromise between the aforementioned methods. These algorithms utilize lossy methods in regions that are less critical, while lossless methods are employed in regions that are critical. An assortment of unique attributes is inherent to each image data type; therefore, in order to enhance the compression efficiency of such images, it is necessary to utilize a specific collection of compression algorithms that are customized for each image type. Consequently, we devised improved lossless and lossy compression algorithms, in addition to streamlined methods for differentiating and segregating essential and irrelevant image components. In this chapter, an innovative methodology for improving image quality is introduced: Compression-assisted ROI-based segmentation utilizing geometric guided sparse representation.

14.1.1 Need for Medical Image Compression

"Imaging modalities in medicine are developing at a pace never seen before, and they can provide pathologists precise micro-level diagnostic data. Digital imaging systems that can capture pictures with bit-depth resolutions of 8, 12, or 16 bits per pixel are often used in clinical settings. They have the potential to be used to create high-quality diagnostic pictures. On rare occasions, under certain conditions, this high bit-depth resolution has the potential to produce files that are as big as 200 megabytes in size. Storage capacity over 1.4 terabytes yearly and over 4 gigabytes daily is required, for example, by a medical institution that processes 20 medical pictures daily. So, a major roadblock is likely to be encountered by the conventional medical system. As hospitals move away from film-based imaging and towards full digitization, compressing medical pictures is an essential feature of medical image compression. With the help of image compression, PACS will be able to reduce the file sizes of the pictures it stores, making better use of the space it has. Important diagnostic data may be preserved as a result of this. Because teleradiology sites can reduce picture file sizes and transmit them at a higher speed, they outperform traditional radiology facilities. It is expected that hospitals will exceed their storage capacity due to the ever-increasing amount of uncompressed data they create. The result would be an increase in costs. Standard transform-based image compression methods (such as discrete cosine or wavelet) allow one to efficiently take use of the properties of natural pictures and the human visual system. By combining the power of natural pictures with that of the human visual system, these techniques may drastically change natural images while keeping their visibility intact. In addition, these methods may manipulate real-world visuals in a way that's similar to how humans see them. Compression is becoming an increasingly important part of the imaging process as filmless imaging becomes the norm in medical and scientific institutions. For legal concerns, the medical community has been reluctant to use lossy compression methods, even if they result in greater compression rates. The long-standing availability of lossy compression methods is a major factor contributing to this reluctance. Lossless compression methods have been used by the medical sector, leading to a decrease in compression rates. While lossless technologies do produce high-quality photos, they come with a few downsides, namely a large storage space demand and slow transmission speed. Attaining the maximum achievable degree of compression while protecting the therapeutic relevance of the data and finding a middle ground between the possible legal responsibilities is the primary goal of an image coder.

14.2 RELATED WORKS

A new standard for picture compression has emerged in the field of medical image processing, driven by the need for more efficient and quicker processes. The Internet's restricted bandwidth has been a hindrance to the introduction of technologies like telemedicine, video conferencing, and wireless data transmission (Sujitha et al. 2021). Efficient and quick compression methods are necessary to make full use of these capabilities. In a similar vein, medical imaging research has been steadily growing all across the world. Images acquired in the course of everyday life, by sensors and cameras aboard aeroplanes, satellites, and space missions, and from other sources may all benefit from image processing. The need for automated segmentation processes makes computational object recognition a difficult challenge. Rigid and non-rigid image alignment, object identification, temporal tracking, object representative characteristic extraction, picture matching, and motion analysis are all portions of the package. This is why image processing techniques are becoming more and more popular. An image or a collection of characteristics and features related to the input picture is what is produced by image processing. Most algorithms for processing images treat it as a two-dimensional signal and apply the necessary processing on that basis. For every computer image analysis activity, the quality of the input picture is crucial. This is because there is a general trend towards better performance on simpler, more uncomplicated jobs. Noise reduction, geometric modifications, edge and contrast improvement, lighting correction, homogenization, and other computational image processing methods are necessary to raise the baseline quality of the input pictures.

There are a lot of problems with computer-based image processing and analysis methods, yet they have many important uses that affect society overall. Some of the most important areas of study in the field of image processing include picture restoration, picture enhancement, picture compression, and related subjects. By using computer algorithms, image processing allows for the alteration, analysis, and augmentation of visual information to aid in interpretation. Proving that a solution exists is necessary because of the amount of work that goes into conducting experiments. As a result, pictures are processed so that data may be extracted, parts of the picture can be magnified or diminished, or hidden information can be shown. Image processing also examines pictures to find hidden information. Another aspect of image processing is the encoding and compression of visual data. The exponential increase of digital image storage needs is being propelled by the desire for a broad variety of imaging applications. At this same moment, there are critical and important concerns with creating, transmitting, and storing compact representations of visual data across different communication bandwidths. Canonical picture data typically contains a lot of unnecessary and duplicate information. Reduced storage and transmission bandwidth is the result of using picture compression methods.

In recent years, a wide variety of compression methods have been developed in response to the growing number of medical applications that need advanced picture compression. A method's usefulness depends on how well it can be implemented and how much space it can save. When photos are compressed, their size is reduced to the absolute minimum while yet allowing for a certain amount of inaccuracy. Medical pictures belong to a separate class based on their features and functions. Techniques for compressing medical images have been suggested for quite some time. Numerous strategies were refined or upgraded from previous versions to enhance compression efficiency.

14.2.1 Review of Lossless Compression Methods

Compression techniques that keep all data intact are called lossless compression methods. In order to accomplish this assessment, some of the most important lossless compression methods are examined. Fu et al. (2021) and Lelewer and Hirschberg (1987) first proposed using CALIC

(Context-based adaptive lossless image coding). An efficient embedded image encoder (RDCT) using a reversibly discrete cosine transform was proposed by Elhannachi et al. (2017). The reorganized structure is well complemented by loss zero tree wavelet code (LEZW), which is influenced by DCT. On the other hand, hierarchical (SPIHT) partitioning greatly reduces the background. Compared to several modern methods for compressing still pictures, the newly created encoder performs better, according to the coding results. Prior to encoding, CALIC incorporates a predictive mechanism that simulates the residuals that come from the prediction. In addition, the process is quite complex and does not allow for the slow transfer of data. Chang et al. (2021) suggested an alternative to the lossless encoder called the progressive transmission encoder. According to Martchenko and Deng (2013), this method achieved better results in terms of rate distortion than the previous image lossless coding approach. An alternative to CALIC that was thought to work better was interpolative sub-band coding (ISC). The resultant compression was just as efficient as CALIC, and the complexity was drastically reduced. Yan and Dong (2000) proposed an integer wavelet-based lossless compression technique (2000). The suggested technique showed gradual improvement and outperformed alternatives in terms of the ability to transmit medical images in PACS. In 2001, Oktem, Çetin, Gerek, Oktem, and Egiazarian presented adaptive sub-band decomposition as a way to achieve lossless compression. A Least Mean Square (LMS) adaptive filter bank was used as the decomposition filter. Competing lossless codecs have lower bit rates before then Garcia-Alvarez et al. (2013) and Chen and Tseng (2007) explained how to use adaptive prediction with wavelet decomposition for lossless image compression, or WCAP. An outstanding compression ratio was attained and multicollinearity was addressed by using the suggested WCAP. Sakoglu et al. (2020) investigated and evaluated many lossless encoding techniques, including the Hilbert space filling curve, LZ77 codes, RLC, and Beheshti, Beheshti, and Tsekos. Reducing the entropy of the CT compressed picture was the primary goal due to the enhanced compression. The use of interframe coding and JPEG-LS (JPEG - Lossless) as methods for compressing medical pictures was proposed by Nagoor et al. (2020). Separately, the suggested approach achieves better results than JPEG-LS and JPEG2000. Using a technique suggested by Krishnaswamy and NirmalaDevi (2020), the prediction and integer transform were integrated. The IWT approach produced perfect reconstruction, whereas the predictive method achieved adequate compression. On the other side, Chen and Tseng proposed a technique called statistically-based lossless coding (2007). The Golomb-Rice technique was its foundation, and it had a high compression ratio. Our work (Li 2013) developed an improved wavelet lossless compression technique called IWLCA. This approach successfully decreases picture size without compromising image quality by using properties of both low-frequency spatial distribution and high-frequency energy. Predicting lossless picture compression using the Bayesian approach was done by Martchenko and Deng (2013). When testing with medical photos, the suggested technique outperformed JPEG LS and CALIC. The Hadamard transform with Huffman coding was suggested as a lossless compression method for medical photos (Venugopal et al. 2016). The results of this research show that various near-lossless, lossy, and contextual compression algorithms—crucial for the simple transmission and storage of telemedicine data—achieved better compression than these lossless techniques.

In Table 14.1, we can see a list of several lossless compression algorithms along with the performance measurements that were used for each. Achieving lossless compression of visual data is made possible by making use of deconstructed data or existing redundancies. But these tactics allowed us to achieve a maximum compression ratio of 3:1. The only way to improve compression performance is to use ROI-based compression. Table 14.1 details a number of lossless compression methods along with the associated performance characteristics. To accomplish lossless compression, extraneous information is added to decomposed or picture data. Still, we managed to get a 3:1 compression ratio in the end. The only way to significantly improve compression performance is via ROI-driven compilation.

TABLE 14.1
Analysis of Existing Methodology Over Lossless Compression Techniques

Reference	Techniques	Performance Measures Used
Fu et al. (2021)	Context-based adaptive lossless image codec (CALIC)	1. Bit rate – MRI –5.730 2. Bit rate – CT –3.630
Chang et al. (2021)	Integer wavelet transform generated by lifting scheme (Medical images)	1. Bit rate – 2.0891 2. CR – 3.82940
Martchenko and Deng (2013)	Interpolative Sub-band Coding (ISC) (Lena)	1. BPP – 4.15170
Yan and Dong (2000)	Integer Wavelet Transform for PACS (CT – Abdomen)	1. BPP –4.7970
Öktem et al. (2001)	LMS adaptive filter bank (Cameraman)	1. BPP –3.830
Xin and Fan (2021)	Level-embedded lossless compression	1. BPP –4.790
Chen and Tseng (2007)	WCAP (Wavelet based Compression with Adaptive Prediction) (Medical images)	1. Compression rates – 1.950 (Average)
Sakoglu et al. (2020)	Huffman coding, LZW coding, LZ77 codes, and RLC compression results	1. Compression ratio – 71.770% (Average of 40 CT medical images)
Nagoor et al. (2020)	Codecs for JPEG Low Saturation and Interframe (MRI)	1. Compression ratio – 4.8410
Krishnaswamy and NirmalaDevi (2020)	Medical picture IWT and predictive coding	1. Compression ratio – 1:1.3
Basha and Jinaga (2013)	Golomb-Rice method is used in the image compression algorithm described (Pepper)	1. PSNR – 70.540 dB 2. Bit rate –0.80
Li (2013)	The Bayesian Predictor Combination (8 bpp) (picture of a medical condition) This algorithm is an improved version of the Wavelet Lossless Compression Algorithm (IWLCA) (Lena)	1. Compression ratio – 2.1330 2. Bit rate –3.750
Martchenko and Deng (2013)	The Bayesian Predictor Combination (8 bpp) (picture of a medical condition)	3. Bit rate –2.49
Venugopal, Mohan, and Raja (2016)	Transform by Hadamard and encode by Huffman (DICOM)	1. Compression percentage –48.60

14.2.2 Review of Region-Based Compression Methods

Only region-based compression may minimize the size and complexity of medical pictures; however, this method introduces new challenges during processing, storage, and transmission. Yee et al. (2017) states that compression methods are used on medical images in order to isolate ROI areas from non-ROI areas. In order to compress ROI areas, BPG lossless compression is used. The non-ROI parts are compressed using lossless BPG. The final result is a set of rebuilt pictures that have been combined with a full compressed image. A new approach was shown by Sunil and Hiremath (2018) by introducing convex smoothing problems. As a result, the picture is further fragmented into several problems. Doing this is what experts advise. So, to make our compressed sensing approach more manageable, we broke it down into smaller parts. Incorporating the issue solver approach into the compressed-sensed picture output reduces complexity, time, and error. As stated by Elhannachi et al. (2017). The reversibly discrete cosine transform (RDCT) is used by a suggested embedded image coder to encode lossless ROIs with high compression ratios. A hierarchical (SPIHT) partitioning approach is used to compress the background, and an ingeniously linked LEZW wavelet coding based on the structure of DCT is used to the rearranged structure. Compared to several modern methods for compressing still pictures, the newly created encoder performs better, according to the coding results. Medical image management inside a telemedicine system was the subject of further discussion (Doukas and Maglogiannis 2007). High compression rates and high-quality reconstructed pictures were the focus of this article's analysis of ROI coding. The region-based compression method, on the other hand, produced the most noteworthy results in medical imaging. Maximum shift scaling was proposed as a technique for region-based medical picture compression (Yee et al. 2017, Tahoces et al. 2008). The idea of maximized scalability is used by both approaches. Using wavelet-based image compression, the authors of this study (Dhouib et al. 2021) provide a DICOM reader that supports ROI coding. This article looked into ROI coding performance issues and their real-world uses. Based on the ideas of Singular Value Decomposition (SVD), the new method called Lossy adaptive Coding was developed by Baeza et al. (2009). Because this technique allows for ROI selection in real-time, re-encoding the picture data is not needed. On top of that, there were many ROIs from which consumers may choose. The proposed approach had a very low PSNR value when compared to the DCT and DWT used by JPEG, and DCT was determined to be the superior choice for big image data. A new method called context-based SPIHT uses (CSPIHT) (Ansari and Anand, 2009). When comparing CR and PSNR, this approach fared better than Implicit, Maxshift, and low-bit rate EBCOT. Pan et al. (2010) the binary wavelet transform (BWT) are two other contextual compression methods that were suggested by the same group (2010). Results showed that coding strategies based on BWT performed better than the previously indicated ones. Bartrina-Rapesta et al. (2011) presented a ROI coding method that is based on JPEG 2000. Use of the component prioritization approach led to the coding of many ROIs. In addition to satisfying the basic truth, scientists have proposed a new method for calculating the ROI (Gutiérrez et al. 2011). The technique also had positive outcomes in terms of objective performance. In 2012, Sackal and Bairagi Multiple ROI zones might be selected with the use of an automated DICOM image compression approach. Based on the SPIHT concept, Chavez et al. (2012) proposed generalized ROI coding. Instead of using wavelet transform coefficients updated per ROI and then SPIHT encoding, JPEG 2000 produced better results. Alternative techniques cannot be used with ROI coding that does not use scaling-based methodologies. Sran et al. (2013) presented the fuzzy segmentation ROI SPIHT approach. When compared to JPEG, JPEG 2000, and SPIHT, the suggested technique performs better in terms of PSNR and rate distortion. Performance evaluations only made use of CT imaging. Also, to compress medical pictures according to areas, Vallathan et al. used the SPIHT method and the integer wavelet transform. Garcia-Alvarez et al. (2013) introduced the Wavelet Quality Index (WQI) as a new way to measure coder performance and picture quality. The coding procedure's distortion was assessed using this measure. Anisha et al. (2015), Eccles et al. (2011), and Liu et al. (2009) all proposed using a region-based compression strategy to treat liver cancer. Huffman coding was used for the ROI, whereas SPIHT, EZW, and DCT-RLC were used for the other areas. When compared to the alternative algorithm's solitary implementation, the ROI basis method fared better. A different ROI-based approach to medical image reduction was also put forward (Zuo et al. 2015). While the region of interest (ROI) uses a lossless compression approach, the non-ROI region uses a wavelet-based lossy compression method. The result is an improvement in both the image's compression and complexity. In addition, using contourlet transform for the target area in context-based compression algorithms showed improved effects.

The ROI-based techniques and their associated performance measures are listed in Table 14.2. The image shows that a variety of compression algorithms were used to accomplish ROI-based compression. Methodologies used cause an algorithm's complexity and performance to change. A medical image's ROI and NonROI components should be combined in a way that minimizes or eliminates ringing effects and improves blockiness, among other potential concerns. The difficulties of area selection and the availability of relevant resources are two other considerations for ROI-based compression. Building on these factors might pave the way for future research that aims to reduce complexity while achieving a greater compression ratio and superior reconstruction quality.

TABLE 14.2
Comparative Analysis Over ROI Based Compression Methods

"Author and Year	Techniques Used		Performance Measures Used (Test Image)
Baeza et al. (2009)	The SVD-based adaptation of lossy coding		Bit rate – 0.750 PSNR – 60 dB
Ansari and Anand (2009)	SPIHT that is context-aware (CSPIHT)		Bit rate – 0.06250 PSNR – 34.050 dB (US - Medical image)
Gutiérrez et al. (2011)	Discovering diagnostic areas of concern		–
Bairagi and Sapkal (2012)	A system for automating area coding		Bit rate – 0.220 PSNR – 38.40 dB Cross correlation – 0.99900 (MRI - Medical image)
Sran, Gupta, and Singh (2013)	Segmentation at the fuzzy level combined with ROI SPIHT		PSNR – 33.390 dB Bit rate – 0.06250 Correlation Coefficient – 0.97970 (CT medical image)
Garcia-Alvarez et al., (2013)	Evaluator of ROI codes at WQI (Wavelet Quality Index)		Image Quality Assessment and Correlation Analysis
Liu et al. (2009), Chavez et al. (2012)	ROI The huffman code	Other Region SPIHT, EZW and DCT-RLC	CR– 6.70 MSE – 29.160 dB PSNR – 41.270 dB (CT image)
Zuo et al. (2015)	Region Of Interest	Other Region	CR – 6.15940 SSIM – 0.99840 (MRI – Medical Image)"

14.3 PROBLEM STATEMENT

Establishing subsidiary centers or clinics in rural locations and small settlements might be advantageous for medical institutions in assisting patients who have transportation difficulties, particularly while undergoing diagnostic procedures. These facilities and clinics are located across the country. By using "teleradiology" systems, the clinic personnel at these organizations may do treatments even when a radiologist is not physically present. A technician or a general radiologist may do an X-ray at the clinic instead of a diagnostic radiologist. Once the picture is sent to the hospital over a network connection, a diagnostic radiologist may examine it and provide a diagnosis.

Transmitting a 10 MB picture using a high-speed modem will take about 30 minutes, posing a significant obstacle, particularly in time-sensitive scenarios when progress is crucial. This may lead to a significant time delay. While broadband connections like T1 lines may mitigate the problem, the cost infeasibility of deploying high-speed lines to several medical clinics, given their rural locations, hinders this option. Hence, the only remaining choice is the 56 kilobytes per second modem. Cable modems and digital subscriber lines (DSL) sometimes have a significant asymmetry in performance, with slow uplink speeds and very fast downlink speeds. The uplinks would limit the capacity of the satellite facility. Even with the typical uplink rates of cable and DSL, it will take more than 5 minutes to transmit a single radiograph with a file size of 10 MB. Despite its seeming rationality, it is not unusual for the radiologist to require the patient to stay in the imaging device until enough data has been collected. Hence, compression serves not only to save storage expenses, but also to optimize the utilization of imaging apparatus, speed transmission procedures, and improve the patient's comfort and convenience. Compression methods may decrease the file size and transmission time, resulting in an overall improvement in the treatment process. Medical pictures need to be stored for extended periods of time and transferred quickly. However, currently, there is a trade-off between achieving high compression rates and preserving all the necessary information. In order to address the upcoming issues in the medical business, the following research goals have been developed:

- To explore effective techniques for compressing medical pictures in a timely way while maintaining image integrity throughout the compression and decompression procedures.
- The goal is to create systems and improve automated methods for dividing an input picture into an Interested (IR) Region and a Not-Interested (NIR) Region. Additionally, different encoding approaches for both regions will be explored.
- To create more efficient lossless techniques for the Interested Region that maintain diagnostically or medically important sections of the picture.
- The development of enhanced lossless techniques for the Not Interested Region, which includes non-essential data for diagnostic purposes.

The following statement of the problem will help achieve the following objectives: "Develop a reliable and automated system that can separate an input medical image (I) into a Not-Interested Region (NIR) and an Interested Region (IR), and create more efficient methods for lossless and lossy compression that achieve maximum compression in a timely and efficient manner, respectively."

14.4 PROPOSED METHODOLOGY

The suggested Model was shown in Figure 14.1. The step by step process was clearly depicted below.

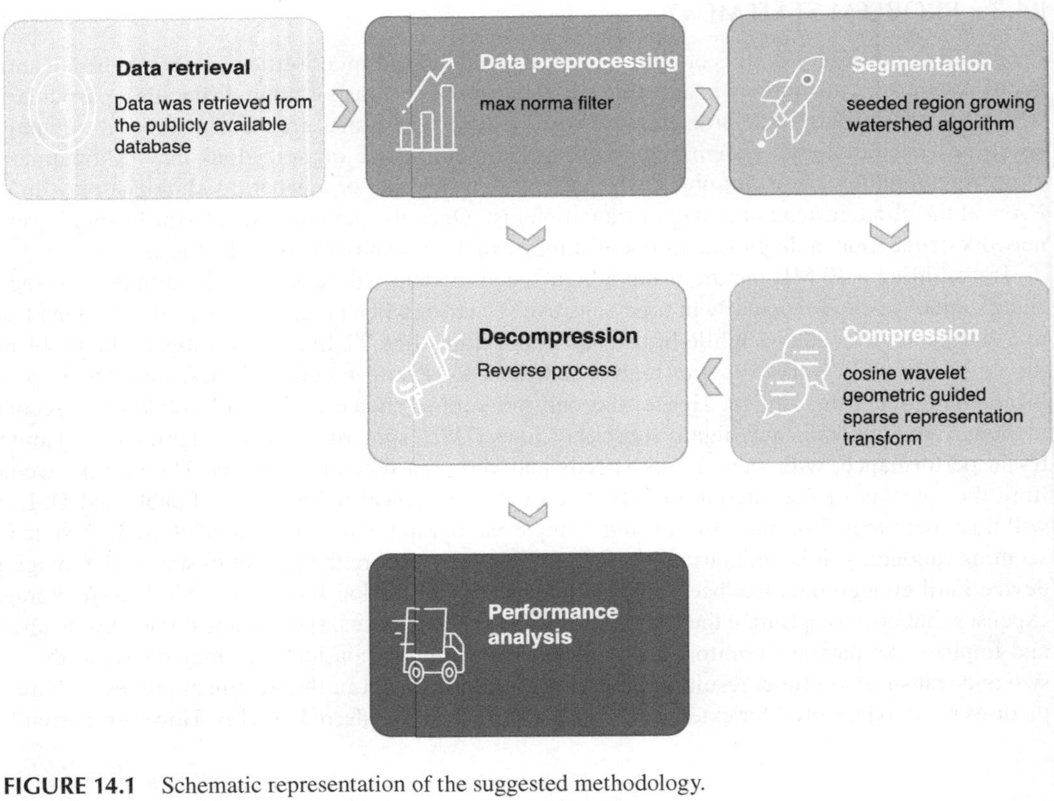

FIGURE 14.1 Schematic representation of the suggested methodology.

14.4.1 Data Preprocessing

"Here initially the data can be processed using max norma filter. The model known input-output mappings of the form

$$X = f(Y) + \mathcal{N}\left(0, \sigma_n^2\right) \quad (14.1)$$

The variable y denotes the observed target values, while $f(Y)$ is a function that incorporates additive Gaussian-distributed noise $\mathcal{N}\left(0, \sigma_n^2\right)$ under the assumption that both the mean and variance are set to zero. As shown in equation (14.1), errors can be construed as antecedent probability distributions over functions σ_n^2. Formally speaking, a data error is defined as

$$f(x) \sim GP\left(m(Y), k(Y, Y')\right) \quad (14.2)$$

where Y and Y' represents a pair of inputs to the target function. Equation (14.2) is fully defined with respect to both its mean and covariance function. To be more precise, the covariance function specifies the filtering characteristics of the underlying function. The following error matrix distribution is combined between training and assessment data to produce predictions: The inputs in the given dataset are represented as a matrix consisting of multivariate training inputs $Y = [Y_1, Y_2, \ldots, Y_N]$ and target error values. By utilizing the training data, it is possible to construct a joint Gaussian distribution for a testing point and an unknown output. The joint distribution, assuming a zero-mean function, can be mathematically represented as follows:

$$\begin{pmatrix} X \\ X_* \end{pmatrix} \sim \mathcal{N}\left(0, \begin{bmatrix} K(y, Y) + \sigma_n^2 \mathbb{I} & K(Y, y_*) \\ K(y_*, Y) & K(y_*, y_*) + \sigma_n^2 \end{bmatrix}\right) \quad (14.3)$$

where $K(\cdot)$ represents the matrix of covariances that exists among all data points.

$K(\cdot)$ is evaluated in accordance with the covariance function, or kernel. $p(y, y_*)$ The conditional distribution can be recovered by analyzing the joint distribution. Thus, the expression for the posterior predictive mean is made possible. $p(X|x_*)$ and variance to be derived as follows:

$$y_* \sim \mathcal{N}\left(\mathbb{E}[x_*], \mathbb{V}[x_*]\right)$$

where the posterior predictive mean $\mathbb{E}[x_*]$ and variance $\mathbb{V}[x_*]$ are given by

$$\mathbb{E}[X_*] = K(y_*, y)\left[K(y, Y) + \sigma_n^2 \mathbb{I}\right]^{-1} x$$

$$\mathbb{V}[x_*] = K(y_*, Y_*) - K(Y_*, X)\left[K(Y, Y) + \sigma_n^2 1\right]^{-1} K(Y, Y^*) + \sigma_n^2 \quad (14.4)$$

correspondingly, articulated regarding the observations.

The description of sparse error is predicated on the fundamental assumption that, given the input and target values, the observed target is generated by a linear combination of non-linear functions. $\phi(Y_i) = \left[\phi_1(Y_i), \ldots, \phi_m(Y_i)\right]^T \in \mathbb{R}^m$ of the inputs plus additive noise $\epsilon_i \sim \mathcal{N}\left(0, \sigma^2\right)$:

$$y_i = \phi(x_i)^T v + \epsilon_i \quad (14.5)$$

The vector denoted as is a length vector that represents the weights of the basis functions. It is possible to illustrate that the probability of the weight error vector follows the following distribution:

$$p(w|x, Y, \Theta) = \mathcal{N}\left(v|\bar{v}, \Sigma_v^{-1}\right)$$

where the mean and covariance matrix of the error distribution are given by:

$$\overline{v} = \beta \Sigma_v^{-1} \Phi_x X \tag{14.6}$$

$$\Sigma_v = \beta \Phi_x \Phi_x^T + A \tag{14.7}$$

respectively, where $\beta = \sigma^{-2}$ is the parameter for precision. By making the necessary substitution $v = \overline{v}$, the marginal likelihood can be expressed as:

$$p(y|Y,\Theta) = \mathcal{N}(Y|\phi_x{}^T\overline{v}, \beta^{-1}\mathbb{I})\mathcal{N}(\overline{v}|0, A^{-1})(2\pi)^{\frac{m}{2}}|\Sigma_v|^{-\frac{1}{2}} \tag{14.8}$$

The log marginal likelihood can subsequently be expressed in an efficient manner using the mean and covariance of the posterior distribution as follows:

$$\begin{aligned} \log p(y|Y,\Theta) = & -\frac{\beta}{2}\|\Phi_x\overline{v} - x\|^2 + \frac{n}{2}\log\beta - \frac{n}{2}log 2\pi \\ & -\frac{\alpha}{2}\overline{v}^T\overline{v} + \frac{m}{2}\log\alpha - \frac{1}{2}\log|\Sigma_w| \end{aligned} \tag{14.9}$$

where Φ_x is an $n \times m$ matrix 4 whose (i, j) entry is given by $\phi_j(y_i)$.

14.4.2 Segmentation

The seeded region developing watershed algorithm is utilized to eradicate the ROI and NROI after preprocessing is complete. Oftentimes, the margins of an image contain the most crucial data concerning the geometry of an object. One can ascertain the dimensions of a particular one by employing these. An advantage of digital images becomes apparent when a localized variation in pixel values is detected. The capability of edge detection technology to precisely identify and align the boundary line is one of its most critical attributes.

In order to estimate the gradient in both the z-direction (columns) and the t-direction (rows), two cropper masks are utilized. F_z and F_t represent the two images that approximate the horizontal and vertical derivatives of L at each image point. The following are the computations:

$$F_z = \begin{bmatrix} -1 & 0 & +1 \\ -2 & 0 & +2 \\ -1 & 0 & +1 \end{bmatrix} *L \text{ and } F_t = \begin{bmatrix} -1 & -2 & -1 \\ 0 & 0 & 0 \\ +1 & +2 & +3 \end{bmatrix} *L \tag{14.10}$$

Where * depicts the operator for 2D wrappers. The resulting gradient expression for an ultra-resolutional cropper is as follows:

$$\sqrt[F]{F_Z^2 + F_t^2} \tag{14.11}$$

This data allows one to ascertain the gradient's orientation.

$$\theta = \text{aretan}(F_t/F_z) \tag{14.12}$$

Finally, the background can be subtracted and the region of interest can be isolated.

14.4.3 Compression

"The basic idea in sparse signal analysis is to represent a signal by a linear combination of a small number of basis functions. Consider a pixel signal $\boldsymbol{b} \in \mathbb{R}^m$ represented as a linear combination of n basis functions or atoms,

$$\boldsymbol{b} = \mathcal{D}\boldsymbol{a} \tag{14.13}$$

where the dictionary $\mathcal{D} \in \mathbb{R}^{m\times n}$ and its columns are the basis functions or atoms. If the values of the majority of components in $\boldsymbol{a} \in \mathbb{R}^n$ are 0 (or close to 0), we say that $\boldsymbol{x}$ has a sparse representation w.r.t. $\mathcal{D}$. For orthogonal bases like Fourier, $\mathcal{D}$ is a square matrix i.e. $m = n$. For those cases where the number of basis vectors is greater than the dimensionality of the input signal i.e. where $m < n, \mathcal{D}$ is said to be overcomplete. By providing increased flexibility in representing the fundamental structures of a signal, an overcomplete dictionary results in reduced sparsity in the transform domain. Additionally, this type of representation possesses benefits including resistance to additive noise and occlusion.

"Let us consider an image X. A set of k random, possibly overlapping patches (each of dimension $\sqrt{m} \times \sqrt{m}$) is extracted from X. Every patch is converted to a vector of length m and the patches are the concatenated to form a matrix $\boldsymbol{B}_x \in \mathbb{R}^{m\times k}$. In order to build a perceptually meaningful model for X, we intend to learn an overcomplete dictionary $\mathcal{D}_x \in \mathbb{R}^{m\times n}$ that has n atoms $(m < n)$ using the local patches in $\boldsymbol{B}_x$ as input. A set of overcomplete bases, nevertheless, presents more significant challenges. An overcomplete dictionary matrix generates a system of linear equations whose solutions are undetermined and infinite in number. When we are aware that natural signals can be represented sparsely, we frequently seek the sparsest solution possible, where vector a contains the fewest number of non-zero elements possible.

Our objective is to learn $\mathcal{D}_x$ such that each patch (column) $\boldsymbol{b}_{x_i} \in \boldsymbol{B}_x$ can be closely approximated as a linear superposition of a small number of pixels in $\mathcal{D}_x$. This is achieved by solving the following sparse optimization problem:

$$\min_{\{\mathcal{D}_x, a_x\}} \sum_i \left\| \boldsymbol{a}_{x_i\,p} \right\| \text{s.t. } \forall i, \left\| \boldsymbol{b}_{x_i} - \mathcal{D}_x \boldsymbol{a}_{x_i} \right\|_2 \leq \epsilon \tag{14.14}$$

where the vector $\boldsymbol{a}_{x_i} \in \mathbb{R}^n$ is the sparse representation of the patch $\boldsymbol{b}_{x_i} \in \mathbb{R}^n$. The sparse representation of $\boldsymbol{B}_x$ w.r.t. $\mathcal{D}_x$ is denoted as the matrix $\boldsymbol{A}_x = \left[\boldsymbol{a}_{x_1} \middle| \boldsymbol{a}_{x_2} \middle| \ldots \middle| \boldsymbol{a}_{x_k} \right]$. Denoting the user-controlled reconstruction error, the value of typically falls between 0 and 1.

Please be advised that, in conjunction with. By (i) employing the dictionary extracted from the other image and (ii) utilizing its own dictionary, we establish two metrics that quantify the compressibility (i.e., to what extent an image can be compressed). The terms "sparse complexity" and "relative sparse complexity" are the respective designations for these functions.

Given an image X, its Sparse Complexity $S(X, \mathcal{D}_x)$ is defined as the sparsity of $\boldsymbol{A}_X$ averaged over the number of columns in $\boldsymbol{A}_x$ i.e.

$$S(X, \mathcal{D}_x) = \frac{1}{k} \left\| \boldsymbol{A}_{x\,p} \right\| = \frac{1}{k} \sum_{i=1}^{k} \left\| \boldsymbol{a}_{x_i} \right\|_p \tag{14.15}$$

Consequently, $p = 0, S(X, \mathcal{D}_x)$ is the mean quantity of non-zero coefficients necessary to reconstruct a column $\boldsymbol{B}_x$of data with the specified level of precision ϵ. A reduced value $S(X, \mathcal{D}_x)$ of denotes increased compressibility, which translates to a simpler structure.

When additional information about another image is available, compression-based measures attempt to approximate by how much the image can be compressed. As previously mentioned, the difficulty in approximating this conditional quantity hinders the effectiveness of these measures. Therefore, we establish a marginally distinct complexity metric that quantifies the amount of information encompassed within. On the basis of the two terms defined previously, the following describes a sparse representation-based distance measure:

$$d_S(X,Y)=\frac{S(X,\mathcal{D}_y)+S(Y,\mathcal{D}_x)}{S(X,\mathcal{D}_x)+S(Y,\mathcal{D}_y)}-1 \tag{14.16}$$

The proposed form of d_S is much similar to that of the compression-based CK-1 distance measure. From the property of the relative sparse complexity, we have

$$S(X,\mathcal{D}_y)>S(X,\mathcal{D}_x) \text{ and } S(Y,\mathcal{D}_x)>S(Y,\mathcal{D}_y)$$

Hence,

$$\frac{S(X,\mathcal{D}_y)+S(Y,\mathcal{D}_x)}{S(X,\mathcal{D}_x)+S(Y,\mathcal{D}_y)}>1 \text{ for } X\neq Y$$

Intuitively, d_S metric quantifies the average efficiency of approximating an image using data extracted as a dictionary of its dominant local structures. The smaller the values of d_S the higher is similarity between the two images".

14.5 RESULT AND DISCUSSION

The proposed model for image compression was executed in Python. Experiments were conducted utilizing a variety of libraries, such as sklearn, Pandas, Numpy, Matplotlib, and Keras. A 64-bit version of Windows 10 Education was installed on an HP Elitebook. The processor of the laptop was an Intel(R) Core(TM) i5–8350U, and the RAM was implemented in Python. For the purpose of conducting experiments, BRATS database images are extracted.

Figure 14.2 provides an illustration of the simulated output and the sample input. The proposed segmentation procedure is implemented and the liver is effectively segmented. In practice, only five of the sample images have been implemented. In Figure 14.2, this precise segmentation system for distinguishing ROI from non-ROI is illustrated.

The author provides several well-known performance matrices that are commonly used to assess the efficacy of a model in the context of anomaly detection applications. Sensitivity, specificity, and accuracy are a few examples.

These performance indicators are defined according to these criteria:

- t_p = true positive
- t_n = true negative
- f_p = false positive
- f_n = false negative
- p = total positive = $t_p + f_n$
- n = total negative = $t_n + f_p$

In addition, significant metrics such as NAE, average difference, compression ratio, PSNR, and cross-correlation are defined as follows:

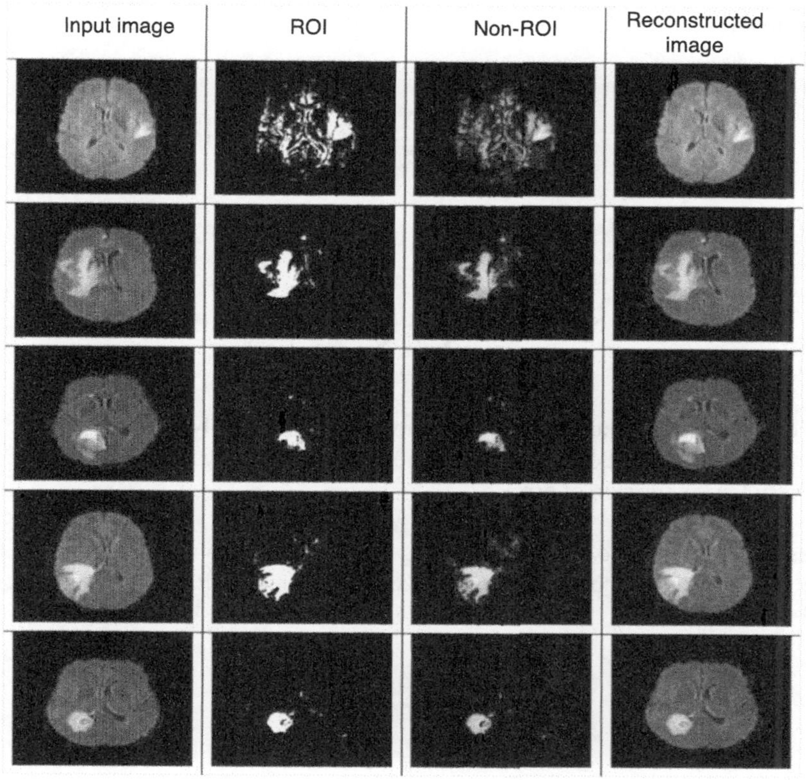

FIGURE 14.2 Sample input and output obtained regarding proposed methodology.

To determine the compression ratio of an image, divide its uncompressed size by its compressed size.

$$\text{Compression ratio} = \frac{\text{Size of original image}}{\text{Size of compressed bit stream}} \tag{14.17}$$

PSNR: The formulas provided below delineate the PSNR description.

$$\text{PSNR} = 10\log\frac{E_{\max}^2 \times D_i[i,j]_w \times D_i[i,j]_h}{\sum \left(O_i[i,j]_{xy} - D_i[i,j]_{xy}\right)} \tag{14.18}$$

where $D_i[i.j]_w$ and denotes the dimensions of the decompressed image in terms of width and height, $O_I[i.j]_{xy}$ is the pixel value of the original image at coordinate, and $(x,y), D_i[i.j]_{xy}$ is the pixel with the highest energy among the image pixels (i.e., for 256 gray-level images).

Coronal cross-section: The cross-correlation between the decompressed and original images is

$$O_I[i.j] \circ D_i[i,j] = \sum_{i=0}^{M-1}\sum_{j=0}^{N-1} O_I[i,j] D_i[i,j] \tag{14.19}$$

Average difference: The average difference (AD) of the input and decompressed image is given by

$$\mathrm{AD} = \frac{1}{MN}\sum_{i=0}^{M}\sum_{j=0}^{N}\left\{O_I[i,j] - D_i[i,j]\right\} \tag{14.20}$$

NAE: The NAE is given by

$$\mathrm{NAE} = \frac{\sum_{i=1}^{M}\sum_{j=1}^{N}\left|\left[O_I(i,j)\cdot D_i(i,j)\right]\right|}{\sum_{i=1}^{M}\sum_{j=1}^{N}\left|O_I(i,j)\right|} \tag{14.21}$$

Figure 14.3 presents the PSNR and compression ratio analysis results of the proposed system. From the result obtained, the suggested methodology have high compression ratio with very low expression of error.

We compress the ROI and the non-ROI by using the existing methodology. To prove the effectiveness of the proposed approach, it can be analyzed with some performance metrics as depicted in Tables 14.3 and 14.4

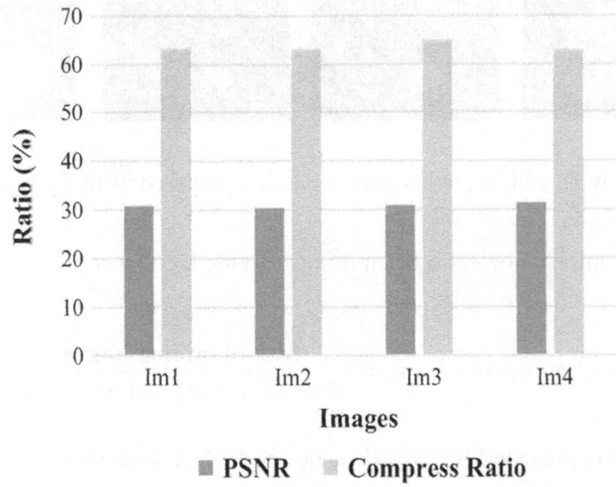

FIGURE 14.3 Calculation of PSNR and compression ratio of the images.

TABLE 14.3
Comparative Analysis of Proposed Against Existing Method for the Compression Stage

	Compression Ratio	PSNR	Cross Correlation	NAE	Average Difference
"Images	Proposed	Proposed	Proposed	Proposed	Proposed
Image 1	3.880	39.730	0.860	0.1340	5.60310
Image 2	1.680	38.650	0.8700	0.138	6.170
Image 3	2.300	44.290	0.870	0.092	4.590
Image 4	2.500	41.980	0.880	0.1280	6.2490
Image 5	2.460	46.690	1.120	0.1010	3.1760"

TABLE 14.4
Comparative Analysis of Proposed Against Existing Method for Segmentation Stage

	PFCM		
Images	**Sensitivity**	**Specificity**	**Accuracy**
Image 1	1	0.993465	0.99369
Image 2	0.9796	0.993048	0.99273
Image 3	1	0.994797	0.99485
Image 4	1	0.991914	0.99212
Image 5	0.981384	0.98254	0.99

TABLE 14.5
Comparative Results from Different Existing Algorithms

Rajliwall et al. (2018)

	Uncompressed		Compressed		
	SNR	**Time (ms)**	**SNR**	**CR**	**Time (ms)**
DCST	8.1730	72.80	4.0120	9.005	54.20
IWT (Typical)	8.6720	72.50	4.2710	8.1750	59.60
IWT (Modified)	7.3210	67.90	3.740	12.23	48.8730
Proposed	7	5.60	3.00	10.90	38.60

From the result obtained from Tables 14.3 and 14.4. The suggested methodology shows higher segmentation and compression ratio than other existing mechanism by obtaining high range of sensitivity, specificity and accuracy ratio with low range of error expression.

As of from the Table 14.5 it was revealed that the suggested methodology outperforms well than other existing mechanism in use. The results are tabulated in Table 14.5; the computational difference is achieved in a greater improvement towards the compression ratio of suggested approach by appending a layered mechanism of clustering pixel to extract a pattern and feature. Thus, the comparative study is made with respect to DCST, IWT (Typical Version) and IWT (Modified Version)".

14.6 CONCLUSION AND FUTURE WORK

The results of this research indicate that when selecting an appropriate filter for an image, it is crucial to consider both the nature and amount of noise that is inherent in the image. Furthermore, the efficacy of de-noising medical images is contingent upon the filtration processes employed as well as the nature of the noise present. In contrast to alternative filters, the one proposed exhibited a significantly superior capability of eliminating the various types of noise. Then, in the second phase, a segmentation-based watershed algorithm for seeded region growth is implemented. Each of these models was constructed utilizing the recommended compression method. With the compression of images, the required quantity of computational complexity is decreased in a brief time period of 38.6 milliseconds. The results obtained from the simulation demonstrate that the proposed method selects the most efficient and resource-conserving technique for compressing the images. As a consequence of this, the approach enhances compression efficacy in comparison to other presently employed methods. Consequently, the implementation of this methodology enhances the efficiency of compression.

Furthermore, the research can be implemented to optimize the compression of surgical videos. The video data is represented as a three-dimensional array comprising color pixels, and it incorporates redundancy in both space and time. Consequently, similarities can be encoded through the registration of differences within a frame, which comprises every pixel representing a singular moment in time. A data frame comprises the entirety of these pixels. Due to developments in compression technology, the process of compressing video files has become uncomplicated, efficient, and effortless. As a consequence, the proposed concepts became applicable and allowed for the expansion of the scope of future research.

REFERENCES

Anisha, PR, CKK Reddy, and LVN Prasad. 2015. "A pragmatic approach for detecting liver cancer using image processing and data mining techniques." *2015 International Conference on Signal Processing and Communication Engineering Systems* (pp. 352–357). IEEE, Vijayawada, India.

Ansari, MA, and RS Anand. 2009. "Context based medical image compression for ultrasound images with contextual set partitioning in hierarchical trees algorithm." *Advances in Engineering Software* 40 (7): 487–496.

Baeza, I, J-A Verdoy, J Villanueva-Oller, and R-J Villanueva. 2009. "ROI-based procedures for progressive transmission of digital images: A comparison." *Mathematical and Computer Modelling* 50 (5–6): 849–859.

Bairagi, VK, and AM Sapkal. 2012. "Automated region-based hybrid compression for digital imaging and communications in medicine magnetic resonance imaging images for telemedicine applications." *IET Science, Measurement & Technology* 6 (4): 247–253.

Bartrina-Rapesta, J, J Serra-Sagristà, and F Aulí-Llinàs. 2011. "JPEG2000 ROI coding through component priority for digital mammography." *Computer Vision and Image Understanding* 115 (1): 59–68.

Basha, S, and BC Jinaga. 2013. "A novel optimized golomb-rice technique for the reconstruction in lossless compression of digital images." *International Scholarly Research Notices* 2013 (1), 539759.

Chang, C-C, X Wang, J-H Horng, and I Echizen. 2021. "Progressive transmission of medical images via a bank of generative adversarial networks." *Journal of Healthcare Engineering* 2021 (1): 9917545.

Chavez, RFL, Y Iano, RS Higa, R Arthur, and O Saotome. 2012. "Generalized region of interest coding applied to SPIHT." *Journal on Selected Areas in Communications*. 40: 42.

Chen, Y-T, and D-C Tseng. 2007. "Wavelet-based medical image compression with adaptive prediction." *Computerized Medical Imaging and Graphics* 31 (1): 1–8.

Dhouib, D, A Naït-Ali, C Olivier, and MS Naceur. 2021. "ROI-based compression strategy of 3D MRI brain datasets for wireless communications." *IRBM* 42 (3): 146–153.

Doukas, C, and I Maglogiannis. 2007. "Region of interest coding techniques for medical image compression." *IEEE Engineering in Medicine and Biology Magazine* 26 (5): 29–35.

Eccles, CL, LA Dawson, JL Moseley, and KK Brock. 2011. "Interfraction liver shape variability and impact on GTV position during liver stereotactic radiotherapy using abdominal compression." *International Journal of Radiation Oncology* Biology* Physics* 80 (3): 938–946.

Elhannachi, SA, N Benamrane, and T-A Abdelmalik. 2017. "Adaptive medical image compression based on lossy and lossless embedded zerotree methods." *Journal of Information Processing Systems* 13 (1): 40–56.

Fu, H, F Liang, B Lei, Q Zhang, J Liang, C Tu, and G Zhang. 2021. "An extended context-based entropy hybrid modeling for image compression." *Signal Processing: Image Communication* 95: 116244.

Garcia-Alvarez, JC, H Führ, and G Castellanos-Dominguez. 2013. "Evaluation of region-of-interest coders using perceptual image quality assessments." *Journal of Visual Communication and Image Representation* 24 (8): 1316–1327.

Gutiérrez, R, F Gómez, L Roa-Peña, and E Romero. 2011. "A supervised visual model for finding regions of interest in basal cell carcinoma images." *Diagnostic Pathology* 6 (1): 1–14.

Krishnaswamy, R, and S NirmalaDevi. 2020. "Efficient medical image compression based on integer wavelet transform." *2020 Sixth International Conference on Bio Signals, Images, and Instrumentation (ICBSII)* (pp. 1–5). IEEE, Chennai, India.

Lelewer, DA, and DS Hirschberg. 1987. "Data compression." *ACM Computing Surveys (CSUR)* 19 (3): 261–296.

Li, J. 2013. "An improved wavelet image lossless compression algorithm." *Optik* 124 (11): 1041–1044.

Liu, J, Z Wang, and R Zhang. 2009. "Liver cancer CT image segmentation methods based on watershed algorithm." *2009 International Conference on Computational Intelligence and Software Engineering, Wuhan, China* (pp. 1–4).

Martchenko, A, and G Deng. 2013. "Bayesian predictor combination for lossless image compression." *IEEE Transactions on Image Processing* 22 (12): 5263–5270.

Nagoor, OH, J Whittle, J Deng, B Mora, and M W Jones. 2020. "Lossless compression for volumetric medical images using deep neural network with local sampling." *2020 IEEE International Conference on Image Processing (ICIP)* (pp. 2815–2819). IEEE, Abu Dhabi, United Arab Emirates.

Öktem, R, AE Çetin, ON Gerek, L Öktem, and K Egiazarian. 2001. "Lossless image compression by LMS adaptive filter banks." *Signal Processing* 81 (2): 447–450.

Pan, H, L-Z Jin, X-H Yuan, S-Y Xia, and L-Z Xia. 2010. "Context-based embedded image compression using binary wavelet transform." *Image and Vision Computing* 28 (6): 991–1002.

Rajliwall, NS, R Davey, and G Chetty. 2018. "Machine learning based models for cardiovascular risk prediction." *2018 International Conference on Machine Learning and Data Engineering (ICMLDE)* (pp. 142–148). IEEE, Sydney.

Sakoglu, U, L Bhupati, N Beheshti, N Tsekos, and L Johnsson. 2020. "An adaptive space-filling curve trajectory for ordering 3D datasets to 1D: Application to brain magnetic resonance imaging data for classification." *International Conference on Computational Science* (pp. 635–646). Springer International Publishing, Málaga, Spain.

Sran, PK, S Gupta, and S Singh. 2013. "Content based medical image coding with fuzzy level set segmentation algorithm." *Proceedings of the Fourth International Conference on Signal and Image Processing 2012 (ICSIP 2012), Volume 1* (pp. 161–171). Springer India.

Sujitha, B, VS Parvathy, EL Lydia, P Rani, Z Polkowski, and K Shankar. 2021. "Optimal deep learning based image compression technique for data transmission on industrial Internet of things applications." *Transactions on Emerging Telecommunications Technologies* 32 (7): e3976.

Sunil, H, and SG Hiremath. 2018. "A combined scheme of pixel and block level splitting for medical image compression and reconstruction." *Alexandria Engineering Journal* 57 (2): 767–772.

Tahoces, PG, JR Varela, MJ Lado, and M Souto. 2008. "Image compression: Maxshift ROI encoding options in JPEG2000." *Computer Vision and Image Understanding* 109 (2): 139–145.

Venugopal, D, S Mohan, and S Raja. 2016. "An efficient block based lossless compression of medical images." *Optik* 127 (2): 754–758.

Xin, G, and P Fan. 2021. "A lossless compression method for multi-component medical images based on big data mining." *Scientific Reports* 11 (1): 1–11.

Yan, Y, and Z Dong. 2000. "An approach to integer wavelet transform for medical image compression in PACS." *Wuhan University Journal of Natural Sciences* 5 (2): 204–206.

Yee, D, S Soltaninejad, D Hazarika, G Mbuyi, R Barnwal, and A Basu. 2017. "Medical image compression based on region of interest using better portable graphics (BPG)." *2017 IEEE International Conference on Systems, Man, and Cybernetics (SMC)* (pp. 216–221). IEEE, Banff, Canada.

Zuo, Z, X Lan, L Deng, S Yao, and X Wang. 2015. "An improved medical image compression technique with lossless region of interest." *Optik* 126 (21): 2825–2831.

15 A Comprehensive Analysis on Advanced Techniques in Healthcare Sensor Data Analytics

S. Chidambaram

15.1 INTRODUCTION

The advent of sensor technology has ushered in a period of unprecedented opportunities to enhance patient care, progress diagnostics, and optimize healthcare operations. Medical sensors continuously generate data streams full of information that, when used wisely, have the potential to revolutionize the way healthcare is provided. As healthcare becomes more digitally connected, wearable devices, implanted sensors, and other monitoring technologies have grown to offer a large ecosystem of health-related data. Real-time patient vital sign monitoring, predictive analytics for early disease identification, and sensor data integration for individualized treatment are three examples of how healthcare sensor data analytics can revolutionize the field.

Applying machine learning algorithms to sensor data analysis is a paradigm shift that allows correlations, trends, and patterns to be found that would not be immediately apparent with more traditional methods. This research aims to explore the potential of machine learning in comprehending sensor data from healthcare providers, focusing on developing models that can assist customized treatment regimens and remote patient monitoring.

However, there are several challenges in applying sensor data analytics in the medical field. Methods to safeguard confidential patient data must be carefully considered in light of security and privacy concerns. Additionally, ethical concerns about data governance and responsible use are critical and call for carefully balancing privacy protection with innovation; by addressing both the technological and moral components, sensor analytics research offered essential insights into integrating healthcare sensor data analytics in modern medical procedures.

15.2 LITERATURE REVIEW

This section surveys clever health monitoring methods using data analytics and deep learning techniques. A novel deep-learning approach is proposed in Pustokhin et al. (2021). In that, data analytics-assisted feature approximation and disease investigative prototype is introduced. Using the "Link-based Quasi Oppositional Binary Particle Swarm Optimization Algorithm," the dimensionality and feature count were minimized while choosing the features to create the best feature set. The Deep Belief Network model is applied, which can be acting as a classifier to use a minor feature set to diagnose the presence of disease. The simulation series was run to highlight the effectiveness of the suggested strategy, which demonstrated enhanced performance in several areas. A monitoring system for patients with cardiac arrhythmias has been created (Moghadas et al. 2020). Electrocardiography is performed for determining the severity of heart disease, and the system's heart rhythm monitoring functionality was tested using conventional sensor modules. The deep learning method is used to categorize and validate the variety of cardiac arrhythmia. To accomplish

 DOI: 10.1201/9781003486640-15

feature learning using sensor data by unsupervised learning, hybrid LSTM architecture is proposed for healthcare (Ye and Yu 2021). The multi-sensor data information was captured using the suggested deep learning architecture. An experimental analysis was conducted on turbofan engines to demonstrate the effectiveness of the proposed method for evaluating the machine's health.

A large data model (Li et al. 2021) is based on artificial intelligence (AI) used in real-world applications and for calculating and forecasting the air eminence shown in the highly temporal-spatial perseverance. Subsequently, the "deployment of mobile pollution sensor platforms" has been integrated to improve accuracy in perception data, health condition assessment, activity tracking, and air quality estimation and forecasting. The investigational examination has identified the created skeleton as the incorporated interdisciplinary approach for managing health and observing air pollution. This model can be used in different fields and nations.

A new system for evaluating the human body has been developed by Zhang et al. (2021) and includes "data collection, transmission, and query and analysis modules". Then, using unsupervised learning, CNN was used to learn the features using the body measurement data. Moreover, an evaluation model for physical assessment was integrated with the Gaussian mixture distribution. In this case, the evaluation model received the learned characteristics as input to produce the physical suitability assessment result. The replication aims to demonstrate the relative's adaptable behavior and lower operational expenses by increasing productivity. An intelligent framework (Syed et al. 2019) for the healthcare sector is applied to monitor the physical actions of older adults which depends on the Internet of Medical Things (IoMT) in conjunction with specific machine learning techniques. Effective decision-making strategies allow for much faster analysis and better treatment recommendations. The map-reduce paradigm was used with the machine learning classifier to identify the motions made on different body parts. The evaluation was conducted to offer excellent efficiency and scalability when comparing the parallel processor to the serial processor.

A novel model called HealthFog (Tuli et al. 2020) incorporates the collaborative approach above the edge computing level and applies it to the real-world problem of automated analysis of heart disease. The method has experienced the concert on the subject of power consumption, network bandwidth, latency, jitter, accuracy and execution time. In an IoT-dependent healthcare approach, a federated learning blockchain for intrusion detection is introduced (Ashraf et al. 2022). To create a workable real-time monitoring system, the novel deep learning approach is proposed in addition to the notion of the Internet of Things (Wu et al. 2023). The designed structure uses wearable medical procedures to calculate vital symbols and integrates several machine-learning algorithms to collect essential data. Deep learning techniques assisted clinicians in assessing patient situations to guarantee appropriate therapy without medical involvement. The developed prototype efficacy has been confirmed by doing a cross-validation test using several measures (Table 15.1).

TABLE 15.1
Description of Performance of Various Healthcare Applications in Big Data Analytics

Authors	Year	Description
Siddiqa et al.	Vol. 71, pp. 151–166, 2016	Examine workable methods for handling large amounts of data, emphasizing processing, storage, pre-processing, and security.
Palanisamy and Thirunavukarasu	Vol. 31, Issue 4, pp. 415–425, October 2019,	There are several analytical paths in the patient-centered healthcare system. They examined a range of big data frameworks in terms of their application domains, data sources, and analytical power.
Ristevski and Chen	Vol. 15(3), 2018.	Incorporates and analyzes a significant quantity of complex heterogeneous data, including biological data, data from electronic health records, and data from genomics, epigenomics, and transcriptomics.

(Continued)

TABLE 15.1 (*Continued*)
Description of Performance of Various Healthcare Applications in Big Data Analytics

Authors	Year	Description
Boja et al.	Vol. 11(1), p. 45, 2014.	Identify the obstacles and difficulties in integrating omics and assist in developing "integromics" in biology and medicine.
Wang and Hajli	Vol. 70, pp. 287–299, 2017.	Suggested a commercial value model utilizing resource-based theory (RBT) and big data analytics.
Wang et al.	Vol. 55(1), pp. 64–79, 2018.	Suggested the use of a big data analytics-enabled transformation model to identify the causal links between IT-enabled transformation processes and extensive data analytics capabilities.
Bajaber et.al.	Vol. 14 (3), 79–405, 2016	The Map Reduce framework has become a prevalent framework, as has Hadoop, its open-source implementation.
Mehta and Pandit	Vol. 114, 57–65, 2018.	NLP in Big Data analytics was explored, along with how it might optimize clinical operations, lower healthcare costs, and improve clinical decision-making.
Sajid and Abbas	Vol. 40(6), 2016.	They are suggested to proactively identify and mitigate these patients' concerns about their data privacy.
Alotaibi et al.	Springer, pp. 267–279, 2020	Big data enabled healthcare supply chains: prospects and difficulties are explored.
Pikkarainen et al.	Vol. 6(1), 55, 2018.	They are highlighting the transformations in a network. The data from various sectors will allow individuals and doctors to interconnect via intellectually adapted facilities.
Usak et al.	Vol. 33, 1–17, 2019.	With the rapid growth of IT-based expertise, effective central management and public health observation can be recognized.

15.3 ARCHITECTURAL FRAMEWORK

Hadoop/Map Reduce is a platform in healthcare organizations that can manages several network nodes and enables parallel processing in a distributed environment. Hadoop and Map Reduce technologies have been successfully applied to many healthcare applications, where they improve the efficiency of different tasks like signal detection methods, lung texture classification, protein structure alignments, image processing, and neural signal processing. The healthcare analytics comprises three primary elements: data aggregation, processing, and visualization as shown in Figure 15.1.

15.3.1 Data Processing

Batch and stream processing methods are used in healthcare data processing. The process of evaluating data in batches includes gathering and storing data without considering reaction time. Batch processing is a widespread use case for Apache Hadoop Map-Reduce architecture. The frameworks Apache Spark and Flink allow both batch and stream processing. It is applicable for handling massive amounts of data in a distributed, parallel fashion. The significant data analytics process is carried out inside this framework using various instruments and strategies.

15.3.2 Data Aggregation

In healthcare, data aggregation refers to collect and combine raw data from many sources. It can be processed and analyzed in a standard format utilizing a data warehouse. Process features include data loading, data transformation, and extraction.

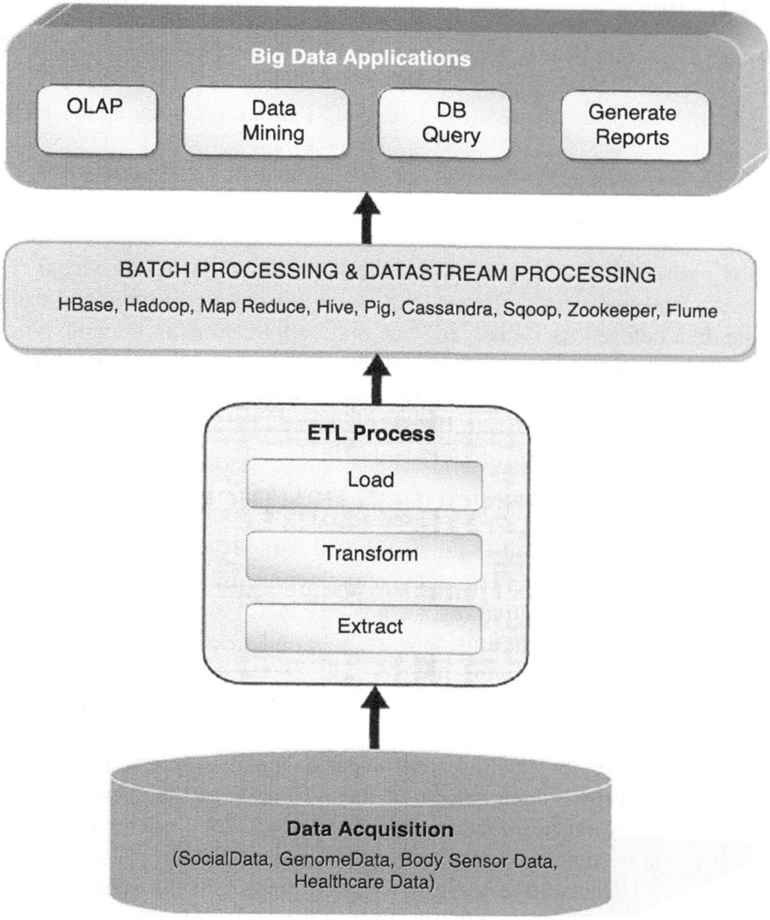

FIGURE 15.1 The structure of big data architecture.

15.3.3 Data Extraction

There is a vast amount of health information that comes from various sources. The primary medical data sources include surveys, hospital records, insurance claims, disease records, surveillance data, experimental test data, and management records. Both structured and unstructured data are available from these sources. The numerical, category, and nominal data types that comprise structured data are easy to deal with and have predetermined structures. A standard format is used for additional processing. Medical data can be in any format, including electronic health records (EHRs), images, sensor data, genetic, biochemical, and clinical text data. These data may be in the DICOM picture format, XML, JSON, or text/ASCII format.

15.3.4 Data Transformation

The acquired raw data are processed through several data filtering processes. It removes unnecessary data and includes steps like noise reduction, normalization, and data modification to apply certain business logic. The data is converted using this procedure into a typical format that is suitable and dependable for advanced research.

15.3.5 Data Loading

In this process, each distinct healthcare system usually requires the creation of a customized relational database with specific data formats and storage techniques for medical data. Modified medical data fit for further analysis are sent to the destination dataset, such as the HDFS and NoSQL databases.

15.3.6 Data Visualization

The specialist is assisted in gaining extra insights from the data by the visual representation of the data. The analytical tool uses software tools, data-mining algorithms, and evaluation to clean and evaluate the data before it is visualized. The main applications of data analytics in the healthcare sector include report creation, online analytical processing, and querying. Proactive messages, real-time warnings, visualization of patient health records, prediction reports, and dashboards tracking patients' daily health status are all displayed using them.

15.4 DATA ANALYTICS TECHNIQUES IN HEALTHCARE

Multidimensional health information in the healthcare industry is gathered from multiple sources, such as biological signals, printed instructions, data from wearables and medical equipment, electronic health records, and medical imaging, such as MRIs, CT scans, and X-rays. Because the data are complex and dynamic, it is intriguing to work with and assess those using traditional methods (Gietzelt et al. 2016).

The healthcare data analytics have been applied for various real time applications. It includes Data mining, machine learning, NLP, Pattern recognition and graph analytics shown in Figure 15.2. Neural network, Support Vector machine, and linear & logistic regression are the important data mining techniques to find the hidden pattern of data. To manage the current issues and the growing demands for healthcare services, telehealth and telemedicine have developed into applications that may be used in many remote health tracking methods to deliver essential facilities and assist with supported living. The machine learning helps to automate the Electronic Healthcare Data Management (HER). It also provides clinical support system and improved disease diagnosis. For that Deep learning and reinforcement learning helps to determine the disease. Patient segmentation, disease identification and drug response prediction are some of the applications of clustering in data analytics.

Visual data analytical tools like SAS Visual Analytics, Tableau, and QlikView can help to understand the data easily by visually. And easy to find the hidden pattern and improve prediction. Based

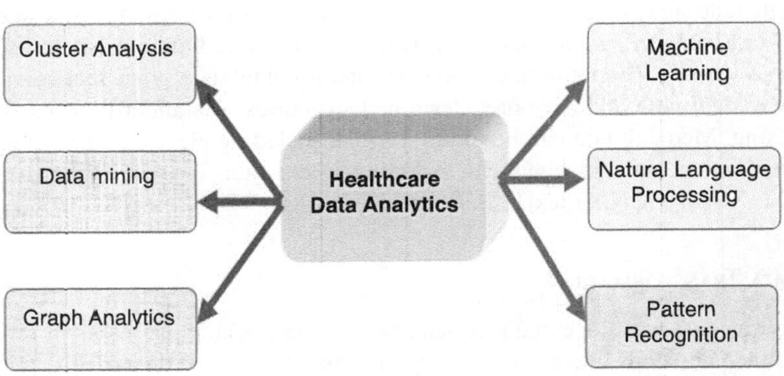

FIGURE 15.2 Various data analytics techniques in healthcare.

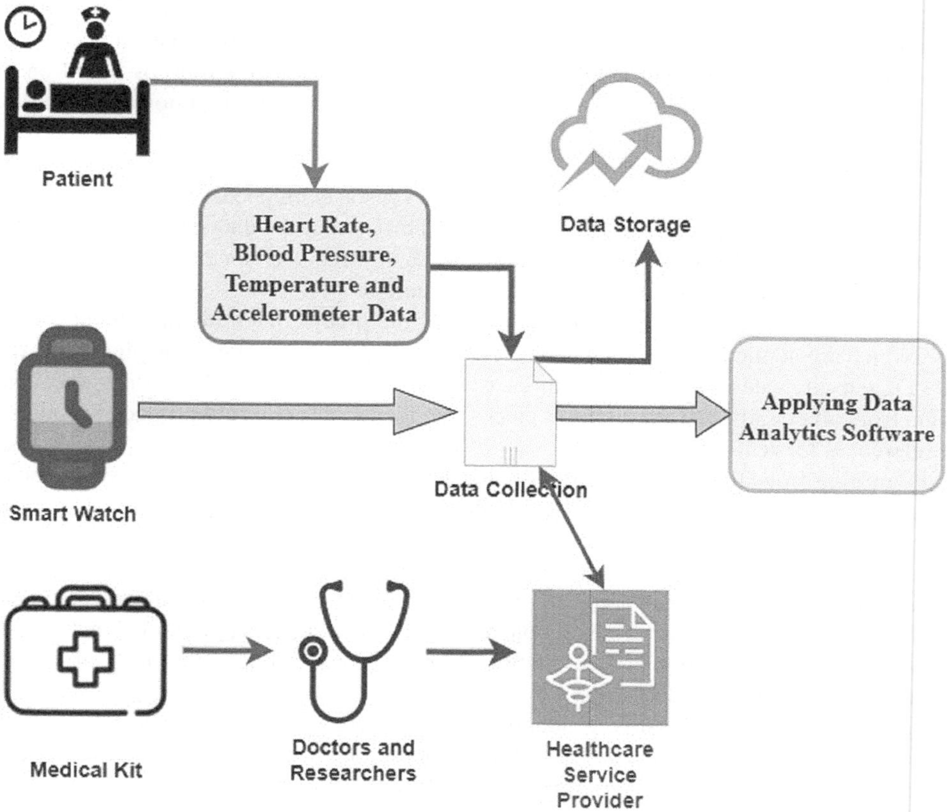

FIGURE 15.3 Procedure of healthcare sensor data analytics.

on the increasing volume of data, infrastructure and maintenance cost is increased. Since, it is necessary to handle all types of data such as structure and unstructured and semi structured form of healthcare data. Latency and security issues also be considered in healthcare data management.

In Figure 15.3, denotes the healthcare data are generated from various sources such as smart watches, medical IoMT sensor components, medical practioners and health care service providers. The gathered data are stored and processed used data analytics approaches. Graph analytics can help to analyze the complex relationship among the healthcare data. Anomaly detection and temporal analysis are the some of the important techniques used. Assistances of consuming real-time stream processing tools like Apache Storm, SQL Stream Blaze, and Apache Flinkincludes real time monitoring of patients and sent the alert during emergency time, fraud detection and resource optimization.

The number of senior persons is rising, which makes it necessary to create healthcare solutions for older people that are affordable, discrete, and simple to use. These devices can create medical equipment, computing systems, software applications based on IoMT, and healthcare services. IoMT-related devices play a critical role in providing helpful monitoring for medical situations such as diabetes, heart attacks, asthma attacks, and other conditions that might potentially save lives. Despite their remote locations, these medical devices can support the healthcare industry's clinical operations and workflow management through sensors and comparable linked devices that guarantee high-quality patient care (Rodrigues et al. 2016).

Predicting diseases and epidemics that can be prevented and improving the standard of treatment in healthcare are two benefits of the extensive data analytics method. Furthermore, proficient schemes and deeply organized architectures are used to analyze data, find patterns, and learn arrangements to mark an actual conclusion for a health condition. This ensures the patient's safety and makes threat prevention possible by precisely noticing at the appropriate time. A collaborative learning strategy is applied for the older adults. Their physical activity is based on big data which can be included in a novel Map-Reduce structure-based health monitoring system to assess enhanced individual suggestions.

The Hadoop Map Reduce techniques were employed. The necessary data were obtained, as stated in the dataset descriptions, through wearable sensor components attached to human body parts such as the "left ankle, right arm, and chest." Throughout the data extraction stage, the large amount of data is divided into smaller portions. Data splitting was done to calculate control time, and the result is that it is difficult to reach the optimum.

These minor chunk records are utilized to select the precise features throughout the mapping phase, which are applied to each map task. Using the suggested classifiers, the physical activities of senior citizens are categorized in the combiner phase. Ultimately, the reducer step concatenates the outputs from all classifiers from different pieces into identical sessions to produce adequate healthcare references for senior citizens.

Data mining in healthcare aims to find patterns in massive databases and extract meaningful information. Using a sizable healthcare data collection, these data-mining techniques are employed to extract new and valuable information. This is a result of the growing volumes of health data. Disease forecasting, bio-signal intense patient care, diagnostic and therapeutic care, and data exploration are all included in such an application. Machine learning is utilized in healthcare to help with data analysis and outcome recommendation. The machine learning applications include personalized patient care, identification and production of medications, evaluation of hospital performance, and prediction of syndrome diagnosis.

Data analysis makes it possible to identify hidden groups and structures inside massive databases. Cluster analysis expedites the patient population identification process in the medical field based on the patient's features, the rigorousness of the condition, and the patient's response to treatment. Cluster analysis can be used to classify patient groups based on risk factors, obesity groups, and demographic groups with specific infection drivers, among other uses, to optimize outcomes. Graph analytics techniques examine data as a graph, where nodes represent individual data components and edges represent those entities' relationships. Using graph analytics based on quality metrics, healthcare fraud risk is evaluated and hospital performance is examined.

The role of Natural Language Processing is the method by which computers can understand spoken and written language from people. It has enormous promise for looking through, evaluating, and comprehending vast amounts of patient data in the healthcare industry. Natural language processing has several applications, including monitoring healthcare costs, delivering efficient patient care, extracting pertinent health-related information from clinical notes, and providing therapies, consultations, and training. The neural network facilitates medical data analysis, modeling, and comprehension. Artificial neural networks have been used to diagnose patients, forecast cancer occurrence, and analyze medical data to design new medications.

15.5 MAP REDUCE FRAMEWORK FOR BIG DATA-BASED HEALTHCARE APPLICATIONS

MapReduce's programming methodology and framework handles big datasets distributed over numerous nodes. Due to the amount of data, processing is split up and completed concurrently by multiple nodes. There are two parts to the process: reduce and Map.

Map Stage: The data deposited in the HDFS is fed into a mapper function once it has been split into smaller, fixed-sized segments. The mapper function creates the structured output data tuples, or key/value pairs, for each component and saves them into a file in the middle format.

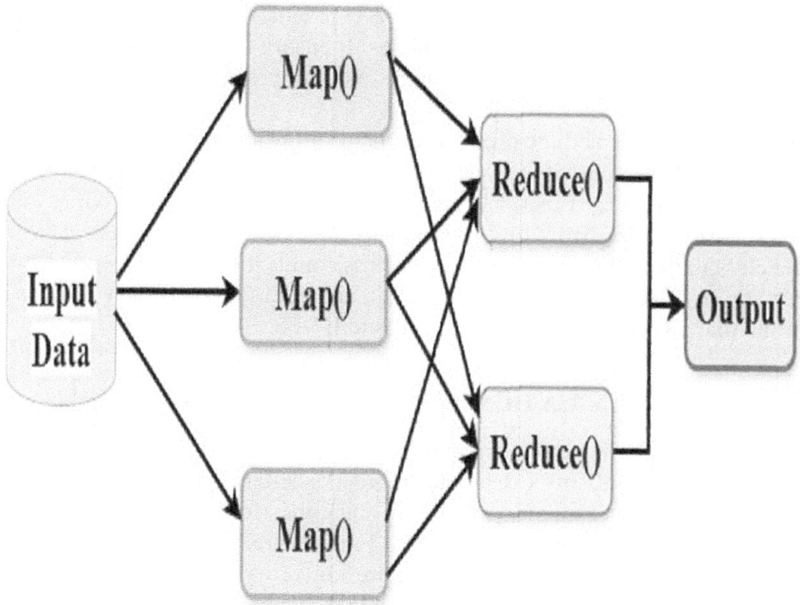

FIGURE 15.4 Sequence of procedures of map reduce framework.

Reduce Stage: The resulting value is shambled to combine and merge the related records into minor ones. The reducer combines the shuffle output by integrating the duplicate keys and outputs, reducing the tuples to a single output file.

From Figure 15.4, there are Two critical aspects of Hadoop Map Reduce are its high scalability and ability to access new data resources. It functions with various kinds of data and guards against illegal access to data. It enhances the security of the system.

Apache Hadoop is a distributed open source framework that practices a cluster of computers to handle massive volumes of data in a similar using the Map Reduce programming methodology.

The following lists Hadoop's two main modules.

Big data is stored using the "Hadoop Distributed File System (HDFS)," which has hundreds of file systems for data storage. The software for analyzing, processing, and retrieving data is called MapReduce. It processes data while retrieving it concurrently and consumes less time.

In the MapReduce Execution phase, Big datasets are processed and produced using an effective programming technique called "MapReduce". Map and reduce are two operations that permit the more extensive parallel calculation. It often follows the "Divide and Conquer" strategy, in which large amounts of data are broken up into smaller pieces and then shuffled and reduced to obtain an estimated output. The steps in this framework are given below.

- With the help of the user programme, several worker processes and a primary process are created.
- The Map is assigned, and tasks for the worker processes are derived from the primary process.
- The files are divided into smaller portions, ranging from 16 MB to 64 MB, using the user programme described in the MapReduce library. These split files are taken into account for the Map assignment.
- The tiny records are transformed into consecutive key-value sets for the Map tasks, and then each input line values are calculated to give the number of times each term occurs.

Hadoop Map Reduce technology provides higher level of handling large volume of data. It provides the cost effective solution for the complex problems. It ensure the availability and faulty tolerance. In order to speed up the analysis process, supports parallel processing. It also supports analysis of variety of data.

The combiner phase (intermediate phase) uses the result from the map stage. The combiner stage uses the established DEL to classify physical activities after obtaining the keys and values via the Map function. Here, the reducer function receives the combined set of all activities and values in the same class. The retrieved data from different chunks are combined with their activities and values under a single class in the reducer method. Every class counts the occurrences of every activity, and the consequences are calculated and lead to the main procedure. The primary process influences the user programme that transmits the obtained results to HDFS.

15.6 ROLE OF DATA ANALYTICS IN HEALTHCARE APPLICATIONS

Big data analytics can help the healthcare industry in many ways. Electronic health records, medical histories, and other records offer data analytics an excellent opportunity to uncover important information. The diversity of data produced at various times from multiple sources is equal. Since the volume of data produced by this industry, data analysts are highly interested in it. Conventional computing methods and systems cannot deliver preventive care programmes or real-time patient monitoring. Thus, intelligent strategies that evaluate incoming data to uncover hidden patterns and provide patient recommendations are required to assist doctors in their practice.

Apache Hadoop, Spark and flink are the powerful framework for speed up the processing of data. It can support batch processing, Stream processing and graph processing. It is suitable for handling streaming of data continuously.

15.6.1 Image-Based Analytics

Physicians are a basis of evidence and mainly use image-based databases for internal imaging. Several imaging techniques are commonly used to diagnose conditions, including mammograms, MRIs, CT scans, positron emission tomography (PET) CT), X-rays, and ultrasound.

Tumors are abnormalities in which cells develop and harden into neoplasms. These abnormalities are commonly detected with brain MRIs and neuro-images. Early detection is crucial for efficient treatment and recovery and to reduce the chance of death. X-rays diagnose fractures, pneumonia, cancer, and other illnesses.

The number of medical records is rising, and the usage of computer-aided diagnosis and analysis is improved. The aim of sophisticated analytical techniques like machine learning and optimization is predictive error reduction through high-performance computers. For countries with low doctor-to-patient ratios, machine-aided diagnosis holds excellent promise.

15.6.2 Signal-Based Analytics

In ubiquitous wearable sensors, period-oriented signals are produced at an occurrence higher than their processing capacity. Wearable technology, such as smart wearable devices, constantly monitors heart rate, pressure level, sleep designs, calories seared, and other information. Analyzing these signals significantly affects pharmacological decisions and medication prescriptions, treatment plans, and routine check-ups. Such signal measurements can obtain relevant information regarding the patient's present state.

The prevalence of heart disease has increased over the last 10 years due to lifestyle changes. ECG signals, which offer a clear picture of cardiac health and may be sent directly to doctors for immediate analysis, can be monitored by carbon nanotubes. A multitude of sensors can generate signals continuously. If a patient's condition warrants it, these signals can be constantly monitored; alternatively, they can be checked during routine check-ups. Imagine the volume of data generated by a person who wears a smartwatch continually. This kind of data is large and varied, much like analytics derived from photos. Each sensor generates data that falls into a specific class.

It is necessary to contextualize such time-stream data to obtain pertinent information regarding the patient's current status. It also increases the difficulty of signal-based data analysis. The situation becomes more complex because real-time stream analytics and diagnostics are required.

15.6.3 Clinical Diagnosis and Research

A clinical diagnosis is made after examining a patient's signs, symptoms, and medical history to rule out any underlying illnesses or disorders. Usually, a preliminary diagnosis is obtained using the patient's historical medical records and current symptoms and traits; no laboratory testing is necessary. The physician may then recommend additional tests to ascertain the precise course of the sickness or to search for variances and misleading indications. A physician practices years of knowledge to make the initial diagnosis, but evaluating the patient's medical history and treatments takes time.

15.6.4 Disease Communication and Avoidance

Certain illnesses are contagious and can spread by contact, either straight or unintended, with the carrier or a diseased individual. To avoid the inception of such problems, it is imperative to investigate the disease's communication route and forecast its spread to design more effective justification strategies and disease organization approaches. By using data analytics, mathematical representations may be developed to estimate the disease's impact and predict when it will spread.

15.7 CHALLENGES OF HEALTHCARE DATA ANALYTICS

The practice of big data analytics has been highly beneficial to the healthcare industry. These advantages include improved clinical results, successful therapies, more personalized patient care, reduced healthcare expenditures, and more effective operational administration of healthcare. Big data has many benefits, but it also has certain drawbacks. One of the main problems in the healthcare industry is the collection of health-related data. The innovative healthcare system uses many wearables and Internet of Things (IoT) devices, constantly generating massive amounts of streaming data. As a result, collecting and interpreting data has grown increasingly challenging. Robust governance systems for data sources are needed to collect data from various sources, which could bring about inaccurate data.

The exponential development of health stream data poses a significant data storage challenge for the healthcare business. Utmost health establishments choose to keep their data locally to retain control over data security and access due to the high expenses associated with maintenance and scale-up. However, it gets harder to scale up internal data storage systems as health data grows accelerating. The privacy and confidentiality of medical data, especially patient health data, are essential to the healthcare industry. When many healthcare providers share data, the need for privacy grows. Informed consent is another issue that data analytics in healthcare must deal with. Because digital healthcare crosses geopolitical boundaries, health services are available domestically and abroad. The healthcare sector encounters considerable challenges in creating uniform laws because of country differences in patient data privacy, medical licensure, and healthcare service marketing and advertising.

15.8 CONCLUSION

Incorporating sensor data analytics into healthcare has proved to be a game-changer and indispensable instrument for boosting productivity, promoting patient outcomes, and furthering medical research. Healthcare practitioners can obtain real-time insights into patients' health statuses by continuously monitoring patients' vital signs, environmental factors, and other pertinent parameters. More proactive and individualized medical actions are made possible by this abundance of data and improving patient care. The Map-Reduce framework can provide better performance for analyzing, processing, and storing large volumes of data in the distributed remote environment for analyzing the patient health data.

REFERENCES

Alotaibi, S., Mehmood, R., & Katib, I (2020). The role of big data and twitter data analytics in healthcare supply chain management. In Mehmood, R., See, S., Katib, I., Chlamtac, I. (eds), *Smart Infrastructure and Applications* (pp. 267–279). Springer, Cham.

Ashraf, E., N. F. F. Areed, H. Salem, E. H. Abdelhay, & A. Farouk (2022). FIDChain: federated intrusion detection system for blockchain-enabled IoT healthcare applications. *Healthcare*, 10(6), 1110. https://www.mdpi.com/2227-9032/10/6/1110

Bajaber, F., R. Elshawi, O. Batarfi, A. Altalhi, A. Barnawi, & S. Sakr (2016). Big data 2.0 processing systems: taxonomy and open challenges. *J. Grid Comput.*, 14 (3), 379–405.

Boja, E.S., C.R. Kinsinger, H. Rodriguez, & P. Srinivas (2014). Integration of omics sciences to advance biology and medicine. *Clinc. Proteomics*, 11, 45.

Gietzelt, M., M. Löpprich, C. Karmen, & M. Ganzinger (2016). Models and data sources used in systems medicine. *Methods Inf. Med.*, 55 (2), 107–113.

Li, V.O.K., J.C.K. Lam, Y. Han, & K. Chow (2021). A big data and artificial intelligence framework for smart and personalized air pollution monitoring and health management in Hong Kong. *Environ. Sci. Policy*, 124, 441–450. https://doi.org/10.1016/j.envsci.2021.06.011

Mehta, N., & A. Pandit (2018). Concurrence of big data analytics and healthcare: asystematic review. *Int. J. Med. Inform.*, 114, 57–65.

Moghadas, E., J. Rezazadeh, & R. Farahbakhsh (2020). An IoT patient monitoring based on fog computing and data mining: cardiac arrhythmia usecase. *Internet Things*, 11. https://doi.org/10.1016/j.iot.2020.100251

Palanisamy, V., & R. Thirunavukarasu (2017). Implications of big data analytics in developing healthcare frameworks, a review. *J. King Saud. Univ. Comput. Inf. Sci.*, 31, 415–425.

Pikkarainen, M.A. (2018). Data as a driver for shapingthe practices of a preventive healthcare service delivery network. *J. Innovation Manage.*, 1, 55–79.

Pustokhin, D.A., I.V. Pustokhina, P. Rani, V. Kansal, M. Elhoseny, G.P. Joshi, & K. Shankar (2021). Optimal deep learning approaches and healthcare big data analytics for mobile networks toward 5G. *Comput. Electr. Eng.*, 95. https://doi.org/10.1016/j.compeleceng.2021.107376

Ristevski, M.C. (2018). Big data analytics in medicine and healthcare. *J. Integr. Bioinforma.*, 15(3), 20170030.

Rodrigues Jr, J.F., F.V. Paulovich, M.C. de Oliveira, & O.N. de Oliveira Jr. (2016). On the convergence of nanotechnology and Big Data analysis for computer-aided diagnosis. *Nanomedicine*, 11(8), 959–982.

Sajid, A., & H. Abbas (2016). Data privacy in cloud-assisted healthcare systems: state of the art and future challenges. *J. Med. Syst.*, 40(6), 155.

Siddiqa, A., I.A.T. Hashem, I. Yaqoob, M. Marjani, S. Shamshirband, A. Gani, et al. (2016). A survey of big data management: taxonomy and state-of-the-art. *J. Netw. Comput. Appl.*, 71, 151–166.

Syed, L., S. Jabeen, & A. Alsaeedi (2019). Smart healthcare framework for ambient assisted living using IoMT and big data analytics techniques. *Future Gener. Comput. Syst.*, 101, 136–151. https://doi.org/10.1016/j.future.2019.06.004

Tuli, S., N. Basumatary, S.S. Gill, M. Kahani, R.C. Arya, G.S. Wander, & R. Buyya (2020). HealthFog: an ensemble deep learning based smart healthcare system for automatic diagnosis of heart diseases in integrated IoT and fog computing environments. *Future Gener. Comput. Syst.*, 104, 187–200. https://doi.org/10.1016/j.future.2019.10.043

Usak, M., M. Kubiatko, & M. Salman (2019). Healthcare service delivery based on the Internet of things: a systematic and comprehensive study. *Int. J. Commun. Syst.*, 33, 1–17.

Wang, Y., L. Kung, W.Y.C. Wang, & C. Cegielski (2018). An integrated big data analytics- enabled transformation model: application to health care. *Inf. Manag.*, 55(1), 64–79.

Wang, Y., & N. Hajli (2017). Exploring the path to big data analytics success in healthcare. *J. Bus. Res.*, 70, 287–299.

Wu, X., C. Liu, L. Wang, & M. Bilal (2023). Internet of Things-enabled realtime health monitoring system using deep learning. *Neural Comput. Appl.*, 35(20), 14565–14576. https://doi.org/10.1007/s00521-021-06440-6

Ye, Z., & J. Yu (2021). Health condition monitoring of machines based on long short-term memory convolutional auto encoder. *Appl. Soft Comput.*, 107. https://doi.org/10.1016/j.asoc.2021.107379

Zhang, N., C. Zhang, & D. Wu (2021). Construction of a smart management system for physical health based on IoT and cloud computing with big data. *Comput. Commun.*, 179, 183–194. https://doi.org/10.1016/j.comcom.2021.08.018

16 Internet of Medical Things in Healthcare
Enhancing Patient Care and Monitoring Through Connected Devices

V. Harish and Dhanushiya D

16.1 INTRODUCTION

Technological developments in today's exponentially growing healthcare sector have transformed the delivery, monitoring, and management of medical services. One of the most prominent transformative innovations is the Internet of Medical Things (IoMT), a network of devices and applications that harness the power of the internet to gather, diffuse, and analyze health-related data (Vishnu et al. 2020). From wearables to trackers to sophisticated medical implants and remote patient monitoring systems, the IoMT is reshaping the future of healthcare delivery by enabling personalized, proactive, and patient-centric care.

The broader Internet of Things (IoT) paradigm deeply roots the concept of IoMT, encompassing the interconnectedness of everyday products through the internet and in the healthcare context (Aceto et al. 2018). IoMT extends this connectivity to medical devices, equipment, and infrastructure, creating a seamless ecosystem where data flows seamlessly between all key stakeholders in the healthcare space (Sonavane et al. 2023). This interconnectedness allows for real-time monitoring of patients' health status, early identification of medical issues, and early interventions, resulting in improved patient satisfaction and enhanced healthcare efficiency.

At the heart of IoMT lies a diverse array of gadgets and applications, each fortified with sensors, connectivity features, and data processing abilities, and they range from simple wearables to sophisticated medical implants, diagnostic equipment, and remote monitoring systems (Dwivedi et al. 2022). With the power of these gadgets, IoMT enables medical staff to capture a wealth of information about patients' health in real-time, including vitals, biometric measurements, medication usage, and activity levels using sensor data Analytics (Adewole et al. 2021).

One of the most notable features of IoMT is its ability to enable remote patient monitoring (Polu and Polu 2019), allowing medical staff to continuously monitor patients' health outside conventional clinical settings (Adeniyi et al. 2021), elderly individuals, and post-operative patients who require ongoing monitoring and support. IoMT not only allows for remote monitoring, but it also lets doctors make medical interventions that are specific to each patient's needs and preferences by looking at the health data that IoMT devices produce (Awotunde et al. 2021), finding clinical trends, and guessing how their health will turn out (Manickam et al. 2022).

IoMT also has a huge potential to improve healthcare in places with few resources and in communities that aren't getting enough care. By using portable, low-cost IoMT devices and telemedicine platforms, healthcare providers can reach people in remote areas and give them access to basic medical services and consultations with specialists (Trayush et al. 2021).

DOI: 10.1201/9781003486640-16

Despite its numerous advantages, IoMT also presents unique hurdles and considerations that require careful examination to ensure its ethical use and optimize its potential in healthcare settings. These roadblocks include patient data privacy (Singh et al. 2020), regulatory compliance, and interoperability issues (Yasmeen et al. 2022). Hospitals should aim to mitigate the various roadblocks before reaping the benefits of IoMT technology. IoMT represents a boon in the medical arena, offering unprecedented opportunities to increase patient service, improve healthcare outcomes, and revolutionize healthcare delivery. By leveraging the power of interconnected medical devices and applications, IoMT has the potential to present a personalized, practical, and patient-first approach, ultimately leading to healthier, happier communities around the world.

16.2 LITERATURE REVIEW

A detailed review of the existing literature on the topic of IoMT was done to understand the current scenario on the topic and some of the key aspects of existing literature are as follows

16.2.1 Definition and Overview

According to a detailed literature review, some of the perspectives on IoMT are as follows:

1. **Network of Medical Devices:** The IoMT refers to a network of interconnected medical devices that collect, share, and analyze patient health data, and these devices can include wearables, implants, diagnostic tools, and hospital equipment (Srivastava et al. 2022).
2. **Healthcare Transformation through Connectivity:** The IoMT represents a paradigm shift in healthcare, leveraging the power of the internet to connect healthcare professionals, patients, and medical devices, enabling remote monitoring, real-time data analysis, and improved healthcare delivery (Osama et al. 2023).
3. **Patient-Centered Data Ecosystem:** The IoMT fosters a patient-centered data ecosystem where individuals have greater control and access to their health information, empowering patients to participate actively in their healthcare decisions (Adarsha et al. 2019).
4. **Bridge between Physical and Digital Health:** The IoMT acts as a bridge between the physical world of medical care and the digital realm of data analysis, facilitating the seamless flow of health data and enabling more data-driven and personalized healthcare approaches (Morphy 2021).
5. **Revolutionizing Disease Management and Prevention:** The IoMT has the potential to revolutionize disease management and prevention by providing continuous health data. It allows for early detection of health issues, proactive interventions, and personalized preventive measures (Jain et al. 2024).

Researchers with different central foci have provided various definitions, leading to a unified definition.

16.2.1.1 Unified Definition of IoMT

"The Internet of Medical Things (IoMT) is a network of interconnected medical devices, wearables, and healthcare IT systems that collect, share, and analyze patient health data in real-time. This connected ecosystem empowers healthcare professionals, patients, and researchers to leverage data for improved healthcare delivery, disease management, preventive care, and ultimately, a more patient-centered approach to health.".

The below given Table 16.1 lists the 5 Whys and 2H for IoMT based on the various definitions studied

TABLE 16.1
5- Why's and 2- How's for IoMT

Aspect	Question	Description
Who	Who benefits from IoMT?	Patients, healthcare providers, caregivers, and researchers.
What	What is IoMT?	IoMT refers to the system of medical gadgets connected through the internet for remote monitoring, data collection, and analysis in healthcare.
When	When is IoMT used?	IoMT is used continuously for real-time monitoring and management of patient health, both in clinical settings and at home.
Where	Where is IoMT deployed?	IoMT is deployed in hospitals and various other medical settings in clinics as well as home as well as in research laboratories and medical device manufacturing facilities.
Why	Why is IoMT important?	IoMT improves patient care, enhances clinical workflows, reduces healthcare costs, and enables personalized medicine through remote monitoring and data analytics.
How	How does IoMT work?	IoMT works by inter linking healthcare gadgets, sensors, gathering and diffusing data to medical staff for analysis and decision-making.
How much	How much does IoMT cost?	The cost of IoMT varies depending on factors such as device complexity, deployment scale, and ongoing maintenance requirements. Initial investments may include device procurement, infrastructure setup, and training costs. However, IoMT can lead to long-term cost savings and optimizing healthcare resource utilization.

16.2.2 Evolution of IoMT in Healthcare

We can connect the evolution of IoMT in the medical sector to the growth of digital health technologies and the increasing prevalence of connected medical devices. The early 2000s saw the emergence of telemedicine and remote patient monitoring systems (Qureshi and Krishnan 2018). These systems typically involve the use of specialized healthcare devices, such as heart rate monitors and glucose meters, linked to centralized monitoring platforms via wired or wireless networks.

As internet connectivity became more omnipresent and affordable, the scope and capabilities of IoMT expanded rapidly, driven by advances in sensor technology, miniaturization, and wireless communication protocols (Pramanik et al. 2020). Wearable devices, such as "fitness trackers, smartwatches, and health monitoring bands," had more acceptance among consumers for various applications such as tracking the movement of people, understanding sleep data, and various other medical metrics, and these consumer-grade wearables paved the way for medical-grade IoMT devices designed specifically for healthcare applications (Kakhi et al. 2022).

The proliferation of gadgets and apps further accelerated the adoption of IoMT by providing convenient platforms for data collection, analysis, and communication. Health and wellness apps, equipped with features for tracking diet, exercise, medication adherence, and vital signs, became widely accepted among consumers looking to take control of their health (Sharma et al. 2021). Healthcare providers also embraced mobile health (mHealth) technologies as tools for engaging patients, monitoring health metrics, and delivering personalized care remotely.

In parallel, advances in medical device technology and healthcare infrastructure paved the way for more sophisticated IoMT solutions designed for clinical settings. Implantable medical devices, such as cardiac monitors, pacemakers, and insulin pumps, became increasingly connected and capable of transmitting real-time data for better management (Ahmed et al. 2024). Diagnostic gadgets, such as MRI machines (Magnetic Resonance Imaging) and X-ray machines, also became equipped with connectivity features to facilitate image sharing, consultation, and collaboration among healthcare professionals.

The rise of cloud computing and big data analytics further transformed the landscape of IoMT by enabling the storage, processing, and analysis of data in real-time. Cloud-based platforms and analytics tools allow healthcare providers to aggregate data from multiple sources, analyze it for insights, and generate actionable recommendations for patient care (Tamiziniyan and Keerthana 2022). Machine learning (ML) algorithms can examine trends in health data to predict disease progression, identify risk factors, and optimize treatment strategies, paving the way for personalized medicine and precision healthcare (Manickam et al. 2022).

Looking ahead, the future of IoMT in the medical arena holds great promise for better patient service, increased healthcare efficiency, and cost reduction. Advances in IoMT tools, such as 5G connectivity and wearable biosensors, will enable faster data transmission, higher data processing speeds, and greater interoperability between devices and systems (Magsi et al. 2018).

16.3 OBJECTIVES OF THE CHAPTER

Based on the detailed review of literature the following objectives have been arrived at

1. To understand the Importance and Benefits of IoMT Adoption in healthcare setting.
2. To understand the key components of IoMT's.
3. To understand the various applications of IoMT in patient care and monitoring.
4. To examine the role of Wearable health and fitness devices in the IoMT space.
5. To examine the application of IoMT in Hospital Settings
6. To understand the Security and privacy challenges in the adoption of IoMT
7. To list the Challenges and future directions of the IoMT in healthcare sector.

16.3.1 Importance and Benefits of IoMT Adoption

Various literature papers highlight the various benefits of IoMT, as indicated in Figure 16.1 below.

1. **Improved Patient Monitoring:** IoMT lets healthcare providers keep an eye on patients' vital signs, medication compliance, and disease progression in real time. This proactive approach to patient monitoring makes it easier to spot health problems early, act on them quickly, and create personalized treatment plans that help patients get better and avoid having to go back to the hospital (Sharmila et al. 2024).
2. **Improved Access to Healthcare:** Telemedicine platforms and remote monitoring solutions enable patients to receive on-time diagnostic assessments and follow-up care from

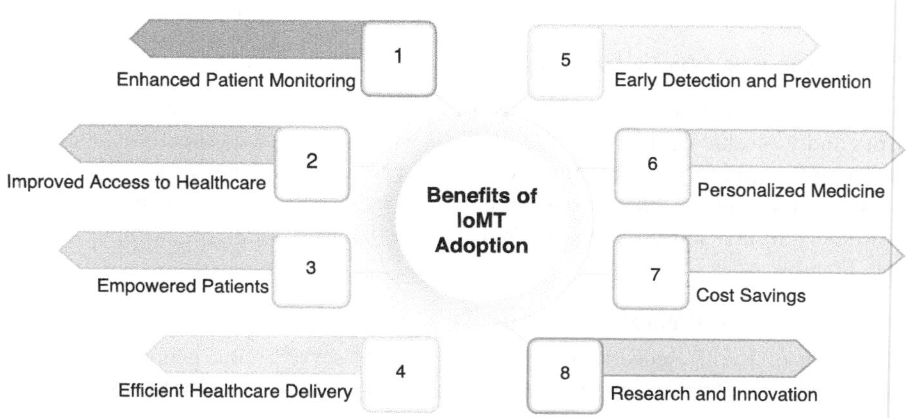

FIGURE 16.1 Benefits of IoMT.

their homes. IoMT primarily aims to provide medical services in underprivileged communities and remote places where traditional medical facilities might not be available or delivered (Dwivedi et al. 2022).

3. **Empowered Patients:** The IoMT empowers patients to take control of their health by providing access to on-time health data and personalized insights, and wearables allow individuals to monitor their vitals, movements, and sleep data, encouraging proactive health management and lifestyle modifications to prevent chronic diseases and maintain optimal health (Wagle et al. 2021).
4. **Efficient Healthcare Delivery:** IoMT streamlines healthcare delivery by optimizing clinical workflows, reducing administrative burdens, and minimizing unnecessary hospital visits. Remote patient data allows medical staff to prioritize resources, allocate personnel, and deliver targeted interventions to patients with the greatest need, leading to better use of medical resources and enhanced patient satisfaction (Monteiro et al. 2023).
5. **Early Detection and Prevention:** IoMT helps find health problems and risk factors early by constantly looking at health data, and ML tools can find patterns, trends, and outliers in health metrics. This lets healthcare providers find new health problems, predict how diseases will progress (Shiraj et al. 2022), and act before they get worse. This proactive approach to healthcare enables early intervention and preventive measures.
6. **Personalized Medicine**: According to Monteiro et al. (2023), IoMT makes custom-made medicine possible by tailoring treatments and plans to each patient's needs. By looking at a patient's health data, such as genetic markers, biomarkers, and daily habits, doctors can create personalized treatment plans, change medications, and suggest lifestyle changes that will improve therapeutic outcomes and reduce side effects.
7. **Cost Savings:** The IoMT has the potential to reduce healthcare costs by preventing hospital readmissions, minimizing emergency room visits, and optimizing resource utilization. Remote patient monitoring systems enable early detection of complications and deterioration in patients' health, enabling timely interventions, and preventing costly medical emergencies (Chaaben 2022). Additionally, by shifting care delivery from hospital settings to home and community-based settings, IoMT can reduce healthcare expenditures associated with hospital stays and inpatient care.
8. **Research and Innovation:** By aggregating and analyzing anonymized health data from diverse sources, researchers can gain insights into disease trends, treatment outcomes, and healthcare disparities, thereby informing evidence-based practice guidelines, clinical decision support systems, and public health interventions (Osama et al. 2023). Furthermore, IoMT fuels innovation in medical device technology, software development, and healthcare delivery models, driving continuous improvement and advancement in the field.

16.3.2 Key Components of IoMT's

The IoMT relies on a variety of components to gather, diffuse, and analyze medical data, including sensors and wearable devices, medical devices with embedded connectivity, cloud computing and data analytics platforms, and communication protocols and networks. These components are critical in enabling the continuous exchange of information between patients and medical staff, ultimately improving patient care and monitoring in healthcare settings, as indicated in Figure 16.2 below.

16.3.2.1 Sensors and Wearable Devices

At the forefront of IoMT, sensors and wearable devices serve as the primary means of capturing health-related data from patients in real-time. These devices typically feature various sensors, including accelerometers, gyroscopes, heart rate monitors, temperature sensors, and GPS (Global Positioning System) trackers, to measure a wide range of physiological parameters, activity levels,

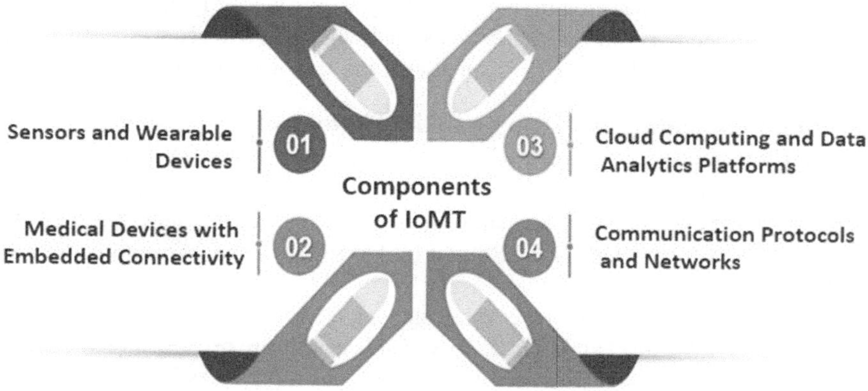

FIGURE 16.2 Components of IoMT.

and environmental factors (Adeniyi et al. 2021). You can wear wearable devices on your body or attach them to clothing or accessories to continuously monitor vital signs and health metrics throughout the day.

One of the key advantages of wearable devices is their ability to provide personalized health insights and actionable recommendations to users. By analyzing the data collected from sensors, wearable devices can track physical activity, sleep patterns, stress levels, and other health indicators, empowering individuals to make informed decisions about their health and well-being (Roy and Nahid 2022). For example, fitness trackers can monitor exercise intensity, calorie expenditure, and sleep quality, while smartwatches can track heart rate, blood pressure, and oxygen saturation levels (Anikwe et al. 2022).

In healthcare settings, wearable devices play a crucial role in remote patient monitoring, chronic disease management, and postoperative care. Patients with chronic conditions, such as diabetes, hypertension, or heart disease, can use wearable devices to monitor their health status and adherence to treatment regimens, enabling healthcare providers to intervene early in cases of abnormalities or deviations from the norm (Hariharan et al. 2021). Telemedicine platforms can also integrate wearable devices to enable virtual consultations, diagnostic assessments, and remote patient support.

16.3.2.2 Medical Devices with Embedded Connectivity

Medical devices with embedded connectivity are another essential component of IoMT, allowing medical equipment and infrastructure to be integrated into the internet-connected ecosystem. These devices encompass a diverse array of medical equipment, including blood glucose meters, blood pressure monitors, pulse oximeters, electrocardiogram (ECG) machines, and imaging devices. Equipped with wireless communication capabilities, these devices enable real-time data transfer to medical staff (Mkwashi and Brass 2022).

Embedded connectivity allows medical devices to communicate with each other, as well as with centralized monitoring systems, electronic health records (EHR) platforms, and cloud-based data repositories (Bhushan et al. 2023). For example, an ECG machine can transmit electrocardiogram readings to a cardiologist for interpretation and diagnosis, while a blood glucose meter can send glucose levels to a diabetes care team for remote monitoring and adjustment of insulin dosages.

Using medical devices that are connected to the internet improves the speed, accuracy, and efficiency of medical delivery by cutting down on mistakes made when entering data by hand, speeding up clinical workflows, and making remote consultations easier. It also lets you keep track of medical equipment usage, maintenance schedules, and performance metrics in real time

(Dwivedi et al. 2022). This makes sure that everything works perfectly and meets regulatory standards. Moreover, embedded connectivity enables medical devices to receive software updates and security patches remotely, enhancing their longevity and resilience to cyber threats.

16.3.2.3 Cloud Computing and Data Analytics Platforms

Cloud computing is what makes IoMT work. It provides a scalable infrastructure and advanced analytics tools for storing, processing, and analyzing huge amounts of health-related data. These platforms use cloud-based storage, processing, and networking technologies to handle the "volume, velocity, and variety" of data (Dilibal 2020) that IoMT devices create, so healthcare providers can act on the data.

Cloud computing platforms offer several advantages for IoMT, including scalability, flexibility, and cost-effectiveness (Wagan et al. 2022), as they enable healthcare organizations to store and access large volumes of health data securely without the need for on-premises infrastructure or expensive hardware investments. Cloud-based alternatives also offer real-time data access from anywhere, at any time, facilitating collaboration among healthcare providers, researchers, and patients.

IoMT relies on data analytics platforms to turn raw data into actionable insights and predictive models. These platforms use advanced analytics tools, like machine learning (ML) and predictive tools, to find patterns, trends, and correlations in health data. This lets medical staff spot problems, predict how diseases will progress, and make personalized treatment plans (Pandey et al. 2023). Furthermore, data analytics platforms enable population health management initiatives by analyzing health data from diverse bases, such as e-records, wearables, and medical claims databases. By analyzing population-level health trends, healthcare organizations can identify opportunities for preventive interventions and allocate resources more effectively (Khatiwada et al. 2024).

16.3.2.4 Protocols and Networks for Communicating

Communication protocols and networks are important parts of IoMT because they make it easier for IoMT devices, healthcare providers, and other stakeholders to send and receive data. These protocols set the rules and conventions for data exchange, making sure that different devices and systems can work together safely and reliably (Pushpalatha et al. 2022). Common communication protocols used in IoMT include "Bluetooth Low Energy" (BLE), Wi-Fi, Zigbee, Z-Wave, Cellular (3G/4G/5G), and LoRaWAN ("Long Range Wide Area Network"), all of which have unique applications and are applicable to different types of IoMT devices and use cases.

Wearables typically use "Bluetooth Low Energy" (BLE) to transmit data to nearby smartphones or gateway devices for short-range, power-efficient communication (Chaaben 2022). BLE enables seamless connectivity between IoMT devices and mobile apps, allowing users to access real-time health data and receive notifications on their smartphones.

Wi-Fi: Medical settings commonly use Wi-Fi, a ubiquitous wireless networking protocol, to connect IoMT gadgets to the internet and centralized monitoring systems (Zikria et al. 2020). Wi-Fi enables the real-time transmission of huge volumes of health data to healthcare providers and carers.

Zigbee: Home healthcare and assisted living environments commonly use Zigbee, a "low-power, low-data-rate" wireless communication protocol, to connect IoMT devices like smart home sensors, remote monitoring systems, and personal emergency response systems (PERS) (Ma et al. 2022). Zigbee enables interoperability between diverse IoMT devices and facilitates remote monitoring and management of patients' health status.

Z-Wave: Designed for home automation, Z-Wave functions on a diverse frequency and optimizes low-power, low-latency communication between IoMT devices (Koutras et al. 2022). Z-Wave enables seamless integration of IoMT devices into home healthcare systems, allowing patients to control and monitor their environment remotely.

Cellular (3G/4G/5G): 3G, 4G, and 5G provide wide-area wireless connectivity for IoMT devices, enabling remote monitoring and communication over long distances. Wearable medical devices and telemedicine platforms commonly adopt cellular technology to transfer health data to healthcare providers and receive timely interventions. They offer high bandwidth, low latency, and broad coverage, making them suitable for IoMT applications in diverse healthcare settings (Markova et al. 2021).

LoRaWAN, also known as the "Long Range Wide Area Network," enables IoMT devices to communicate over long distances with minimal power consumption, making it ideal for applications in remote or resource-constrained environments (Matni et al. 2020).

Overall, communication protocols and networks are critical enablers of IoMT, providing the foundation for seamless connectivity, data exchange, and interoperability between IoMT devices and healthcare systems. By leveraging a combination of wireless communication protocols, healthcare providers can build scalable, reliable, and secure IoMT solutions that improve patient care, enhance clinical workflows, and drive innovation in healthcare delivery.

16.3.3 Applications of Sensor Data Analytics in IoMT in Patient Care and Monitoring

The integration of sensor data analytics (SDA) within the framework of the IoMT represents a significant stage in the healthcare segment by leveraging advanced sensor technologies and data analytics, IoMT has the potential to revolutionize patient care, streamline medical workflows, and improve healthcare outcomes. While the IoMT refers to the interconnected ecosystem of medical devices, wearables, and sensors that collect and exchange health-related data over the internet, Sensor data analytics, on the other hand, involves the systematic analysis of data collected from these sensors to derive meaningful insights and together, they enable a new paradigm in healthcare, characterized by real-time monitoring, predictive analytics, and personalized treatment.

The SDA and IoMT has revolutionized patient care and monitoring by enabling the development of innovative healthcare solutions that leverage connected devices and digital technologies. From remote patient monitoring systems to early warning systems for health deterioration, sensor analytics IoMT applications are significantly improving the quality of patient care. This section will explore five key applications of Sensor analytics IoMT in patient care and monitoring, as illustrated in Figure 16.3 below.

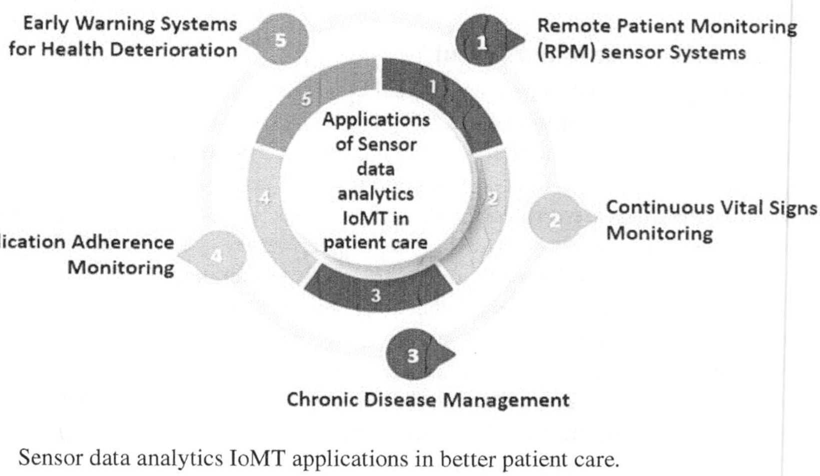

FIGURE 16.3 Sensor data analytics IoMT applications in better patient care.

16.3.3.1 Remote Patient Monitoring (RPM) Sensor Systems

RPM systems allow medical staff to constantly check patients' vitals from a distance, eliminating the requirement for in-person visits. RPM systems classically consist of wearables and telemedicine platforms that enable real-time data transmission using SDA and communication between patients and healthcare providers (Jeba Kumar et al. 2021), and these systems are predominantly helpful for chronic patients, elderly individuals, and post-operative patients who require ongoing monitoring and support.

Wearables in an RPM system continuously gather physiological data from patients, such as "heart rate, blood pressure, blood glucose levels, and activity levels" (Sadhu et al. 2022), wirelessly transmitting this data to a centralized monitoring platform or cloud app for analysis of anomalies, trends, and patterns using SDA. Healthcare providers can access the patient's data remotely through a secure web portal or mobile app, allowing them to track changes in health status, monitor treatment effectiveness, and intervene in cases of emergencies or abnormalities (Razdan and Sharma 2022).

RPM systems offer several advantages over traditional healthcare delivery models, such as enhanced patient care, reduced medical costs by enabling remote monitoring through SDA and virtual consultations, and minimizing the requirement for medical staff visits and expenses for patients.

16.3.3.2 Continuous Vital Signs Monitoring

Continuous vital signs monitoring involves the real-time measurement and tracking of key physiological parameters, such as "heart rate, respiratory rate, blood pressure, temperature, and oxygen saturation levels" using SDA (Rubi and Dhivya 2022). IoMT devices, such as wearable sensors, medical-grade monitors, and bedside monitors, allow patients' vital signs to be continuously monitored using SDA.

Continuous vital signs monitoring is essential for detecting changes in patients' health status, identifying signs of deterioration, and initiating timely interventions to prevent adverse outcomes and SDA can assist in achieving the same (Balasubramanian et al. 2021). For example, continuous monitoring of heart rate and rhythm can detect arrhythmias, ischemia, and other cardiac abnormalities early, allowing healthcare providers to intervene with appropriate treatments, such as medications or cardioversion. Similarly, continuous monitoring of blood pressure can identify hypertensive crises or hypotensive episodes, prompting adjustments in medication dosages or fluid management.

Continuous vital sign monitoring is particularly valuable in "intensive care units (ICUs) and emergency departments," where patients require close monitoring and rapid intervention. Medical staff can continuously track vitals with IoMT devices like wearable patches, wireless monitors, and bedside sensors, and receive real-time alerts when they detect abnormalities using SDA (Lu et al. 2021) and this proactive monitoring approach enables early detection of deteriorating health.

16.3.3.3 Chronic Disease Management

It involves treating patients with chronic medical conditions such as diabetes, hypertension, heart disease, chronic obstructive pulmonary disease (COPD), and asthma using IoMT technologies (Bendre and Khurge 2022) by allowing remote nursing, self-management, and personalized interventions tailored to individual patients' needs and preferences.

In chronic disease management, IoMT devices such as glucometers, blood pressure monitors, spirometers, and peak flow meters allow patients to keep track of their health data from home and provide data to medical staff for review and analysis (Rajamohan et al. 2022). This approach permits medical staff to assess patients' obedience to treatment regimens, monitor disease progression, and adjust medications or interventions as needed.

Moreover, IoMT devices and SDA can facilitate patient education, self-management, and behavior modification by giving on-time advice and reminders (Rayan et al. 2022). For example, mobile apps remind patients to take their medications, monitor their diet and exercise habits, and provide educational resources on managing their condition.

16.3.3.4 Monitoring Medication Adherence

Medication adherence monitoring involves tracking patients' adherence to prescribed medication regimens and identifying barriers to compliance with medications. This is a common problem in healthcare (Ghozali 2023), with increasing medical costs and higher rates of hospital admissions and adverse events. IoMT technologies offer innovative solutions for medication adherence monitoring, enabling medical staff to screen patients' medication-taking behavior and intervene when adherence issues arise.

IoMT devices, like smart pill dispensers, medication reminder apps, and connected pill bottles, track patients' medication usage in medication adherence monitoring and send alerts or notifications when patients miss or delay doses using SDA (Karagiannis et al. 2022). These SDA devices can also record the date, time, and dosage of each medication taken by the patient, providing a comprehensive overview of their adherence patterns over time. Healthcare providers can access this data remotely through a secure online portal or mobile apps.

Medication adherence monitoring technologies can also incorporate feedback mechanisms to encourage and reward adherence behaviors (Kelly et al. 2020). For example, smart pill dispensers may emit audible or visual reminders when medications are due, and a few devices may even provide positive reinforcement messages or incentives for adherent behavior using SDA. Additionally, IoMT platforms can generate adherence reports and trend analyses, which healthcare providers can use during patient consultations to discuss adherence challenges, address medication misconceptions, and develop strategies for improving adherence (Bharati et al. 2021). By leveraging IoMT technologies for medication adherence monitoring, healthcare providers can effectively personalize interventions, identify adherence patterns, and address barriers to medication adherence.

16.3.3.5 Early Warning Systems for Health Deterioration

Early warning systems for health deterioration use IoMT technologies to find signs that a patient's condition is getting worse and to take action quickly to avoid bad outcomes. These systems usually use predictive analytics algorithms, machine learning models, and real-time monitoring data to spot small changes in a patient's health status (Toor et al. 2020) that could mean their condition is about to get worse or is already getting worse.

IoMT devices continuously monitor patients' vitals in an early warning system, generating a stream of real-time data that analysts analyze for anomalies, deviations from baseline, and patterns indicative of deterioration (Rajasekar et al. 2024) and apply advanced analytics, like trend analysis and risk stratification, to identify patients at risk of deterioration and generate alerts or notifications for healthcare providers adopting SDA devices.

Healthcare providers can seamlessly receive alerts and notifications by integrating early warning systems into existing clinical workflows, including "electronic health records" (EHR) systems, nurse call systems, and bedside monitors (Mitra et al. 2022). For example, an early warning system may trigger an alert when a patient's heart rate exceeds a predefined threshold or when oxygen saturation levels drop below a certain level, prompting nurses or clinicians to assess the patient's condition and initiate appropriate interventions.

Studies have shown that the implementation of early warning systems for health deterioration reduces the incidence of adverse events, such as cardiac arrests, sepsis, and respiratory failure, in hospital settings. These systems enable early detection of patient deterioration, facilitating timely interventions, preventing clinical deterioration, and improving patient outcomes. Moreover, early warning systems can enhance patient safety, optimize resource utilization, and reduce healthcare costs by minimizing the need for emergency interventions and intensive care admissions.

The applications of SDA as a part of IoMT in patient care and monitoring are diverse and transformative, offering innovative solutions for remote monitoring, chronic disease management, medication adherence monitoring, and early detection of health deterioration. By leveraging IoMT technologies, healthcare providers can deliver personalized, proactive, and patient-centered care,

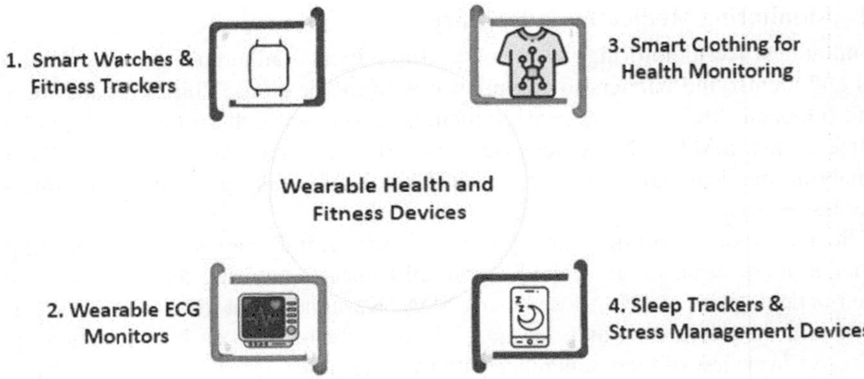

FIGURE 16.4 Types of wearable health and fitness devices.

improving treatment outcomes, enhancing patient satisfaction, and reducing healthcare costs. As IoMT evolves, its potential to revolutionize patient care and monitoring will only grow, driving innovation and advancements in healthcare delivery worldwide.

16.3.4 Wearable Health and Fitness Devices

Wearables have, over the years, become progressively popular, offering individuals the capability to look into various characteristics of their health and well-being in real-time. These devices, which include smartwatches, fitness trackers, wearable ECG monitors, smart clothing, sleep trackers, and stress management gadgets, assist people with valuable insights into their movement, vital signs, sleep patterns, and stress levels. This section will explore the key features and benefits of each type of wearable health and fitness device as given in Figure 16.4 below.

16.3.4.1 Smart Watches and Fitness Trackers

Smart watches and fitness trackers are among the most widely used wearable health and fitness devices, offering a wide range of features to help users track and improve their overall health and well-being. These devices typically include sensors for monitoring heart rate, steps taken, calories burned, distance travelled, and sleep quality. They also often feature GPS tracking, activity recognition, smartphone connectivity for notifications, and app integration (Perumal 2023).

Smart watches and fitness trackers are versatile devices that cater to users with varying fitness goals and lifestyle preferences, as they provide real-time feedback on their activity levels, encouraging them to stay active throughout the day and achieve their fitness targets. Additionally, many smart watches and fitness trackers offer advanced features such as heart rate variability monitoring, guided workouts, and personalized coaching to help users optimize their workouts and improve their overall fitness (Yadav et al. 2024).

One of the key benefits of smart watches and fitness trackers is their ability to provide insights into users' sleep patterns and quality of sleep. By monitoring metrics such as sleep duration, sleep stages, and sleep disturbances, these devices can help users identify factors that may be affecting their sleep and make lifestyle changes to improve sleep quality. Additionally, some smart watches and fitness trackers offer features such as silent alarms and sleep tracking, which can help users establish healthier sleep habits and wake up feeling refreshed.

16.3.4.2 Wearable ECG Monitors

Wearable ECG monitors are specialized devices designed to continuously monitor the electrical activity of the heart. Typically, these devices wear a small, portable sensor on the chest or wrist, which wirelessly connects to a smartphone or other mobile device. Wearable ECG monitors provide users with real-time feedback on their heart rhythm, allowing them to detect irregularities such as arrhythmias, atrial fibrillation, and other cardiac abnormalities (Rubi and Dhivya 2022).

The primary use of wearable ECG monitors is the early detection of potentially life-threatening heart conditions by continuously monitoring the heart's electrical activity. These devices can detect abnormalities that may not be evident during routine medical check-ups or intermittent monitoring (Pushparaj and Saini 2023). Early detection of cardiac arrhythmias and other heart conditions can help users seek timely medical intervention, prevent complications, and improve overall cardiac health.

16.3.4.3 Smart Clothing for Health Monitoring

Smart clothing is a relatively new category of wearable health and fitness devices that integrates sensors and electronics into garments such as shirts, bras, socks, and shorts. These garments contain embedded sensors that monitor various physiological parameters. Marr (2020) intended smart clothing to be comfortable, lightweight, and unobtrusive, making it suitable for everyday wear.

One of the primary benefits of smart clothing is that it provides continuous, non-invasive monitoring of vital signs without the need for additional accessories or devices (Liu et al. 2020), and by embedding sensors directly into the garment's fabric, smart clothing can track users' health metrics discreetly and accurately without interfering with their daily activities. This makes smart clothing particularly well-suited for applications such as remote patient monitoring, elder care, and sports performance monitoring.

16.3.4.4 Sleep Trackers and Stress Management Devices

They are wearable health and fitness devices designed to help users monitor and manage their sleep and stress, and these devices typically use multiple sensors, such as "accelerometers, heart rate monitors, and skin conductivity sensors," to track users' sleep quality, sleep duration, and stress levels throughout the day (Rachakonda et al. 2020). They also often include features such as guided breathing exercises and relaxation tools to help users improve their sleep quality.

One of the primary benefits of sleep trackers and stress management devices is their ability to provide consumers with valuable data on their sleep habits and stress levels, enabling them to make changes. These devices, by monitoring metrics such as sleep duration, sleep stages, and heart rate variability, can help users identify factors (Imtiaz 2021) that may be contributing to poor sleep and high stress levels, such as caffeine consumption, screen time, or work-related stress. Additionally, sleep trackers and stress management devices can provide users with personalized recommendations and feedback to help them establish healthier sleep habits and coping strategies.

Wearable health and fitness devices offer users a convenient and effective way to monitor and manage various dimensions of their fitness and well-being. From smart watches and fitness trackers to wearable ECG monitors, smart clothing, sleep trackers, and stress management devices, these devices provide users with valuable insights into their activity, vitals, sleep schedule, and stress levels, empowering them to make informed decisions about their health and lifestyle.

16.3.5 Application of IoMT in Hospital Settings

The incorporation of IoMT devices in hospitals has revolutionized healthcare delivery by enhancing efficiency, improving patient care, and optimizing clinical workflows. From integration with Electronic Health Records (EHR) to real-time location systems (RTLS) for asset tracking, smart infusion pumps, and IoMT-enabled surgical and diagnostic equipment, IoMT technologies (Rana et al. 2022) offer a wide range of benefits for hospitals and medical staff, and this part will look into the key applications and benefits of IoMT in hospital settings as given in Figure 16.5 below.

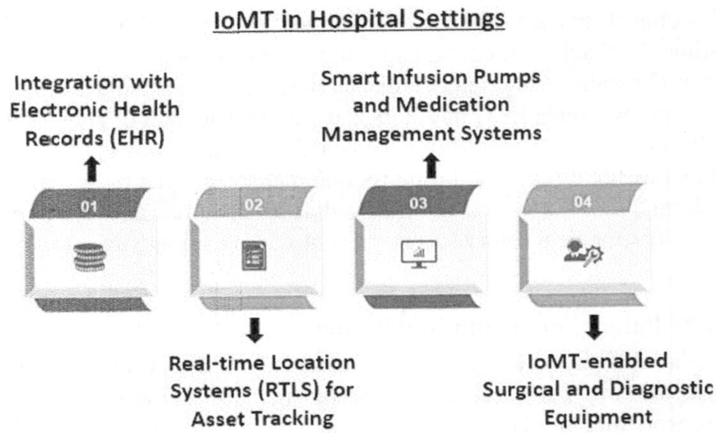

FIGURE 16.5 IoMT application in hospital settings.

16.3.5.1 Integration with Electronic Health Records (EHR)

The integration of IoMT devices with Electronic Health Records (EHR) systems, such as wearable sensors, medical monitors, and diagnostic equipment, is a primary application of IoMT in hospital settings. These devices generate vast amounts of patient data that healthcare providers can seamlessly access in real-time (Girardi et al. 2020). This integration enables healthcare providers to access up-to-date patient information, track changes in health status, and make informed clinical decisions.

By integrating IoMT devices with EHR systems, hospitals can improve the accuracy and completeness of patient records, reduce duplicate data entry, and streamline clinical documentation processes (Vaiyapuri et al. 2021). Healthcare providers can access patient data from any location, at any time, using web-based EHR platforms or mobile applications, enabling more efficient care coordination and collaboration among multidisciplinary care teams. Additionally, the integration of IoMT devices with EHR systems facilitates automated data capture, trend analysis, and decision support, enhancing the quality and safety of patient care.

16.3.5.2 Real-Time Location Systems (RTLS)

Real-time Location Systems (RTLS) are another key application of IoMT in hospital settings, enabling hospitals to track the location and movement of assets, equipment, and personnel in real-time. RTLS solutions typically use a combination of technologies, such as radio frequency identification (RFID), Bluetooth Low Energy (BLE), and Wi-Fi, to provide accurate indoor positioning and tracking capabilities.

Hospitals use RTLS solutions to locate medical equipment like infusion pumps and defibrillators, as well as high-value assets like wheelchairs, stretchers, and mobile carts. By providing real-time data, RTLS solutions help hospitals optimize asset utilization, reduce equipment loss or theft, and improve staff efficiency by reducing the time spent searching for equipment (Banat 2020).

Furthermore, RTLS solutions can improve patient safety by ensuring that critical equipment is readily available when needed and automating asset maintenance and inspection processes. For example, RTLS-enabled smart infusion pumps can automatically alert staff when maintenance is due, track medication usage and dosages in real-time, and provide insights into infusion pump utilization patterns to optimize inventory management and staffing levels.

16.3.5.3 Using Smart Infusion Pumps and Medication Management Systems

They are IoMT-enabled devices that automate and enhance medication administration processes in hospital settings. These devices integrate with EHR systems to provide clinicians with real-time access to patient medication orders, dosing guidelines, and alerts for medication errors or adverse drug interactions (Arthi et al. 2022).

Advanced technology, including "dose error reduction systems" (DERS), drug libraries, and barcode scanning capabilities, equips these pumps to ensure the safe and accurate delivery of intravenous medications. These pumps can automatically calculate infusion rates based on multiple factors like patient weight, age, and medical condition, thereby reducing the risk of medication errors and adverse drug events (Kaur et al. 2022). Additionally, smart infusion pumps can generate electronic medication administration records (eMARs) and audit trails for documentation and regulatory compliance purposes.

Medication management systems, such as automated dispensing cabinets (ADCs) and pharmacy robotics, automate medication dispensing, storage, and inventory management processes in hospital pharmacies. These systems use IoMT technologies to track medication usage, expiration dates, and stock levels in real-time, ensuring that medications are readily available when needed and reducing the risk of medication shortages or stockouts. Moreover, medication management systems can integrate with EHR systems to provide clinicians with access to patients' medication histories, allergies, and drug interactions, enabling more informed prescribing decisions (Shanmugam and Azam 2023).

16.3.5.4 IoMT-Enabled Surgical and Diagnostic Equipment

IoMT technologies are also changing hospital surgical and diagnostic tools, making care faster, more accurate, and more tailored to each patient. Surgical robots like the da Vinci Surgical System use advanced robotics, AI, and IoMT sensors to improve surgical precision, dexterity, and visualization, which lowers the risk of complications and improves patient outcomes (Razdan and Sharma 2022).

Furthermore, diagnostic imaging equipment, such as MRI machines, CT scanners, and ultrasound devices, is increasingly being equipped with IoMT capabilities to enable real-time image acquisition, processing, and interpretation. These IoMT-enabled imaging systems can automatically adjust imaging parameters based on patient characteristics, optimize image quality, and reduce radiation exposure, thereby improving diagnostic accuracy and efficiency.

IoMT technologies offer numerous benefits for hospitals and healthcare providers, including improved clinical workflows, enhanced patient care, and increased operational efficiency. From integration with EHR systems to real-time location tracking, smart infusion pumps, and IoMT-enabled surgical and diagnostic equipment, IoMT is transforming hospital settings and revolutionizing the delivery of healthcare. As IoMT continues to evolve, its potential to improve patient outcomes and drive innovation in healthcare delivery will only continue to grow.

16.3.6 Security and Privacy in the IoMT

While IoMT has various benefits, including improved patient care, enhanced monitoring capabilities, and increased efficiency (Hireche et al. 2022). However, along with these benefits come significant security and privacy concerns. As IoMT devices collect, transmit, and store patient data, it is important to protect them and ensure patient privacy and confidentiality. This section will look at key security and privacy considerations in IoMT and strategies for mitigating associated risks, as shown in Figure 16.6 below.

16.3.6.1 Data Encryption and Secure Communication Protocols

Data encryption is a fundamental security measure for protecting sensitive patient information transmitted between IoMT devices, healthcare providers, and data repositories. Encryption techniques, such as Advanced Encryption Standard (AES) and Transport Layer Security (TLS), encrypt data in transit and at rest, rendering it unreadable to unauthorized parties. Furthermore, the implementation of secure communication protocols like HTTPS, MQTT, and CoAP guarantees the secure transmission of data across networks, preventing any potential interception or manipulation by malicious actors (Bhushan et al. 2023).

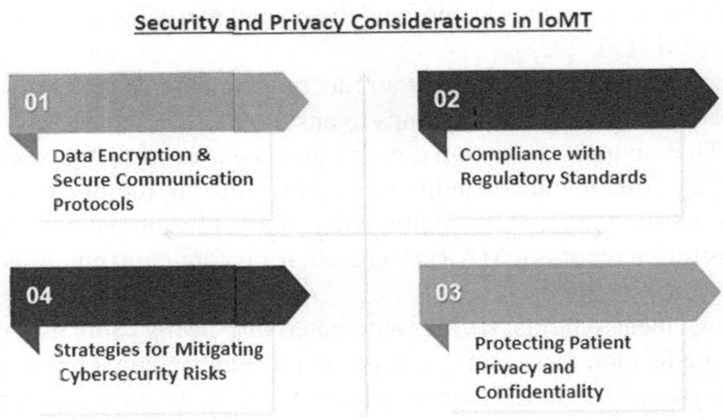

FIGURE 16.6 Security and privacy in IoMT.

Implementing end-to-end encryption and strong authentication mechanisms, such as public-key infrastructure (PKI) and multi-factor authentication (MFA), further enhances security by verifying the identity of users and devices and preventing unauthorised access to sensitive data. By encrypting data and using secure communication protocols, healthcare organizations can guard patient data from unlawful access, interception, and tampering, safeguarding patient privacy and confidentiality.

16.3.6.2 Compliance with Regulatory Standards

Compliance with regulatory standards, such as the "Health Insurance Portability and Accountability Act" (HIPAA) in the United States and countries such as India and the "General Data Protection Regulation" (GDPR) in the European Union, is indispensable for ensuring the security and privacy of patient data in IoMT systems and is important to protect patient data (Tyagi et al. 2023).

Healthcare firms must make sure that their IoMT systems comply with relevant regulatory standards and guidelines to avoid potential legal and financial consequences (Morphy 2021), and this includes having scheduled and random risk audits and providing staff training on safe best practices and compliance requirements. By following the prescribed regulatory standards, medical firms can demonstrate their obligation to protect patient data and confidentiality, as well as build trust with patients and stakeholders.

16.3.6.3 Protecting Patient Privacy and Confidentiality

It is one of the most paramount aspects of IoMT, as healthcare data often contains sensitive information, including personal identifiers, the history of the patient, and treatment records. Hospitals must adopt stringent access controls, data minimization practices, and anonymization techniques to ensure that data is limited only to authorised individuals (Searle and Gururaj 2023).

Furthermore, healthcare organizations should have clear policies for managing patient data to ensure that patient information is managed in a safe way, and this includes encrypting data stored on IoMT devices and servers, implementing access controls and audit trails, and securely disposing of data when it is no longer needed. By prioritizing patient privacy and confidentiality, healthcare organizations can mitigate the risk of data breaches, identity theft, and unauthorized disclosure, maintaining patient trust and confidence in the healthcare system.

16.3.6.4 Strategies for Mitigating Cybersecurity Risks

IoMT systems face significant cybersecurity risks due to their frequent internet connectivity, making them susceptible to various cyber threats such as malware, ransomware, and phishing attacks. Healthcare organizations must implement comprehensive cybersecurity measures (Rahman and Jahankhani 2021) to protect against these threats, including network segmentation, intrusion detection and prevention systems (IDPS), and regular security assessments and penetration testing.

Additionally, healthcare organizations should educate staff and end-users about cybersecurity best practices, such as creating strong passwords, recognizing phishing attempts, and avoiding the use of unsecured networks (Kalinaki et al. 2023). Implementing security awareness training programs can help raise awareness about potential threats and empower employees to identify and respond to security incidents effectively.

Furthermore, healthcare organizations should establish incident response plans and procedures for responding to security breaches and data breaches promptly, and by implementing proactive cybersecurity measures and incident response protocols, healthcare organizations can minimize the impact of security breaches and protect patient data from unauthorized access or disclosure.

Security and privacy considerations are paramount in IoMT, as hospitals and clinics must ensure the confidentiality of patient data while leveraging IoMT technologies to improve patient care and outcomes. By employing safe security measures, confirming regulatory standards, protecting patient privacy and confidentiality, and mitigating cybersecurity risks, medical firms can reap the benefits of IoMT.

16.4 CHALLENGES AND FUTURE DIRECTIONS OF THE IoMT

The IoMT holds immense potential to revolutionize medical services through RMS, personalized treatments, and improved patient outcomes. However, to fully reap the benefits of IoMT, we must address several challenges, with ongoing research and innovation shaping future directions in this field. This section will discuss the key challenges facing IoMT, as well as future directions and emerging trends, as shown in Figure 16.7 below.

16.4.1 Interoperability Issues and Standardization Efforts

One of the primary challenges facing IoMT is interoperability, as IoMT devices often use proprietary protocols and formats that hinder seamless data exchange and integration with existing healthcare systems (Yasmeen et al. 2022). Efforts to standardize data formats, communication protocols, and interoperability frameworks are essential to enabling seamless integration of IoMT devices into healthcare ecosystems.

Standardization bodies, such as the "Institute of Electrical and Electronics Engineers" (IEEE), the "International Organization for Standardization" (ISO), and the "Healthcare Information and Management Systems Society (HIMSS), are developing standards and guidelines for interoperability and data exchange in IoMT (Shiraj et al. 2022). These efforts aim to define common data models,

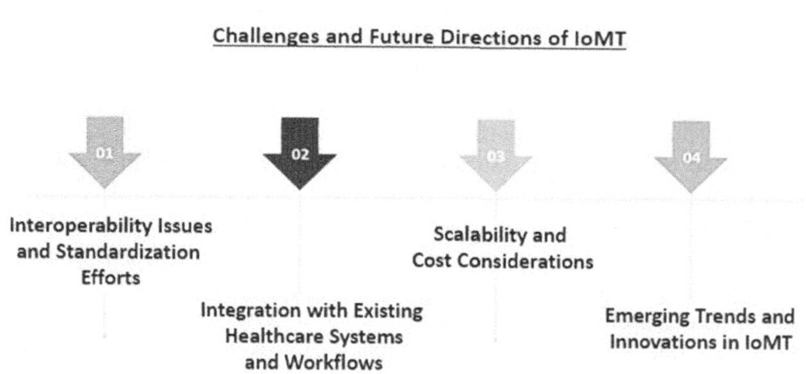

FIGURE 16.7 Challenges and future directions of IoMT.

communication protocols, and interfaces to facilitate interoperability between IoMT devices, electronic health records (EHR) systems, and other healthcare IT systems.

Future directions in IoMT include the development of open standards and interoperability frameworks that enable plug-and-play integration of IoMT devices into existing healthcare systems. By adopting open standards and interoperability frameworks, medical firms can reduce integration costs, improve data exchange, and enhance collaboration among stakeholders.

Another challenge facing IoMT is the integration of IoMT devices into existing medical systems and workflows. Firms must navigate complex regulatory requirements, data privacy concerns, and workflow disruptions when implementing IoMT solutions, which can hinder adoption and scalability (Dwivedi et al. 2022).

Future directions in IoMT include the development of interoperable IoMT platforms that integrate seamlessly with existing healthcare systems, such as EHR systems, clinical decision support systems, and telehealth platforms. These platforms leverage application programming interfaces (APIs) and middleware to facilitate data exchange and workflow integration, enabling healthcare providers to access IoMT data within familiar workflows and interfaces.

Additionally, future IoMT solutions will focus on user-centered design principles to ensure that IoMT devices are intuitive, easy to use, and seamlessly integrate into clinical workflows. By prioritizing usability and workflow integration, healthcare organizations can minimize disruption and maximize the value of IoMT solutions, leading to better adoption and acceptance among clinicians and staff.

Future directions in IoMT include developing scalable and cost-effective IoMT architectures and deployment models that leverage cloud computing, edge computing, and distributed processing capabilities. These architectures enable healthcare organizations to scale IoMT deployments rapidly and cost-effectively by leveraging elastic computing resources and pay-as-you-go pricing models.

Furthermore, future IoMT solutions will focus on maximizing the value of data generated by IoMT devices through advanced analytics, artificial intelligence (AI), and machine learning (ML) techniques. By analyzing IoMT data in real-time and deriving actionable insights, healthcare organizations can optimize resource allocation, improve clinical decision-making, and enhance patient outcomes, ultimately driving greater value from IoMT investments.

16.4.2 Emerging Trends and Innovations in IoMT

Several emerging trends and innovations are shaping the future of IoMT, including wearable biosensors, implantable devices, remote patient monitoring systems, and telemedicine platforms. These innovations are enabling new use cases and applications in areas such as chronic disease management, remote patient monitoring, and personalized medicine.

Future directions in IoMT include the development of advanced biosensors and wearable devices that can monitor a wide range of physiological parameters, biomarkers, and health metrics in real-time. These devices will enable continuous, non-invasive monitoring of patients' health status, allowing for early detection of health issues, proactive interventions, and personalized treatments.

Additionally, future IoMT solutions will leverage emerging technologies such as 5G, edge computing, and blockchain to enhance connectivity, security, and data privacy in IoMT deployments. These technologies will enable faster data transmission, lower latency, and greater resilience to cyber threats, ensuring the reliability and integrity of IoMT systems.

IoMT holds immense promise to alter healthcare services by ensuring remote monitoring, personalized treatments, and improved patient outcomes. However, to fully realize the potential of IoMT, we must address several challenges such as interoperability issues, integration with existing medical services, scalability and cost considerations, and privacy and security concerns.

16.5 CONTRIBUTIONS OF THE STUDY

There are numerous implications of this article which are listed as follows

Implication for Healthcare Professionals:

- The study gives the readers the various importance and benefits of IoMT adoption in hospitals.
- Healthcare professionals can have a general understanding on the IoMT's key components and the usage of these components.
- The study attempts to consolidate the various applications of IoMT in patient care and monitoring which can help healthcare practioners to have the idea on the various applications of IoMT.
- The study gives an overall view on the various wearable health and fitness devices as a part of the IoMT in Hospital Settings and their benefits and applications.
- The article also indicates the various security and privacy considerations in the IoMT space and gives the healthcare professionals on potential hazards of adopting IoMT.

Implications for Future Research:

There are various implications for future research such as

- Explore how IoMT can be customized for managing different chronic conditions, mental health, and care for specific populations (elderly, children) and at specific healthcare settings.
- Investigate integrating IoMT with prominent and recent technologies such as AI, big data analytics, and blockchain to personalize care, predict health risks, and enhance data security.
- Explore and address data security, interoperability, digital divide, and algorithmic bias to ensure equitable access, privacy, and fair healthcare delivery.
- Analyze cost-effectiveness, return on investment, and sustainable business models for implementing IoMT solutions in healthcare.
- Focus on user-friendly IoMT devices and explore how IoMT can empower patients to manage their health and participate in decision-making.
- Research how IoMT, combined with advanced technologies, can transform healthcare delivery towards a more preventive, personalized, and patient-centered model.

16.6 CONCLUSION

The IoMT signifies a profound shift in healthcare delivery, presenting unparalleled prospects to improve patient care, improve clinical outcomes, and streamline healthcare workflows. By integrating connected devices, sensors, and data analytics, IoMT enables real-time monitoring, personalized treatments, and proactive interventions, fundamentally altering the landscape of healthcare delivery. Throughout this comprehensive exploration of IoMT, several key findings and insights have emerged. IoMT offers various benefits, including remote patient monitoring, continuous vitals measurement, chronic disease management, medication adherence monitoring, and early warning systems for health deterioration. Key components of IoMT encompass sensors and wearable devices, medical devices with embedded connectivity, cloud computing and data analytics platforms, and communication protocols and networks. IoMT is used in many areas of healthcare, such as hospitals, clinics, nursing homes, and home healthcare. It makes it easy to connect to electronic health records (EHR), real-time location systems (RTLS) for tracking assets, smart infusion pumps, and surgical and diagnostic equipment that is IoMT-enabled.

Security and privacy considerations stand as paramount in IoMT, necessitating data encryption compliance with regulatory standards (such as HIPAA and GDPR), protection of patient privacy and confidentiality, and strategies for mitigating cybersecurity risks. The challenges and future directions of IoMT include interoperability, integration with existing healthcare systems and workflows scalability and cost considerations, and emerging trends and innovations. Healthcare providers are encouraged to embrace IoMT technologies to enhance patient care, optimize clinical workflows, and improve outcomes. Investing in interoperable IoMT solutions, prioritizing patient privacy and data security, and integrating IoMT devices into clinical workflows are recommended strategies to maximize their value. The advancements in IoMT solutions will become more interoperable, scalable, and cost-effective, driving greater adoption and acceptance among healthcare providers and patients. IoMT will play a crucial role in addressing healthcare challenges such as chronic disease management, aging populations, and rising healthcare costs. In conclusion, IoMT represents a transformative force in healthcare delivery, offering unprecedented opportunities to improve patient care, enhance clinical workflows, and drive innovation. Addressing challenges such as interoperability, data privacy, and cybersecurity, and embracing emerging trends and innovations are essential steps in realizing the full potential of IoMT. Collaboration among healthcare providers, policymakers, and industry stakeholders is crucial to accelerate the adoption of IoMT and create a healthier, more connected future for all.

REFERENCES

Aceto, G., Persico, V., & Pescapé, A. (2018). The role of information and communication technologies in healthcare: taxonomies, perspectives, and challenges. *Journal of Network and Computer Applications*, 107, 125–154.

Adarsha, A. S., Reader, K., & Erban, S. (2019). User experience, IoMT, and healthcare. *AIS Transactions on Human-Computer Interaction*, 11(4), 264–273.

Adeniyi, E. A., Ogundokun, R. O., & Awotunde, J. B. (2021). IoMT-based wearable body sensors network healthcare monitoring system. In Marques, G., Bhoi, A. K., & Hareesha, K. S. (eds) *IoT in Healthcare and Ambient Assisted Living. Studies in Computational Intelligence* (vol. 933, pp. 103–121). Springer, Singapore.

Adewole, K. S., Akintola, A. G., Jimoh, R. G., Mabayoje, M. A., Jimoh, M. K., Usman-Hamza, F. E., …, & Ameen, A. O. (2021). Cloud-based IoMT framework for cardiovascular disease prediction and diagnosis in personalized E-health care. In Arun Kumar, S., & Subhas, C. (eds) *Intelligent IoT Systems in Personalized Health Care* (pp. 105–145). Academic Press.

Ahmed, S. F., Alam, M. S. B., Afrin, S., Rafa, S. J., Rafa, N., & Gandomi, A. H. (2024). Insights into Internet of Medical Things (IoMT): data fusion, security issues and potential solutions. *Information Fusion*, 102, 102060.

Anikwe, C. V., Nweke, H. F., Ikegwu, A. C., Egwuonwu, C. A., Onu, F. U., Alo, U. R., & Teh, Y. W. (2022). Mobile and wearable sensors for data-driven health monitoring system: state-of-the-art and future prospect. *Expert Systems with Applications*, 202, 117362.

Arthi, K., Chidhambararajan, B., & Revathi, A. R. (2022, December). A deep investigation of architectural elements and computing technologies for internet of medical things. In *2022 6th International Conference on Electronics, Communication and Aerospace Technology* (pp. 556–563). IEEE, Coimbatore, India.

Awotunde, J. B., Ogundokun, R. O., & Misra, S. (2021). Cloud and IoMT-based big data analytics system during COVID-19 pandemic. In Chinmay, C. & Siddhartha, B. (eds) *Efficient Data Handling for Massive Internet of Medical Things: Healthcare Data Analytics* (pp. 181–201). Springer International Publishing, Cham.

Balasubramanian, V., Sulthana, R., Stranieri, A., Manoharan, G., Arora, T., Srinivasan, R., … & Menon, V. G. (2021, October). A secured real-time IoMT application for monitoring isolated COVID-19 patients using edge computing. In *2021 IEEE 20th International Conference on Trust, Security and Privacy in Computing and Communications (TrustCom)* (pp. 1227–1234). IEEE, Shenyang, China.

Banat, D. (2020). Conditions of cost-effectiveness for the use of real-time location systems (RTLS) in medical facilities and the benefits of effective implementation process. *Edukacja Ekonomistów i Menedżerów*, 58(4), 21–34.

Bendre, V., & Khurge, D. (2022). Introduction to smart healthcare using IoMT. In Shinde, S.V., Mahalle, P. N., Bendre, V., & Castillo, O. (eds), *Disruptive Developments in Biomedical Applications* (pp. 109–125). CRC Press, London.

Bharati, S., Podder, P., Mondal, M. R. H., & Paul, P. K. (2021). Applications and challenges of cloud integrated IoMT. In Hassanien, A. E., Slowik, A., Khamparia, A., Gupta, D. & Shankar, K. (eds) *Cognitive Internet of Medical Things for Smart Healthcare: Services and Applications* (pp. 67–85). Springer, Cham.

Bhushan, B., Kumar, A., Agarwal, A. K., Kumar, A., Bhattacharya, P., & Kumar, A. (2023). Towards a secure and sustainable internet of medical things (IoMT): requirements, design challenges, security techniques, and future trends. *Sustainability*, 15(7), 6177.

Chaaben, A. B. (2022). A survey of different IoMT protocols for healthcare applications. *Research Berg Review of Science and Technology*, 2(1), 41–57.

Dilibal, Ç. (2020, October). Development of edge-IoMT computing architecture for smart healthcare monitoring platform. In *2020 4th International Symposium on Multidisciplinary Studies and Innovative Technologies (ISMSIT)* (pp. 1–4). IEEE, Turkey.

Dwivedi, R., Mehrotra, D., & Chandra, S. (2022). Potential of Internet of Medical Things (IoMT) applications in building a smart healthcare system: a systematic review. *Journal of Oral Biology and Craniofacial Research*, 12(2), 302–318.

Ghozali, M. T. (2023). Implementation of the IoT-based technology on patient medication adherence: a comprehensive bibliometric and systematic review. *Journal of Information and Communication Technology*, 22(4), 503–544.

Girardi, F., De Gennaro, G., Colizzi, L., & Convertini, N. (2020). Improving the healthcare effectiveness: the possible role of EHR, IoMT and blockchain. *Electronics*, 9(6), 884.

Hariharan, U., Rajkumar, K., Akilan, T., & Jeyavel, J. (2021). Smart wearable devices for remote patient monitoring in Healthcare 4.0. In Hemanth, D. J., Anitha, J., & Tsihrintzis, G. A. (eds), *Internet of Medical Things: Remote Healthcare Systems and Applications* (pp. 117–135). Springer, Cham.

Hireche, R., Mansouri, H., & Pathan, A. S. K. (2022). Security and privacy management in Internet of Medical Things (IoMT): a synthesis. *Journal of Cybersecurity and Privacy*, 2(3), 640–661.

Imtiaz, S. A. (2021). A systematic review of sensing technologies for wearable sleep staging. *Sensors*, 21(5), 1562.

Jain, S. S., Kothari, S. M., & Agrawal, S. K. (2024). The role of IoMT technologies in revolutionizing healthcare: a comprehensive overview. In Sushmita Sunil Jain, Saurabh Manoj Kothari, & Satyam Kumar Agrawal (eds) *WSN and IoT* (1st edition, pp. 187–202). CRC Press.

Jeba Kumar, R. J. S., Roopa Jayasingh, J., & Telagathoti, D. B. (2021). Intelligent transit healthcare schema using internet of medical things (IoMT) technology for remote patient monitoring. In Jude Hemanth, D., Anitha, J., & Tsihrintzis, G. A. (eds) *Internet of Medical Things: Remote Healthcare Systems and Applications* (pp. 17–33). Berlin, Heidelberg.

Kakhi, K., Alizadehsani, R., Kabir, H. D., Khosravi, A., Nahavandi, S., & Acharya, U. R. (2022). The internet of medical things and artificial intelligence: trends, challenges, and opportunities. *Biocybernetics and Biomedical Engineering*, 42(3), 749–771.

Kalinaki, K., Fahadi, M., Alli, A. A., Shafik, W., Yasin, M., & Mutwalibi, N. (2023). Artificial intelligence of internet of medical things (AIoMT) in smart cities: a review of cybersecurity for smart healthcare. In Lucky Imoize, A. & Balas, V. E. (eds) *Handbook of Security and Privacy of AI-Enabled Healthcare Systems and Internet of Medical Things* (pp. 271–292). CRC Press, London.

Karagiannis, D., Mitsis, K., & Nikita, K. S. (2022). Development of a low-power IoMT portable pillbox for medication adherence improvement and remote treatment adjustment. *Sensors*, 22(15), 5818.

Kaur, M., Sugadev, M., Kaur, H., Mahmood, M. R., & Maheshwari, V. (2022). Healthcare internet of things: a new revolution. In Md Rashid Mahmood, Rohit Raja, Harpreet Kaur, Sandeep Kumar, & Kapil Kumar Nagwanshi (eds) *Ambient Intelligence and Internet of Things: Convergent Technologies* (pp. 301–337). Scrivener Publishing LLC., Massachusetts.

Kelly, J. T., Campbell, K. L., Gong, E., & Scuffham, P. (2020). The internet of things: impact and implications for health care delivery. *Journal of Medical Internet Research*, 22(11), e20135.

Khatiwada, P., Yang, B., Lin, J. C., & Blobel, B. (2024). Patient-generated health data (PGHD): understanding, requirements, challenges, and existing techniques for data security and privacy. *Journal of Personalized Medicine*, 14(3), 282.

Koutras, D., Stergiopoulos, G., Dasaklis, T., Kotzanikolaou, P., Glynos, D., & Douligeris, C. (2020). Security in IoMT communications: a survey. *Sensors*, 20(17), 4828.

Liu, J., Liu, M., Bai, Y., Zhang, J., Liu, H., & Zhu, W. (2020). Recent progress in flexible wearable sensors for vital sign monitoring. *Sensors*, 20(14), 4009.

Lu, Z. X., Qian, P., Bi, D., Ye, Z. W., He, X., Zhao, Y. H., … & Zhu, Z. L. (2021). Application of AI and IoT in clinical medicine: summary and challenges. *Current Medical Science*, 41(6), 1134–1150.

Ma, S. C., Alkhaleefah, M., Chang, Y. L., Chuah, J. H., Chang, W. Y., Ku, C. S., … & Chang, L. (2022). Inter-multilevel super-orthogonal space–time coding scheme for reliable zigbee-based IoMT communications. *Sensors*, 22(7), 2695.

Magsi, H., Sodhro, A. H., Chachar, F. A., Abro, S. A. K., Sodhro, G. H., & Pirbhulal, S. (2018, March). Evolution of 5G in Internet of medical things. In *2018 International Conference on Computing, Mathematics and Engineering Technologies (iCoMET)* (pp. 1–7). IEEE, Sukkur, Pakistan.

Manickam, P., Mariappan, S. A., Murugesan, S. M., Hansda, S., Kaushik, A., Shinde, R., & Thipperudraswamy, S. P. (2022). Artificial intelligence (AI) and internet of medical things (IoMT) assisted biomedical systems for intelligent healthcare. *Biosensors*, 12(8), 562.

Matni, N., Moraes, J., Pacheco, L., Rosário, D., Oliveira, H., Cerqueira, E., & Neto, A. (2020, June). Experimenting long range wide area network in an e-health environment: discussion and future directions. In *2020 International Wireless Communications and Mobile Computing (IWCMC)* (pp. 758–763). IEEE, Limassol, Cyprus.

Markova, V., Ganchev, T., Pencheva, E., & Atanasov, I. (2021, October). Intelligent architecture for real-time personal health monitoring in the context of 3G/4G/5G networks. In *2021 29th National Conference with International Participation (TELECOM)* (pp. 53–56). IEEE, Bulgaria.

Marr, B. (2020). *Tech Trends in Practice: The 25 Technologies That are Driving the 4th Industrial Revolution.* John Wiley & Sons, Massachusetts.

Mitra, A., Roy, U., & Tripathy, B. K. (2022). IoMT in healthcare industry – concepts and applications. In Tripathy, B. K., Lingras, P., Kar, A. K., & Chowdhary, C. L. (eds), *Next Generation Healthcare Informatics* (vol. 1039, pp. 121–146). Springer, Singapore.

Mkwashi, A., & Brass, I. (2022). The future of medical device regulation and standards: dealing with critical challenges for connected, intelligent medical devices. In *PETRAS National Centre of Excellent in IoT Systems Cybersecurity*. Elsevier, London.

Monteiro, A. C. B., França, R. P., Arthur, R., & Iano, Y. (2023). An overview of the Internet of medical things (IoMT): applications, benefits, and challenges. In Rajkumar Buyya, Muhammad Imran Tariq, Valentina Emilia Balas, Guojun Wang, & Radu Prodan (eds) *Security and Privacy Issues in Internet of Medical Things*, 83–98. Elsevier, United Kingdom.

Morphy, R. (2021). *Fundamental Security for IoT and IoMT Devices within Health Care in the Absence of Industry Standards* (Doctoral dissertation, Capella University).

Osama, M., Ateya, A. A., Sayed, M. S., Hammad, M., Pławiak, P., Abd El-Latif, A. A., & Elsayed, R. A. (2023). Internet of medical things and healthcare 4.0: trends, requirements, challenges, and research directions. *Sensors*, 23(17), 7435.

Pandey, R., Maurya, P., & Chiong, R. (eds.). (2023). *Data Modelling and Analytics for the Internet of Medical Things*. CRC Press, USA.

Perumal, U. (2023). Smart health care for monitoring elderly people using IoMT and Ml. *Journal of Data Acquisition and Processing*, 38(2), 4865.

Polu, S. K., & Polu, S. K. (2019). IoMT based smart health care monitoring system. *International Journal for Innovative Research in Science & Technology*, 5(11), 58–64.

Pramanik, P. K. D., Solanki, A., Debnath, A., Nayyar, A., El-Sappagh, S., & Kwak, K. S. (2020). Advancing modern healthcare with nanotechnology, nanobiosensors, and internet of nano things: taxonomies, applications, architecture, and challenges. *IEEE Access*, 8, 65230–65266.

Pushpalatha, N., Anbarasu, P., & Venkatesh, A. (2022). Communication protocols for IoMT-based healthcare systems. In Prasanth, A., Lakshmi D, Rajesh Kumar, D., Balamurugan, B., & Sherimon P.C. (eds) *Cognitive Computing for Internet of Medical Things* (pp. 59–75). Chapman and Hall/CRC, USA.

Pushparaj, A. K., & Saini, G. (2023). AI-based ECG signal monitoring system for arrhythmia detection using IoMT. In Raj, B., Gupta, B. B., Yamaguchi, S. & Sandeep Singh, G. (eds) *AI for Big Data-Based Engineering Applications from Security Perspectives* (p. 85). CRC Press, USA.

Qureshi, F., & Krishnan, S. (2018). Wearable hardware design for the internet of medical things (IoMT). *Sensors*, 18(11), 3812.

Rachakonda, L., Bapatla, A. K., Mohanty, S. P., & Kougianos, E. (2020). Sayopillow: blockchain-integrated privacy-assured IoMT framework for stress management considering sleeping habits. *IEEE Transactions on Consumer Electronics*, 67(1), 20–29.

Rahman, M., & Jahankhani, H. (2021). Security vulnerabilities in existing security mechanisms for iomt and potential solutions for mitigating cyber-attacks. In Hamid Jahankhani, Stefan Kendzierskyj, & Babak Akhgar (eds) *Information Security Technologies for Controlling Pandemics* (pp. 307–334). Springer, London.

Rajamohan, K., Rangasamy, S., Nayak, S., Anuradha, R., & Chellasamy, A. (2022). Revolutionizing healthcare: decentralized data management of IoT devices using blockchain technology. In Bharat Bhushan, Nitin Rakesh, Yousef Farhaoui, Parma Nand, & Bhuvan Unhelkar (eds) *Blockchain Technology in Healthcare Applications* (pp. 153–174). CRC Press, USA.

Rajasekar, S. J. S., Thangavelu, S., & Perumal, V. (2024). An AI-powered IoMT model for continuous remote patient monitoring using COVID early warning score (CoEWS). In Saravanan, K. & Aboobucker, I. (eds) *Internet of Medical Things in Smart Healthcare* (pp. 39–55). Apple Academic Press, London.

Rana, A., Chakraborty, C., Sharma, S., Dhawan, S., Pani, S. K., & Ashraf, I. (2022). Internet of medical things-based secure and energy-efficient framework for health care. *Big Data*, 10(1), 18–33.

Rayan, R. A., Tsagkaris, C., & Zafar, I. (2022). IoT for better mobile health applications. In Kumar, P., Obaid, A. J., Cengiz, K., Khanna, A., & Balas, V. E. (eds), *A Fusion of Artificial Intelligence and Internet of Things for Emerging Cyber Systems* (vol. 210, pp. 1–13). Springer, Cham.

Razdan, S., & Sharma, S. (2022). Internet of medical things (IoMT): overview, emerging technologies, and case studies. *IETE Technical Review*, 39(4), 775–788.

Roy, T., & Nahid, M. M. (2022, March). The IoMT and cloud in healthcare: use, impact and efficiency of contemporary sensor devices used by patients and clinicians. In *Proceedings of the 2nd International Conference on Computing Advancements* (pp. 426–434), Warsaw, Poland.

Rubi, J., & Dhivya, A. J. A. (2022). Wearable health monitoring systems using IoMT. In Hemalatha, R. J., Akila, D., Balaganesh, D., & Paul, A. (eds), *The Internet of Medical Things (IoMT) Healthcare Transformation* (pp. 225–246). Scrivener Publishing LLC, Massachusetts.

Sadhu, P. K., Yanambaka, V. P., Abdelgawad, A., & Yelamarthi, K. (2022). Prospect of internet of medical things: a review on security requirements and solutions. *Sensors*, 22(15), 5517.

Searle, R., & Gururaj, P. (2023). Protecting patient confidentiality in the internet of medical things through confidential computing. *Journal of Data Protection & Privacy*, 5(4), 347–362.

Shiraj, T. B., Mortuza, A., Rahman, K. M. A., & Karim, T. (2022). Non-communicable disease detection based on early symptoms using machine learning approach enabling smart healthcare model (IoMT). *Journal of FST*, 1(01), 85.

Sharma, D., Nawab, A. Z. B., & Alam, M. (2021). Integrating M-health with IoMT to counter COVID-19. In Raza, K. (ed) *Computational Intelligence Methods in COVID-19: Surveillance, Prevention, Prediction and Diagnosis* (pp. 373–396), Springer, Singapore.

Sharmila, E. M. N., Rama Krishna, K., Prasad, G. N. R., Anand, B., Kwatra, C. V., & Kapila, D. (2024). IoMT – applications, benefits, and future challenges in the healthcare domain. In Satya Prakash Yadav, Sudesh Yadav, Pethuru Raj and Victor Hugo C. de Albuquerque (eds) *Advances in Fuzzy-Based Internet of Medical Things (IoMT)* (pp. 1–23), Wiley, Massachusetts.

Shanmugam, B., & Azam, S. (2023). Risk assessment of heterogeneous IoMT devices: a review. *Technologies*, 11(1), 31.

Shiraj, T. B., Mortuza, A., Rahman, K. M. A., & Karim, T. (2022). Non-communicable disease detection based on early symptoms using machine learning approach enabling smart healthcare model (IoMT). *Journal of FST*, 1(1), 85.

Singh, R. P., Javaid, M., Haleem, A., Vaishya, R., & Ali, S. (2020). Internet of medical things (IoMT) for orthopaedic in COVID-19 pandemic: roles, challenges, and applications. *Journal of Clinical Orthopaedics and Trauma*, 11(4), 713–717.

Sonavane, A., Khamparia, A., & Gupta, D. (2023). A systematic review on the internet of medical things: techniques, open issues, and future directions. *CMES-Computer Modeling in Engineering & Sciences*, 137(2), 1525–1550.

Srivastava, J., Routray, S., Ahmad, S., & Waris, M. M. (2022). Internet of medical things (IoMT)-based smart healthcare system: trends and progress. *Computational Intelligence and Neuroscience*, 1, 7218113.

Tamiziniyan, G., & Keerthana, A. (2022). Future of healthcare: biomedical big data analysis and IoMT. In Hemalatha, D. Akila, D. Balaganesh, & Anand Paul (eds) *The Internet of Medical Things (IoMT) Healthcare Transformation* (pp. 247–267), Scrivener Publishing, Massachusetts.

Tyagi, A. K., George, T. T., & Soni, G. (2023). Blockchain-based cybersecurity in internet of medical things (IoMT)-based assistive systems. In Vijeyananthan, T. (ed) *AI-Based Digital Health Communication for Securing Assistive Systems* (pp. 22–53). IGI Global, UK.

Toor, A. A., Usman, M., Younas, F., M. Fong, A. C., Khan, S. A., & Fong, S. (2020). Mining massive E-health data streams for IoMT enabled healthcare systems. *Sensors*, 20(7), 2131.

Trayush, T., Bathla, R., Saini, S., & Shukla, V. K. (2021, March). IoT in healthcare: challenges, benefits, applications, and opportunities. In *2021 International Conference on Advance Computing and Innovative Technologies in Engineering (ICACITE)* (pp. 107–111). IEEE, Greater Noida, India.

Vaiyapuri, T., Binbusayyis, A., & Varadarajan, V. (2021). Security, privacy and trust in IoMT enabled smart healthcare system: a systematic review of current and future trends. *International Journal of Advanced Computer Science and Applications*, 12(2).

Vishnu, S., Ramson, S. J., & Jegan, R. (2020, March). Internet of medical things (IoMT)-An overview. In *2020 5th International Conference on Devices, Circuits and Systems (ICDCS)* (pp. 101–104). IEEE, Coimbatore, India.

Wagan, S. A., Koo, J., Siddiqui, I. F., Attique, M., Shin, D. R., & Qureshi, N. M. F. (2022). Internet of medical things and trending converged technologies: a comprehensive review on real-time applications. *Journal of King Saud University-Computer and Information Sciences*, 34(10), 9228–9251.

Wagle, A. A., Isakadze, N., Nasir, K., & Martin, S. S. (2021). Strengthening the learning health system in cardiovascular disease prevention: time to leverage big data and digital solutions. *Current Atherosclerosis Reports*, 23, 1–8.

Yadav, A. S., Srivastava, G., & Singh, S. (2024). Wearable technologies in AI and smart healthcare. In Deepshikha Agarwal, Khushboo Tripathi, and Kumar Krishen (eds) *Concepts of Artificial Intelligence and its Application in Modern Healthcare Systems* (pp. 233–249). CRC Press, USA.

Yasmeen, G., Javed, N., & Ahmed, T. (2022). Interoperability: a challenge for IoMT. *ECS Transactions*, 107(1), 4459.

Zikria, Y. B., Afzal, M. K., & Kim, S. W. (2020). Internet of multimedia things (IoMT): opportunities, challenges and solutions. *Sensors*, 20(8), 2334.

Index

N

O

P

R

S

T

U

V

W

X